14. Practical Physiotherapy with Older People
    Lucinda Smyth et al.
15. Keyboard, Graphic and Handwriting Skills
    Helping people with motor disabilities
    Dorothy E. Penso
16. Community Occupational Therapy with Mentally Handicapped Adults
    Debbie Isaac
17. Autism
    Professional perspectives and practice
    Edited by Kathryn Ellis
18. Multiple Sclerosis
    Approaches to management
    Edited by Lorraine De Souza
19. Occupational Therapy in Rheumatology
    An holistic approach
    Lynne Sandles
20. Breakdown of Speech
    Causes and remediation
    Nancy R. Milloy
21. Coping with Stress in the Health Professions
    A practical guide
    Philip Burnard
22. Speech and Communication Problems in Psychiatry
    Rosemary Gravell and Jenny France
23. Limb Amputation
    From aetiology to rehabilitation
    Rosalind Ham and Leonard Cotton
24. Management in Occupational Therapy
    Zielfa B. Maslin
25. Rehabilitation in Parkinson's Disease
    Edited by Francis I. Caird
26. Exercise Physiology for Health Professionals
    Stephen R. Bird
27. Therapy for the Burn Patient
    Annette Leveridge
28. Effective Communication Skills for Health Professionals
    Philip Burnard
29. Ageing, Healthy and in Control
    An alternative approach to maintaining the health of older people
    Steve Scrutton
30. The Early Identification of Language Impairment in Children
    Edited by James Law
31. An Introduction to Communication Disorders
    Diana Syder

32. Writing for Health Professionals
    A manual for writers
    Philip Burnard
33. Brain Injury Rehabilitation
    A neuro-functional approach
    Gordon Muir Giles and Jo Clark-Wilson
34. Living with Continuing Perceptuo-motor Difficulties
    Theory and strategies to help children, adolescents and adults
    Dorothy E. Penso
35. Psychology and Counselling for Health Professionals
    Edited by Rowan Bayne and Paula Nicholson
36. Occupational Therapy for Orthopaedic Conditions
    Dina Penrose
37. Teaching Students in Clinical Settings
    Jackie Stengelhofen
38. Groupwork in Occupational Therapy
    Linda Finlay
39. Elder Abuse
    Concepts, theories and interventions
    Gerald Bennett and Paul Kingston
40. Teamwork in Neurology
    Ruth Nieuwenhuis
41. Eating Disorders
    A guide for health professionals
    Simon B.N. Thompson
42. Community Mental Health
    Practical approaches to long-term problems
    Steve Morgan
43. Acupuncture in Clinical Practice
    A guide for health professionals
    Nadia Ellis
44. Child Sexual Abuse
    A guide for health professionals
    Celia Doyle

Forthcoming titles

Forensic Psychiatry for Health Professionals
Chris Lloyd
Research Methods for Therapists
Avril Drummond
Speech and Language Problems in Children
A practical guide
Dilys A. Treharne

Spinal Cord Injury Rehabilitation

THERAPY IN PRACTICE SERIES

Edited by Jo Campling

This series of books is aimed at 'therapists' concerned with rehabilitation in a very broad sense. The intended audience particularly includes occupational therapists, physiotherapists and speech therapists, but many titles will also be of interest to nurses, psychologists, medical staff, social workers, teachers or voluntary workers. Some volumes are interdisciplinary, others are aimed at one particular profession. All titles will be comprehensive but concise, and practical but with due reference to relevant theory and evidence. They are not research monographs but focus on professional practice, and will be of value to both students and qualified personnel.

1. Occupational Therapy for Children with Disabilities
   Dorothy E. Penso
2. Living Skills for Mentally Handicapped People
   Christine Peck and Chia Swee Hong
3. Rehabilitation of the Older Patient
   Edited by Amanda J. Squires
4. Physiotherapy and the Elderly Patient
   Paul Wagstaff and Davis Coakley
5. Rehabilitation of the Severely Brain-Injured Adult
   Edited by Ian Fussey and Gordon Muir Giles
6. Communication Problems in Elderly People
   Rosemary Gravell
7. Occupational Therapy Practice in Psychiatry
   Linda Finlay
8. Working with Bilingual Language Disability
   Edited by Deirdre M. Duncan
9. Counselling Skills for Health Professionals
   Philip Burnard
10. Teaching Interpersonal Skills
    A handbook of experiential learning for health professionals
    Philip Burnard
11. Occupational Therapy for Stroke Rehabilitation
    Simon B.N. Thompson and Maryanne Morgan
12. Assessing Physically Disabled People at Home
    Kathy Maczka
13. Acute Head Injury
    Practical management in rehabilitation
    Ruth Garner

Spinal Cord Injury Rehabilitation

Karen Whalley Hammell

Occupational Therapist, Saskatchewan, Canada

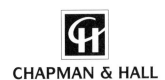

CHAPMAN & HALL

London · Glasgow · Weinheim · New York · Tokyo · Melbourne · Madras

Published by Chapman & Hall, 2–6 Boundary Row, London SE1 8HN, UK

Chapman & Hall, 2–6 Boundary Row, London, SE1 8HN, UK

Blackie Academic & Professional, Wester Cleddens Road, Bishopbriggs, Glasgow G64 2NZ, UK

Chapman & Hall GmbH, Pappelallee 3, 69469 Weinheim, Germany

Chapman & Hall USA, One Penn Plaza, 41st Floor, New York NY 10119, USA

Chapman & Hall Japan, ITP-Japan, Kyowa Building, 3F, 2–2–1 Hirakawacho, Chiyoda-ku, Tokyo 102, Japan

Chapman & Hall Australia, Thomas Nelson Australia, 102 Dodds Street, South Melbourne, Victoria 3205, Australia

Chapman & Hall India, R. Seshadri, 32 Second Main Road, CIT East, Madras 600 035, India

First edition 1995
© 1995 Chapman & Hall

Typeset in 10/12pt Palatino by Florencetype Ltd, Stoodleigh, Devon
Printed in Great Britain by St Edmundsbury Press, Bury St Edmunds, Suffolk

ISBN 0 412 47680 0   1 56593 195 5 (USA)

A catalogue record for this book is available from the British Library

Library of Congress Catalog Card Number: 94-71813

∞ Printed on permanent acid-free text paper, manufactured in accordance with ANSI/NISO Z39 48–1992 (Permanence of Paper).

To Ike

Contents

Preface   xiii
Acknowledgements   xv
Author's note   xvi

Introduction   1
   Client-centred practice   1
   International Classification of Impairments,
     Disabilities and Handicaps   2
   Canadian model of occupational performance   2
   Independence   3
   References   4

1 Rehabilitation and self-determination   5
   Introduction   5
   Medical model of rehabilitation   7
   Educational approach to rehabilitation   9
   Model of occupational performance and the
     assessment process   10
   Goal setting   13
   Establishing objectives   15
   Identifying attainment of objectives   17
   Accountability   18
   Compliance and control   19
   Active participation: the activated patient and
     empowerment in rehabilitation   20
   Learned/taught helplessness   22
   Locus of control   22
   Motivation   24
   Relationship between client and therapist   26
   Conclusion   29
   Acknowledgement   30

References   30
Further reading   32

2 **Education as the key to rehabilitation**   33
   Introduction   33
   Learning process   34
   Theories of learning   35
   How do people 'learn best'?   36
   Application of learning theory in rehabilitation 37
   Compliance and control   38
   Learning and empowerment   39
   Problem-solving and learning   40
   Peer learning   42
   Barriers to learning   43
   Learning needs and Maslow's hierarchy   45
   Setting goals   47
   Family involvement in the learning process   48
   Summary   49
   References   50

3 **Spinal cord injury: aetiology, incidence and**
   impairments   52
   Historical perspective   52
   Incidence and prevalence   53
   Aetiology of traumatic injury   54
   Prevention of traumatic injury   56
   Impairment   60
   Emergency management   69
   Specialized spinal injury units   71
   References   72

4 **Acute care and reduction of disability**   74
   Acute care   75
   Disability reduction: acute and long-term
      management   93
   Survival and mortality   111
   References   113

5 **Engagement in self-care activities**   118
   Introduction   118
   Functional levels   119

Implications of level of injury 121
Central cord syndrome 124
Self-care skills 125
Personal care 125
Functional mobility 141
Community management 157
Discharge planning 165
Re-admission to hospital 167
References 169

6 **Management of high lesions** 174
Introduction 175
High-lesion quadriplegia and rehabilitation 177
Definition 178
Early intervention 178
Occupational therapy 185
Self care: personal care 198
Functional mobility: wheelchairs 203
Environmental control systems: self-care,
  productivity and leisure 209
Telephones 213
Computers: productivity and leisure 213
Workstations 215
Robotics 216
Community re-entry and community
  management 216
Employment 219
Acknowledgement 220
References 220
Further reading 222

7 **Psychological adaptation** 224
Introduction 224
Psychological theories 225
Personality theories 234
Sociological theories 235
Implications for rehabilitation personnel 236
Model for rehabilitation 238
Acknowledgement 241
References 241
Further reading 245

8 Living with a spinal cord injury: productivity,
   leisure and socialization   246
   Introduction   246
   Productivity   247
   Leisure   258
   Social support   267
   Cultural environment   270
   Women and spinal cord injury   271
   Children and spinal cord injury   274
   Adolescents and spinal cord injury   276
   The elderly and spinal cord injury   277
   Independent Living Movement   279
   References   283

9 Long-term issues and ageing   288
   Introduction   288
   Sexuality, sexual function and fertility   288
   Marriage and the family   292
   Independent living options   295
   Informal carers and personal care attendants   296
   Attendant management   299
   Diet and nutrition   300
   Pain   302
   Ageing with a spinal cord injury   304
   Self-neglect and suicide   311
   Continuing care services   313
   Quality of life   317
   References   322

10 The way forward   327
   Prevention   327
   Rehabilitation research   327
   Community-based services   329
   Advocacy and social change   333
   References   337

Bibliography   338
Appendix A: Resource list   339
Appendix B: Suppliers   340
Index   342

Preface

Knowledge of spinal cord injury is largely restricted to specialized units, yet most people who sustain these injuries are treated in general hospitals and not in special centres. Additionally, some units are becoming unable to cope with long-term care problems, with the result that even people who were initially treated at a spinal unit may come to depend upon general hospitals and community services for their future needs. Life expectancies following spinal cord injury now approach those of the general population, hence many healthcare professionals will have the opportunity – and responsibility – of working with people who have sustained spinal cord trauma.

It is thus imperative that knowledge be disseminated more widely so that needless complications can be avoided and all people with spinal cord damage, from whatever cause, can receive excellent care.

In the past, therapists and other health practitioners have focused upon a medical model of service delivery, with emphasis upon the physical components of a disabling condition, self-care skills and mobility. This model has been rejected by many therapists who have found its approach to be too narrow and of limited perspective in achieving a fulfilling adult life in the community. More importantly, it has been rejected by people with disabilities who have experienced frustrations with rehabilitation programmes focused solely upon physical goals, while ignoring more complex and meaningful psychosocial and occupational issues.

This book presents an approach to rehabilitation that is based on a client-centred model of practice. The rehabilitation process is explored from the perspective of the model of occupational performance, and the interaction between the spinal cord injured person and his environment is examined.

In line with this approach, the first chapters present a concept of empowerment in rehabilitation and an educational view of the process of learning to live with a suddenly acquired disability. The medical aspects of spinal cord injury follow, with a study of aetiology, impairments, acute care, disability reduction and engagement in self-care activities.

The management of high lesions in a rehabilitation context is examined separately, as this is a highly specialized area and one that is largely ignored, both in therapy literature and in professional practice.

The final chapters focus upon psychological issues, and upon aspects such as productivity, leisure and socialization, which are important both in early phases of management and in the long term.

I have endeavoured throughout to provide comprehensive references. Much excellent material has been published concerning spinal cord injury and this work attempts to facilitate access to some of this information.

Although this book is focused upon people with spinal cord injuries, it is hoped that the principles of rehabilitation philosophy outlined will be applied to other client groups, who must learn to live with an acquired disability in the context of their unique environments.

It is possible to achieve quality of life and a high degree of satisfaction with life following a spinal cord injury. There is considerable responsibility on rehabilitation professionals to ensure that their programmes and interventions are enabling each client to attain his or her goals and to achieve again a life that has purpose, fulfilment and quality.

Karen R. Whalley Hammell
Oxbow, Saskatchewan, Canada
May 1994

Acknowledgements

Thanks are due to Jo Campling, editor of the *Therapy in Practice* series, for her encouragement and faith in my project; and to the team at Chapman & Hall, for the professional assistance they have provided throughout.

I wish also to thank Simon Tuck, for the drawing of quadriplegic arm positioning and my parents, Harry and Roma Whalley, who first introduced me to concepts of social justice and who continue to provide me with encouragement and support.

It is also essential to thank all those people with spinal cord injuries who have shared their experiences and aspirations with me and who have taught me what it means to live with a spinal cord injury.

Above all, I must acknowledge my debt of gratitude to my husband, Ike Hammell, not only for his unwavering encouragement, support and motivation but also for his practical help.

Author's note

The spinal cord injured individual is referred to throughout the text as 'he'. This is for clarity and convenience but does also reflect the larger percentage of males than females (82% versus 18%, respectively) who sustain a spinal cord injury. This is not intended to discredit the experience of women with spinal cord injuries.

The term **quadriplegia** (from the Latin) has been used, rather than the more traditional British term **tetraplegia** (from the Greek), to describe the involvement of all four limbs, the chest and trunk. This is in line with the designation of the British Library's Cataloguing-in-Publication Data and the Uniform Data Set for Medical Rehabilitation (SUNY, 1990).

Members of the healthcare team are often referred to in the text as **therapists**. This is used as a broad term, unless specified (occupational therapist, physiotherapist), as each member of the rehabilitation team may be regarded as a therapist, namely someone with special skills in health care, obtained through education and experience (Anderson and Anderson, 1990).

The terms **patient** and **client** are used interchangeably – but awkwardly. In acute care, the medical model is appropriate in addressing issues surrounding physiological stabilization and the term 'patient' may be relevant. In rehabilitation, the medical model is no longer appropriate in addressing the issues that surround learning to live with a disability, participating fully in the community, engaging in meaningful occupation and addressing adult, psychosocial issues, values and goals. The person with a spinal cord injury must be part of a co-operative team effort and as such, 'client' may seem more appropriate – although passivity is still implied. In a team, everyone has contributions: the occupational therapist, physiotherapist, psychologist, social worker, surgeon, physician, nurse and, most importantly, the person with the spinal cord injury and his family. As such, all the team members could more accurately be regarded as peers, each making a unique and valuable contribution to achieving the goals of the client.

REFERENCES

Anderson, K.N. and Anderson, L.E. (1990) *Mosby's Pocket Dictionary of Medicine, Nursing and Allied Health*. C.V. Mosby, St Louis, MO.

SUNY (1990) *Guide for Use of the Uniform Data Set for Medical Rehabilitation, Including the Functional Independence Measure (FIM)*. Research Foundation, State University of New York, Buffalo, NY.

Introduction

Current rehabilitation literature is generally divided between practical 'how to' manuals for the physical management of spinal cord injuries; and those theoretical texts that discuss the assumptions and philosophies which underpin our professions and our practice.

'Spinal cord injury rehabilitation' is an attempt to combine contemporary rehabilitation and occupational therapy philosophy with a practical example of how this can, and should be made to work in actual clinical practice. It is hoped that students in particular will value the opportunity to examine theory as it relates to one particular client group.

The book is grounded upon four key concepts:

1. client-centred practice
2. the International Classification of Impairments, Disabilities and Handicaps (ICIDH)
3. the Canadian model of occupational performance
4. 'independence'.

CLIENT-CENTRED PRACTICE

Professional practice that is client-centred rather than therapist-centred recognizes the need to engage the client throughout the therapeutic process as an important and active participant. This framework supports the notion that clients are responsible for maintaining their own health. It focuses on client-identified problems, on the client's own environment and incorporates the roles and role expectations of the client (CAOT, 1991; Law *et al.*, 1991).

Client-centred practice does not allow the therapist to surrender responsibility. Rather, it requires more emphasis upon 'process' – interaction, negotiation, communication, education and exchange of information.

INTERNATIONAL CLASSIFICATION OF IMPAIRMENTS, DISABILITIES AND HANDICAPS

In this classification (WHO, 1980), the World Health Organisation defines **impairment** as an abnormality or loss of psychological, physiological or anatomical structure or function. In the current work, the impairment will be a spinal cord injury and its physiological sequelae.

A **disability** is defined as a restriction or inability to perform an activity due to the impairment. 'Disabilities' in this context may include such aspects as loss of ability to walk, to grasp or to breathe independently.

The WHO defines **handicap** as the disadvantage that may result from impairment and disability which limits fulfilment of roles, such as physical independence, mobility, occupation, social integration and economic self-sufficiency. Handicap cannot be viewed solely as a personal limitation which is susceptible to personal, individual intervention, but rather as the disadvantage that occurs when the abilities and needs of the individual are not matched by the demands and resources of the environment (social, cultural, physical, political, economic and legal environment).

The constitution of Disabled Peoples' International defines 'handicap' as the loss or limitation of opportunities to take part in the normal life of the community on an equal level with others due to physical and social barriers (DPI, 1985).

Hence, with appropriate political and social environmental interventions, a disability does not have to result in handicap.

CANADIAN MODEL OF OCCUPATIONAL PERFORMANCE

The model of occupational performance (CAOT, 1991) provides a useful framework for addressing the personal issues of an 'impairment' and the multiple factors that contribute to 'disability', while encouraging examination of aspects in the client's environment which may either conspire to create handicap or may facilitate independent living and a personally fulfilling lifestyle. The ICIDH is conceptually compatible with the model of occupational performance (Townsend *et al.*, 1990).

The model of occupational performance accepts the premise that engagement in purposeful activity is a critical determinant of quality of life. The essence of occupational performance is believed to reside in an integrated and balanced approach to:

- self-care
  - –personal care
  - –functional mobility
  - –community management
- productivity
  - –paid/unpaid work
  - –household management
  - –play/school
- leisure
  - –quiet recreation
  - –active recreation
  - –socialization (Law *et al.*, 1991).

Satisfactory performance in these areas will be dependent upon the integration of four performance components: the physical, sociocultural, mental–emotional (cognitive, affective and volitional) and spiritual/philosophical components.

The model recognizes that the individual affects, and is affected by, the social, cultural and physical aspects of the environment. There has recently been further recognition of the impact of the economic, political and legal environment upon the individual and upon his opportunities for full community participation (CAOT, 1991; Law *et al.*, 1991).

INDEPENDENCE

One of the primary goals of rehabilitation is to enable a regaining of **independence**. Unfortunately, the concept of independence has frequently assumed an extremely narrow definition – that of physical independence in activities such as personal care and mobility.

Chambers Twentieth Century Dictionary (1972 edn) offers the following definitions of independence:

- not subordinate
- completely self-governing
- thinking or acting for oneself.

It is this larger definition of independence that is assumed in this work. An independent individual is one who can take responsibility, solve problems, establish plans and work towards them and, if needed, direct others in his care. This is the form of independence which I believe to be the goal of the rehabilitation process.

Although much has been said about independence in relation to rehabilitation, most medical rehabilitation programs both fail to encourage independence and to prepare persons with disabilities to develop their maximum potential for productivity, quality of life, and social participation after hospitalization. (Tate *et al.*, 1992)

REFERENCES

CAOT (1991) *Occupational Therapy Guidelines for Client Centred Practice*, Canadian Association of Occupational Therapists and Health Services Directorate, Health Services Promotion Branch, Health and Welfare Canada, Toronto, Ont.

DPI (1985) *Disabled Peoples' International Constitution*, 1, DPI Development Office, Winnepeg, Man.

Law, M., Baptiste, S., Carswell-Opzoomer, A. *et al.* (1991) *Canadian Occupational Performance Measure*, Canadian Association of Occupational Therapists, Toronto, Ont.

Tate, D.G., Maynard, F. and Forchheimer, M. (1992) Evaluation of a medical rehabilitation and independent living program for persons with spinal cord injury, *Journal of Rehabilitation*, **58**(3), 25–8.

Townsend, E., Ryan, B. and Law, M. (1990) Using the World Health Organisation's International Classification of Impairments, Disabilities and Handicaps in Occupational Therapy. *Canadian Journal of Occupational Therapy*, **57**(1), 16–25.

WHO, (1980) *International Classification of Impairments, Disabilities and Handicaps: a Manual of Classification Relating to the Consequences of Disease*, World Health Organisation, Geneva.

1

Rehabilitation
and self-determination

*Compliance with externally imposed routines does
not teach independence, problem solving and coping
with a disability* (Trieschmann, 1986)

INTRODUCTION

Expert medical care is essential in the early management of
spinal cord injury to ensure survival and to prevent unnecessary
complications. Once the acute stage has passed, however, medicine can offer no cure and it is up to each individual to learn to
live with the resulting disability in the context of his own
environment. In examining the rehabilitation process following
spinal cord injury much discussion will centre upon the unique
nature of the injury, its idiosyncracies and its sequelae.
However, it is pertinent to examine first what is implied by the
term **rehabilitation**.

Rehabilitation has frequently been defined in terms of the
process of restoring an individual to his maximum potential in
all areas of life – physical, intellectual, emotional and social.
However, it is unlikely that many people in society actually
achieve their maximum potential in any one of these areas;
fewer still in all four. The inherent risk in such a definition of
rehabilitation lies in the adoption of assumptions concerning
maximum potential. There has been a temptation to close the
file on an individual who has achieved those goals which
Western society values – independence (in self-care activities)
and productivity (return to work). These are superficial indicators of rehabilitation outcome which can mask the considerable difficulties that may continue to prevent quality living for

the individual, such as full social and community integration or personally fulfilling activities.

Rehabilitation has also been viewed as the process of teaching skills to achieve the highest possible level of physical independence. Success in such activities of daily living as transfers and self-care skills has been regarded as evidence of successful rehabilitation. For some people this may indeed have been the case; however, this vision of rehabilitation also has inherent problems. A predominant focus upon physical independence has excluded people with the most profound functional losses caused by high cervical cord lesions (C4 and above) from many rehabilitation services. The potential achievement of independence in self-care activities has been an admission criteria for some rehabilitation services and those who will not be able to gain physical independence (but who could direct others in their care and achieve an independent lifestyle) have received little or no help in their process of adaptation, in learning new skills or accessing appropriate equipment. Unless a new perspective is taken of what independence and rehabilitation really mean, these individuals may continue to be viewed as having 'no rehabilitation potential'.

Another problem with adhering to the view of rehabilitation as a process of maximizing independence is that many people do not live independently but in a state of interdependence. Research studies suggest that people with spinal cord injuries actually spend less time in self-care tasks than do able bodied people (Yerxa and Baum, 1986) indicating perhaps, that interdependence is indeed occurring, and that energy is being conserved for more personally meaningful activities. It has been suggested that a truly self-reliant person is not as independent as cultural stereotypes suppose but rather is able to rely on others he trusts when appropriate. Further, some people with spinal cord injuries may be completely physically independent in a barrier-free environment but not in an inaccessible physical and social milieu. This raises the issue of whether each individual client should be learning to adapt to his surroundings or whether it is the hostile environment itself which needs to be changed. Independence cannot be viewed purely in physical/functional terms but must be seen also in relation to decision-making and problem-solving skills (see Introduction).

Independence is not so much a physical state but a state of mind – an attitude. A further problem that arises is the definition of **success**. Measurement of outcome following a rehabilitation programme has tended to focus on the attainment of physical skills, as these are easy to identify. However, this demands the question of whether physical skills alone determine successful re-integration into the community and to adaptation to life in an altered form. Satisfying relationships, fulfilment in occupations and a meaningful interaction with the social and physical environment depend upon much more than the ability to transfer and dress independently. It is proposed therefore that the aims of the rehabilitation team should not only focus upon the acquisition of skills to enable a person to get out of bed in the morning but to assist him in finding his own reason for so doing (Trieschmann, 1988). Cyr (1989) studied people who had been discharged following rehabilitation after spinal cord injuries. All subjects experienced medical sequelae related to their cord injuries but there were also complaints of pain, depression, loneliness, lack of sexuality counselling, poor re-socialization; and a lack of accessible housing, public buildings and public transportation. Achievement of optimal outcome may thus be seen to reside not solely within the individual but in his interactions with his environment. Outcome measurement must reflect this reality.

For the purpose of this book, rehabilitation will be taken to imply a programme of interventions which empower the individual with a spinal cord injury to achieve satisfaction in productive activity and a personally fulfilling, socially meaningful and functionally effective interaction with the world (Banja, 1990).

MEDICAL MODEL OF REHABILITATION

Rehabilitation services originally developed from the medical, or sickness, model of healthcare delivery, in which a medical problem is identified, a diagnosis is applied and treatment is prescribed and provided. The medical model is based upon mechanistic principles. The human body is examined to determine what is not functioning. The physician or surgeon, having identified a problem, administers his or her choice of treatment. The patient's role is to submit to the authority of the more knowledgeable figure and to follow advice and instructions. Rehabilitation, however, is not primarily concerned with the treatment of disease or injury but addresses the sequelae or effects of that disease or injury. Neither is it appropriate for the client to relinquish control of decision making but rather he must seize the responsibility for his healthcare, decision making and problem solving. There is a conflict of philosophies for rehabilitation professionals who work in facilities that advocate a medical model of treatment.

Working in an institution, the dominant medical model tends to superimpose its philosophy upon the people who work within it, dictating the orientation of the service and setting the context for therapy intervention. When confronted with a prevailing conceptual framework which is incongruent with that of rehabilitation, the lack of professional autonomy often results in provision of a therapy service which is best described as 'technical' (Feaver and Creek, 1993). Therapists cannot focus their assessment on dysfunction since, in rehabilitation, dysfunction alone does not determine the goals of intervention. Rather, they must assess and enhance potential abilities and focus on the client's goals.

The medical model is an inappropriate model in the management of chronic disability. There is a lack of consumer participation which conflicts with the need to empower individuals to be responsible for their own care. The medical model is focused upon intervention for individual deficits rather than upon broader, environmental intervention and is thus particularly unsuited to the management of a traumatic disability such as spinal cord injury.

The medical model of rehabilitation may be aptly seen in the treatment of a condition such as bursitis. A medical problem is identified – localized swelling, pain on pressure and movement. A medical diagnosis of 'bursitis' is given and physiotherapy units of treatment are applied, such as ultrasound and specific exercises. The patient assumes a passive role, having scant knowledge or expertise to contribute to the dilemmas regarding possible medications, surgical options or other treatment modalities. His role is to comply with the treatment and follow the advice he is given. His problem, however, is small, localized and will not require any substantial alterations in his lifestyle, his life goals or his life choices.

In the earliest acute care of someone who has sustained a spinal cord injury, such a model is also appropriate. The patient is unlikely either to have knowledge and skill in the field of spinal cord medicine, or to be in a physical or psychological position to make informed choices concerning his treatments.

However, although a crisis situation and early acute care can competently be managed by such a model, the rehabilitation of a person with a spinal cord injury is unlikely to be so successful. The individual may have to make major adjustments in his life, he must learn to be responsible for his own health status, learn new skills and learn to solve problems creatively. At this stage, Trieschmann (1988) proposes that the client can no longer be the passive recipient of units of treatment but must become an active participant in his own rehabilitation process. The individual will not learn creative independence by co-operation and compliance with the goals set by others. The 'age of disabling professions' has been described by Illich *et al.* (1977) as being when people had 'problems', experts had 'solutions' and scientists measured 'abilities' and 'needs'. This aptly describes the medical model of care.

EDUCATIONAL APPROACH TO REHABILITATION

A rehabilitation process that enables an individual to learn to live with his acquired disability in his own environment will be a dynamic process in which the individual must be an active participant.

People are best able to learn when they are helped to define their own problems, decide on a course of action and evaluate the consequences of their decisions. This learning process will provide the means to solve problems creatively, to address the client's own concerns and to address situations not encountered during the formal rehabilitation programme. It clearly cannot be achieved if the rehabilitation process consists of a 'conveyor belt' approach to treatment, one in which the client follows a tried-and-true routine of self-care skills, mat work, wheelchair mobility and transfers (see Chapter 2).

MODEL OF OCCUPATIONAL PERFORMANCE AND THE ASSESSMENT PROCESS

The model of occupational performance incorporates the basic elements of current philosophy upon which occupational therapy practice is based. The assumption of the model is that the essence of a healthy and functioning person is the balanced integration of the mental (cognitive, affective, volitional), physical, sociocultural and spiritual/philosophical selves. These components predicate the performance of occupations: self-care activities (personal care, functional mobility, community management), productivity (paid/unpaid work, household management, play/school) and leisure (quiet recreation, active recreation, socialization). The individual is affected by engagement with the social, cultural and physical aspects of the environment. There is a further recognition that performance of occupations, such as recreation, mobility, paid or unpaid work, socialization and community management are also impacted by the political, legal and economic environments (CAOT, 1991; Law *et al.*, 1991).

It follows that the assessment process will be determined by the chosen model of care. Evaluation of grip strength, range of motion and other performance components focus on factors related to impairments and fit well within the predominant medical model. It is important to recognize that therapists tend to treat what they measure. If they assess only performance components, these most likely will be the primary focus of intervention. This will be congruent with a programme such as physiotherapy which measures outcomes related to disabilities (e.g. strength, range of motion and mobility). It is incongruent with the priorities espoused by occupational therapists who are ostensibly concerned with the reduction of handicap and the wider issues of engagement in productive occupations and activities in the community.

Although performance components may indeed be usefully assessed and measured, assessment will not focus solely upon the components of occupational performance but upon those aspects of performance itself which are impacted by the injury and are of concern to the individual (Law *et al.*, 1991).

Individualized evaluation will, by definition, use a client-centred process to set goals and evaluate change. This will incorporate the problems that are of prime concern to the client in the context of his environment and role expectations.

> If the person is no longer the problem definer, it is unlikely that he or she will be the problem solver either. This disparity can reduce the client's self-determination and sense of control over health, often leading to what may appear as non compliance. If the therapy goals are set by the client through a process of client-centred assessment, the potential for active participation is enhanced.   (Pollock, 1993)

Although therapists have become adept at compiling range of motion measurements, activity of daily living scores and other assessments of disability, it takes far more skill to facilitate the client's identification of his own problem areas. People with disabilities, and indeed, some therapists, are questioning the role and bias of current activity of daily living scales. Scoring systems represent value judgements concerning how an activity 'should' be performed, reflecting mainstream values and making a statement concerning individual rights and choices. If a technical aid is used to enable a daily living task to be accomplished, for example, a low score is usually allocated to the activity. Someone with high-lesion quadriplegia, who lives an independent lifestyle by managing and directing others in his care, will usually receive no score at all (Law, 1993). Hence the assessment tools used by therapists may reflect value judgements which are not shared by our clients. Someone who receives assistance in dressing will attain a low activity of daily living score yet may have made the choice to conserve time and energy for more productive activities. Should this choice be labelled 'dependence'?

Many professionals consider any assistance with self-care activities to be indicative of a degree of handicap (Whiteneck *et al.*, 1992). However, this must clearly be determined by the individual – his roles, values and sociocultural environment. Hence a system of assessment is required which will consider the client's satisfaction with his performance of activities, one which does not assume the values of the professional. Interventions can then be directed towards real, rather than perceived problems.

Problem-oriented assessments have become popular among professionals. However, these almost exclusively reflect 'problems' as these are perceived by the professionals, from their cultural and socioeconomic belief and value systems. These cannot, therefore, form the basis for intervention – by any discipline, during the rehabilitation process.

The assessment process should enable the therapist to gain an understanding of how the client perceives his problems as they relate to satisfaction in occupational performance. Use of a client-centred assessment tool such as the Canadian Occupational Performance Measure (COPM; Law *et al.*, 1991) will provide a basis for establishing goals and objectives which are relevant and meaningful to the client, rather than those which are dictated by the therapist. The COPM encompasses the occupational performance areas of self-care, productivity and leisure as primary outcomes, while recognizing the performance components that are essential to the process of occupational performance. It incorporates the roles and role expectations of the client and the importance of performance areas to the client. It measures client-identified problems, focuses upon the client's own environment and considers the client's satisfaction with present performance (Law *et al.*, 1991).

The framework of the therapy programme cannot be directed solely towards the client's physical status but rather, towards his life. If therapists do indeed base their intervention upon the findings of assessments, those assessments must consider the broad implication of spinal cord injury for the individual. Therapists may be afraid that their clients will identify only one area of dissatisfaction with occupational performance – regarding mobility and the desire to walk. Therapy programmes which concentrate upon range of motion exercises, functional electrical stimulation of muscles, standing regimes and caliper walking, without explicitly stating their purpose, may inadvertently foster unrealistic goals for functional mobility. In reality, many people with spinal cord injuries do indeed recognize their limitations and, although expressing the desire to walk, will actively pursue other goals. Use of a client-centred assessment such as the COPM can help the client and therapist to work together to identify client concerns in many areas of living and to direct interventions towards those aspects which are amenable to change.

GOAL SETTING

Long-term goals define an end product, a final outcome. Initially, this will be the outcome of the rehabilitation programme but will also comprise future aspirations such as return to further education, achieving financial independence or starting a business. The values and choices of the client will dictate the long-term goals – and thus the short-term goals which are the building blocks towards the long-term goals. Collaborative goal setting by client and therapist ensures that the rehabilitation programme is directed towards mastering skills that the client values and is likely to use. Each member of the team can then work with the client in establishing realistic objectives to try to reach these goals.

Management of healthcare needs is not a goal in itself. Obsessive emphasis upon successful health management and prevention of complications may reinforce a view that spinal cord injury is an illness, will require lifelong nursing care and that concerns about health should predominate. Although careful management and prevention of complications are undoubtedly essential, both to survival and quality of life, those elements must be viewed more in terms of allowing the person to achieve other, more meaningful goals and activities than as goals in themselves. Good health maintenance practices should become as automatic and unconscious as they are for other adults, so that attention can be directed towards goals more conducive to a fulfilling lifestyle. Using Maslow's hierarchy of human needs as a model (Maslow, 1970) one would hope that more energy and drive is directed towards creativity (self-actualization, cognitive and aesthetic needs), self-esteem (being productive and feeling self-respect) and social needs (friendship, social bonds, love relationships) than towards basic needs such as safety and physical, bodily functions.

Salutary lessons can be learned from an early study that examined the occupational therapy goals of people with paraplegia or quadriplegia and those of their occupational therapists. The therapists and their clients identified quite different goals, the variance between the quadriplegic clients and their therapists being especially marked (Taylor, 1974). As active participation of clients in their treatment is considered to be important, the establishment of objectives related to the client's own goals would appear to be fundamental. Clearly these goals will be more easily identified if the client has been involved in the assessment process.

Ozer (1988) outlines a procedure that ensures client partici-pation in the planning process. He suggests that the pro-fessional commences by asking open-ended questions, such as 'What do you hope to gain from your physiotherapy pro-gramme?' The client explores his options and selects his prime concerns. If this approach fails to elicit an appropriate response, the therapist can take a multiple-choice line of questioning from which the client selects an answer. Should this fail to achieve its objective, the therapist can force a choice by recommending an answer and requiring the client to agree or disagree. Ozer proposes that the planning process should always allow maxi-mum choice to enhance client participation and only if this fails should the multiple-choice or forced-choice options be tried. At no time is 'no choice' advocated, whereby the therapist pre-scribes a goal, predetermines the action planned and the client complies. Ozer advocates maximum client participation in the planning process so that eventually the client will both deter-mine the 'question' and find his own answer.

Establishing goals encourages a positive vision of the future, with options for purposeful activity, occupation, performance of self-care, leisure and socialization. Goals may be revised or modified but provide a sense of purpose and direction for the rehabilitation programme. Collaborative goal setting allows the client to convey his hopes and aspirations while enabling the therapist to understand his world and to work with the client in establishing goals which are likely to be accomplished. Overestimating potential produces frustration and disappoint-ment. Underestimation may be self-fulfilling, hence reducing the level and scope of activity that may be achieved.

The collaborative nature of client-centred goal planning can-not be overemphasized. The therapist has a responsibility to gain an understanding of the client's life roles, demands and interests, while conveying the likely functional potential which the individual may attain. By explaining the implication of the level of neurological damage, functional expectations and skills which it may be possible to achieve, the therapist provides information upon which the client can base informed decisions. The choice of goals is the prerogative of the client hence the therapist cannot impose limits or values. However, it is unfair to convey the impression that all goals are possible to those who try hard enough; it is additionally unreasonable to funding agencies to expend unlimited time to achieve unlikely goals. Collaborative goal setting will thus recognize the client's rights to autonomy and self-determination (the rights they had before entering the rehabilitation facility – the rights of all adults in society) while establishing time frames within which goals are to be completed (Somers, 1992).

In an era of financial restraint and accountability, it should be recognized that such an approach does not demand more staff input. It demands more relevant staff input. The skills of the therapist are used to the maximum in establishing goals that are relevant to the client and to his particular life situation and time is not wasted in pursuit of skills that have no relevance for the individual.

It is important to differentiate between a goal and an objective. The aim of increasing upper limb strength, for example, is not a goal. It could be defined as an objective, that is, a measurable and specific activity designed to achieve the goal of self-propulsion in a wheelchair. A goal states the purpose of a programme – for example, to enable a person with C4 quadriplegia to feed himself independently. The objective should state the specific action planned and the outcome expected (CAOT, 1991).

ESTABLISHING OBJECTIVES

An **objective** is a specific, measurable activity which is designed to achieve a goal (CAOT, 1991). Determining a mutually agreed objective between therapist and client can fulfil the following functions.

- It clarifies the intention of the therapy service, thus minimizing frustration from unmet agendas.
- It establishes a framework within which action may be planned.
- It defines expected results, thereby establishing realistic expectations.
- It helps to identify what resources (material and human) will be necessary to accomplish the goals.
- It facilitates an evaluation of the service.

From the earliest phase of treatment, the therapist must focus on an information-giving rather than a decision-making role. This helps to encourage a non-dependent relationship in which the client develops informed decision-making skills. Priority in setting objectives to meet goals is a function of the individual, his values, his life demands, his resources in four component areas (physical/functional, mental/emotional, spiritual/ philosophical and sociocultural) and the therapist's expertise and resources (CAOT, 1991).

An individual with a high spinal cord lesion may, for example, have the long-term goal of returning to university. He may therefore have established the short-term goal of accessing the computer so that he can complete his course work. In establishing objectives, the client and his therapist will need to do the following.

1. Define a problem – perhaps the inability to access a computer keyboard using the hands.
2. Analyse the problem – some keys ('control', 'shift' and 'alternate') must be held down in unison, therefore a mouthstick alone is inadequate.
3. Develop alternative choices – either use:
   (a) pneumatic controls (sip and puff, breath, 'suck and blow'), using military Morse code (see Chapter 6);
   (b) use a snap on/off device to hold down one key while another is struck;
   (c) use an installed computer programme that allows keys to be struck in sequence rather than in unison.
4. Decide upon the best solution. All three methods may be tried, prices compared and the compatibility with the computer system of choice determined.

The degree of value to the client and his unique needs and lifestyle will be the most important consideration in solution selection. If, for example, he wishes to access the computer from his bed as well as a chair, the pneumatic input, although the most expensive, will also be the most appropriate.

Therapists cannot define 'standard practice' for a condition and follow this. Individualized rehabilitation programmes will instead incorporate the unique factors that consitute the complex issues of community living for each individual, such as work situation, family, psychological make-up and socio-economic background. To ensure relevance, achievability and comprehensiveness, goals and objectives must constantly be re-appraised.

IDENTIFYING ATTAINMENT OF OBJECTIVES

Identification of the attainment of an objective is a measurement of outcome, which assesses the results of therapy services in promoting effective change in the client's functional status (CAOT, 1991). Quality assessment outcome measures consider the consequences, results and impact of therapy intervention. To evaluate the worth of a rehabilitation programme, some form of outcome measure must be devised. The therapy programme centres upon the attainment of mutually established objectives and it is important to be able to identify when these objectives have been achieved.

The effectiveness of a therapy programme is determined primarily by goal accomplishment. The client's status in relation to the goals and objectives which he has set should be re-assessed at regular intervals. Regular assessment of goals and of the attainment of the objectives which have been mutually agreed in reaching those goals, will not only help to ensure the relevance and meaning of the objectives but also the satisfaction of their achievement. Rehabilitation is a long and arduous process, entailing great effort and personal commitment on the part of the client. Frustrations may occur if it is felt that nothing constructive is being accomplished.

In addition to providing the client with evidence of objective and goal attainment, therapist satisfaction is also increased if it is evident that progress is being made. This may be especially relevant in the treatment of people with spinal cord injuries, where no cure is possible and rehabilitation is geared toward adaptation rather than restoration. If objectives were established that were specific, measurable activities, then it must also be possible to identify when these objectives have been reached.

The development of sensitive outcome measures – that is, a means of assessing the impact of intervention – can facilitate the achievement of objectives not only for the client but for the profession.

This may be by:

- improving the quality of care by providing information on client outcomes that can be used in future programme planning;
- demonstrating the effectiveness of the therapy programme to funding agencies;
- demonstrating the effectiveness of the therapy programme to other members of the healthcare team;
- clarifying the roles of the various therapy disciplines (CAOT, 1991).

It is unfortunate that quality of life – our ultimate rehabilitation goal – involves so many areas of performance and holds such personal meaning that accurate outcome analysis is extremely difficult. Therapists must not reduce their vision of holistic programme planning to establish only those objectives that can most easily be attained and measured. Comprehensive patient-care planning cannot be allowed to be compromised to facilitate the achievement of a list of established, documented objectives. It would indeed be unfortunate if the aspects of rehabilitation that are most predictive of quality living – those relating to social engagement, performance of occupations, leisure activities, independent lifestyle and environmental interaction – were once again ignored because their outcomes are not as easy to measure objectively. If therapists can design and use outcome measures to evaluate mutually determined objectives such as these, then truly a service of excellence will have been achieved.

ACCOUNTABILITY

Demands for accountability are forcing therapists to establish objectives and to measure accomplishments within predetermined time frames. In many countries, accountability has been a comparatively recent requirement, whereby therapy practitioners have identified the need to demonstrate the effectiveness of their interventions. Unless objectives have been clearly defined there will be no means of measuring whether they have been achieved. It is incumbent upon the therapist to ensure not only that objectives are established which are compatible with the goals and philosophies of the client but also that the attainment of these objectives is clearly identifiable. In this way, it is more likely that the client will derive satisfaction from his treatment programme. It is also possible for the therapist to evaluate the results of intervention and hence to ensure its ongoing appropriateness. It is tempting to establish objectives that can be attained by everyone at a certain level of spinal cord lesion, rather than making the individual's goals and objectives part of a personal rehabilitation programme, as this would greatly facilitate the development of outcome measures.

Functional assessment instruments and outcome measures typically address impairments and disabilities but seldom address handicaps. Rehabilitation outcome measures have hence not concentrated upon the very arena which rehabilitation services ostensibly address. In an attempt to ensure accountability, outcome measures have been designed to track such elements as units of treatment, numbers of people seen each day for therapy, number of orthoses fabricated, numbers of educational sessions held and the numbers of clients who achieve independent dressing and transferring. Few studies examine the social situation of patients following discharge, yet a study of psychosocial outcome helps to map the effects of rehabilitation. Rehabilitation outcome measures have focused predominantly on performance components (such as range of motion or strength) or upon physical function (mobility and self-care measures) whereas research and evaluation of more holistic client care to date has centred solely upon North American practice of occupational therapy. Quality of life and satisfaction with life – surely important goals for rehabilitation – have rarely been studied following discharge, yet would seem to be the prime outcome measure required in rehabilitation research. Hence therapists risk becoming accountable to their funding agencies but not to their clients.

COMPLIANCE AND CONTROL

Hospital staff and rehabilitation personnel have a great affection for patient compliance with routines, treatments, policies and orders. There has traditionally been an unresisted temptation to mould the patient to suit the regimens of the facility and to view with disfavour individuals who would not co-operate with the rules and regulations imposed upon them. Oliver (*et al.*, 1988) studied the experiences of people discharged from a National Spinal Injuries Centre. Several individuals described a rehabilitation process so regimental that it was as if the rehabilitation system was 'engraved in tablets of stone', so inflexible that the patients were expected just to 'slot in'. Others described the rehabilitation process as a conveyor belt – they were put on to it and had no choices or input into decision making. It is easy to understand how such a system would be conducive to the development of outcome measures, much harder to comprehend how it could actually facilitate a positive outcome in anything more than physical skills.

Compliance may not always be in the best interests of the person with a spinal cord injury. Compliance is not an attribute that best serves the individual in his efforts to achieve his goals and 'co-operation' does not predict independent living success after discharge but rather the reverse may be true. Compliance with externally imposed routines does not teach independence, facilitate problem-solving skills or encourage self-directive behaviour (Tucker, 1984; Trieschmann, 1986).

The most positive documented response to the rehabilitation programme in Oliver's study came from a client whose therapist had the confidence to relinquish power and control and to view instead their participation as a partnership. Although claiming to have been a 'difficult patient' (because he had a clear idea of what he wanted to accomplish) this man commented that his therapist 'did it absolutely right' – they had worked together to solve his problems.

It is difficult to achieve independence when the client is required to act dependently and gratefully have all his decisions made for him.

ACTIVE PARTICIPATION: THE ACTIVATED PATIENT AND EMPOWERMENT IN REHABILITATION

Recent thought among rehabilitation researchers and philosophers has focused upon the need to **empower** or **activate** patients to enable them to seize responsibility and initiative for their own rehabilitation plans. Banja (1990) offers the notion of empowerment as a key concept in articulating the value of rehabilitation. He challenges rehabilitation professionals to provide an integrated and holistic programme of interventions that empowers the disabled person to achieve a personally fulfilling, socially meaningful and functionally effective interaction with the world. The activated patient, rejects the passivity of the 'sick role' and assumes responsibility for his own care. Such individuals ask questions, seek explanations, state their preferences and expect their opinions to be heard. These are the very skills that a person with a spinal cord injury will need to negotiate environmental barriers, avoid preventable medical complications and solve problems following discharge. These are hence the behaviours which will need to be encouraged – not quashed – during the rehabilitation process. As a result of this active behaviour, the client is more knowledgeable about, committed to and satisfied with his treatment regimen. By the interactive process of asking questions and sharing personal treatment goals, there is a greater exchange of information and an expanded knowledge base. As a consequence, the client will develop more realistic expectations, more confidence in his abilities to implement appropriate courses of action and more faith in the competence of his therapists and healthcare team (Steele *et al.*, 1987). Although research indicates that younger and better educated patients are more inclined to endorse active participation in treatment planning, it is suggested that rehabilitation professionals examine ways of including all patients in an active role, to empower them to take responsibility for their own care and to pursue activities likely to enhance health, quality living and the fulfilment of personally meaningful goals.

Therapists may experience role satisfaction from a relationship in which the patient is willingly dependent and respects the therapist's knowledge, skills and dedication. Facilitation instead of a productive relationship which is non-dependent and which requires the client to assume problem-solving responsibility and significant decision making may take a conscious effort on the part of the therapist.

The vocational potential of the person with a spinal cord injury will depend upon his ability to analyse and solve problems, to plan and to execute the plan, to apply skills and technologies, to maintain health and physical capabilities and to interact with, and engage, the physical and social environment

(Kanellos, 1985). All these activities stress action and involvement – the positive outcomes of a rehabilitation programme that emphasizes 'activity' and 'involvement' from the earliest phases of treatment.

LEARNED/TAUGHT HELPLESSNESS

The theory of learned helplessness states that, unless a person feels able to exert some control over the events around him, he will cease making the effort to try to do so (Seligman, 1975). The initial incident that caused the damage to the spinal cord is likely to have been traumatic and accidental – beyond the control of the individual. Treatment in intensive care units and acute care settings may reinforce the sense of helplessness, lack of control and removal of the right to determine the outcome of one's life. A traumatic spinal cord injury and its early treatment is one of the most extreme examples of an event over which a person has no control. The treatment environment may reinforce the sense of powerlessness and helplessness. The client is unable to do anything to alter the situation or to resolve it. However, it is proposed that even in critical care nursing, the primary goal of management is to promote the patient's independent thought and restore a sense of control and self-esteem through self-directing behaviour (Mahon-Darby *et al.*, 1988). A client-centred, goal-directed rehabilitation programme will have no relevance if the individual has learned that he is powerless to control events or outcomes. This could best be described as 'taught' helplessness.

By providing early opportunities for a person to control his environment, by enabling him to set his own goals, choose activities, order his priorities and monitor his progress in an interactive partnership, the person with a spinal cord injury can practice the skills he will need during rehabilitation and after discharge and avoid a tendency towards taught helplessness.

LOCUS OF CONTROL

Rotter (1966) hypothesized that those people who believe that the events which happen to them are the result of luck, chance, fate or powerful people have an external **locus of control**. Their view of life's events is that of circumstances beyond or outside their control. Conversely, the theory states that those people who believe they have a high degree of personal control over both the things that happen to them and over their environmental interactions, have an internal locus of control. The critical issue in this hypothesis is not the actual reality of control but rather the person's belief about his control over events. Hence, someone with a high cord injury and little physical control over events and rewards may still have an internal locus – a belief or expectancy of control. Although it is likely that harmonious living may entail use of different expectations in different circumstances – a more complex equation than a simple polarity of expectations, it is clear that an internal locus of control is associated with more assumption of responsibility for self-care, for health promoting behaviours and for meaningful and productive lifestyles. Studies have indicated that people with an external locus of control experience more distress following a spinal cord injury, even when injured longer, and they exhibit less adaptive behaviours. However, it is suggested that beliefs about health control are learned and can be modified to the extent that patients can learn to use their rehabilitation and healthcare personnel as resources and understand how their own actions are responsible for maintenance of good health.

External expectancy of control is closely affiliated with learned helplessness. There is a belief that the individual has no control over what happens to him and, further, he may not believe that his efforts in rehabilitation will reward him with greater function or abilities. It is incumbent upon the healthcare and rehabilitation teams to reinforce control-eliciting behaviour, to encourage independence of thought and to enhance self-esteem by a milieu that rewards self-directive, assertive behaviour. Johnston *et al.* (1992) describe an intervention study aimed at changing perceived control in patients with physical disabilities. Internal control was found to be increased simply by providing additional information to physiotherapy clients about their own role and potential impact upon treatment outcomes. This area could usefully be researched further to determine the interventions that may effect change in control beliefs and to establish whether this effect is lasting and produces greater client involvement and enhanced rehabilitation outcomes.

MOTIVATION

A complex concept, motivation has traditionally been viewed as a feature of personality – an inner drive that enables an individual to establish important goals and work hard towards them. Viewed from the perspective of the medical model, lack of motivation is seen as a defect in the individual, a problem that prevents the smooth functioning of a carefully regulated rehabilitation regimen. The unmotivated patient is seen as a time waster and a failure in the system. If he does not resolve his problems, he is sent for counselling. In the following example, the individual lady (a 'case') is failing to meet the goals that have been established by others on her behalf.

> A case. . .was referred for psychiatric consultation because the spinal cord injured patient, a 52 year old computer operator, was failing to meet either the short- or long-term goals **established for her** by our hospital's rehabilitation unit.
>
> (Steinglass *et al.*, 1982)

It is tempting to consider whose values, needs and priorities had influenced the establishment of such goals and whether a re-evaluation of these goals would have been more appropriate than seeking psychiatric intervention. Problems may not always be found to reside in the client!

More recently, researchers have begun to examine the environment as a critical element in the assessment of motivation. According to contemporary philosophy, unmotivated individuals are the ones for whom rehabilitation is offering no rewards for which they choose to work. Hence examination will need to be made of team policies, regimens and behaviour as they impact upon the client.

The theory of learned helplessness is applicable to motivation, as the person who has learned that his own actions can have no bearing on his circumstances or outcome will not see any benefit in working towards a goal or reward or towards improving his situation. Research indicates that a sense of powerlessness is associated with a negative rehabilitation outcome.

Similarly, locus of control constructs have relevance to motivational theory. Someone with an internal locus of control is more likely to believe he will be rewarded by hard work, gaining knowledge and establishing goals. If an individual has learned that his health and situation are controlled by other, powerful people and that he can contribute nothing towards achieving positive outcomes, he is likely to become focused upon an external expectancy of control and to fail to pursue an active, goal-directed rehabilitation programme.

Motivation may be significantly influenced by the attitudes of influential others, notably rehabilitation and healthcare staff, family and friends. If these people perceive the spinal cord injury to be a great tragedy, with no hope for a future life of meaning and worth, this will clearly have a negative impact upon the individual and upon his commitment to his rehabilitation programme. The client may not feel motivated to learn self-care skills, for example, if he feels that he has no goals or possibilities for meaningful and fulfilling life in the future. 'The practical implications of client goal choice as a potent motivational construct may . . . be blunted by differences in client-staff perspectives toward goals . . . Treatment environments can override client goals and result in ineffective rehabilitation' (Cook, 1981).

Motivation may thus be viewed as a complex interaction of internal, individual factors and elements in the environment. Motivation should not be equated with co-operation. Frequently, an uncooperative individual has been labelled as unmotivated. He may in reality be rejecting the definition that others have made of his problems and their perceptions of what his goals and activities should be.

Motivational levels will be low if it is perceived that there are few rewards in a life with a spinal cord injury which would justify the hard work and commitment required to achieve them. Motivational levels will be low if the **change cost** – the amount of physical or psychological effort required to effect change – is disproportionate to the client's value of the outcome. This implies that a rehabilitation goal which has low value to the client and his subjective evaluation of its importance to his life will be likely to produce poor motivation and a negative outcome (Jordan *et al.*, 1991). In establishing collaborative goals that are meaningful to the client and worth his considerable change costs, it is essential that the rehabilitation staff understand the client's own health concerns, his values, his goals for independent living and the impact the spinal cord injury has upon his lifestyle. This re-alignment of the assessment process may do much to focus the motivation of the client and the co-operation of the therapist.

RELATIONSHIP BETWEEN CLIENT AND THERAPIST

A client who held negative attitudes towards disability before injury and who has feelings of low self-esteem and self-worth following injury is likely to have these perceptions reinforced by rehabilitation staff who adopt aloof, remote relationships with their clients.

Handicap has been described as a social and environmental concept, influenced by the values, attitudes, expectations and actions of others (Sim, 1990). Health professionals have the capacity (and hence the responsibility) of increasing the client's sense of self-worth and of reducing the process of stigmatization which may accompany disability.

Clearly, exhibition of revulsion or distaste will be hurtful to the client, just as the compassion which tends towards pity will reinforce a sense of inferiority. However, even the professional detachment, objectivity and distance (so much admired in the recent history of therapists' training, and indeed in the medical model of care) will tend to diminish rapport between client and therapist and decrease the opportunities for collaboration. Further, it prevents the therapist from developing a fuller understanding of the client's own perspective of the impact of the injury on his lifestyle and may accentuate the sense of social distance between the aloof professional and the degraded client.

Peloquin (1990) outlines three roles typically assumed by therapists in their relationships with their clients. The therapist as **technician** confuses efficiency and excellence in technical performance with caring, valuing technique over relationship and appearing to the client as cold, aloof and uncaring. The client is unlikely to be able to form a working partnership with such an individual or to be willing to be open about his fears and concerns. Although nurses, for example, have been taught to maintain a certain professional demeanour and distance from their patients, it is found that non-traditional staff–patient relationships are more instrumental in facilitating re-integration into the community for people with spinal cord injuries. A relationship of sharing transcends negative stereotypes about disability and sets an example of comfortable partnerships and relationships that will help families and friends model their own responses to disability and hence to the disabled individual.

The therapist as **parent** has a more personal rapport with the client – but as a paternalistic, nurturing figure – a stance that may produce dependency in the client. Further, the client may rebel against a figure who determines and enforces goals and rules and who undermines the client's autonomy.

The therapist as **covenantor/friend** provides a relationship with the client that has a sense of reciprocity of giving and receiving. The relationship is characterized by trust, commitment and respect. Within the context of this relationship, Peloquin suggests that the therapist collaborates and co-operates with the patient's self-actualization. This is the relationship that is likely to enable a client to use his therapist as a resource, to set mutual goals, to solve problems and to reinforce internal locus of control and self-esteem. The therapist assigns equal value to caring and competence.

The interaction that takes place between the client and the therapist should be as concerned about teaching the therapist about the experience of having a spinal cord injury and about paraplegia and quadriplegia as it is involved with the therapist teaching the client about how to function with a spinal cord injury. This challenges the therapist to relinquish his or her authority as an expert and to achieve a more equal relationship, one that allows the client to convey his own perspectives on his problems and enables the professional to enter the world of those who live with disabilities.

Although therapists ostensibly strive to foster independence in their clients, the traditional roles of the detached expert professional and the inferior, co-operative and compliant patient may have achieved the exact opposite. One researcher found that every client with a spinal cord injury exhibited more independent behaviour in the hallways and cafeteria of the rehabilitation centre than they did in interactions with professionally oriented rehabilitation activities on the ward, in occupational therapy or in physiotherapy (Willems, 1972).

Researchers have also observed the tendency for staff to spend too much time in conference talking **about** patients and not enough time talking **with** patients.

Historically, we have worried that becoming involved with
the people we serve will ruin or taint our ability to function
professionally. However . . . I have become convinced that to
be "impersonal" is to become a nonperson and that it undermines the essence of one individual's ability to help another.
(Trieschmann, 1988)

Many people with spinal cord injuries have formed close
relationships with members of staff which persist after discharge. These may range from strong friendships to intimate
and marital relationships. Given the usual ages of these clients
and of the staff, the intensity of the shared commitment to the
long rehabilitation process and the breaking down of barriers
that a partnership entails, such relationships can be considered
neither surprising, nor deviant. Although such relationships
will clearly not be actively encouraged, they must be expected
and accepted as part of the normal adult experience and part of
the 'price' of patient–client partnerships and of interactions built
on trust, respect and empowerment. Indeed, people with spinal
cord injuries who are treated in local District General Hospitals
(i.e. the majority) may already have close friendships with
their staff.

How long should a patient be considered a 'patient'? Brown
(1992) proposes that, as patients with spinal cord injuries may
return for many years for rehabilitation services, the therapeutic relationship can never be viewed as ending, hence no
deeper relationship can be legitimate. She states that: 'Generally, one would not expect an able bodied person to be attracted
to someone who may not be able to walk, control his bladder
and bowel functioning or father children', or who may experience sexual problems. This is a surprising observation in an era
when bowel and bladder functions can usually be controlled
without any 'accidents' and when numbers of men with spinal
cord injuries are enjoying mutually satisfying sexual relationships – and fathering children. Most particularly, this is a
remarkably negative viewpoint from a healthcare professional
who is ostensibly concerned with fostering self-esteem, a
positive self-image and with viewing the disabled person not
as invalid but as a worthy, valued and valid individual.
Rehabilitation professionals can scarcely expect society at
large to assume a more positive attitude towards people with

disabilities, if they themselves view people who have physical limitations in a stigmatizing and negative light. Unfortunately, this has been the viewpoint of more than one professional and explains much of the reason why people with disabilities have felt devalued, inferior and degraded in their interactions with these staff members, who perversely, have chosen to earn their livings in the rehabilitation industry. Behaviours stem from values and attitudes.

From Brown's standpoint, a person with spinal cord injury remains always stigmatized, always devalued – in fact, always a patient. According to this philosophy, spinal cord injury is equated with an illness, from which one never recovers rather than as an injury from which one undergoes a process of re-learning before resumption of adult roles and activities.

Relationships form whenever people work closely together, for example, between co-workers in offices, in operating theatres, in universities and the military. These special relationships may be a cause for concern in any workplace, just as they may in a rehabilitation centre. If health professionals intend to work alongside their clients for many months in an atmosphere of mutuality, equality and learning, it cannot be surprising if friendships develop. The various departments in the rehabilitation facility will need to decide in advance how these relationships are to be managed and to recognize that patients, once discharged, are private citizens, leaving the patient role and returning to their former roles as lawyers, business people, parents, teachers – in fact, normal people!

CONCLUSION

This chapter has examined aspects of professional competence and patient empowerment, in which the professional becomes a resource, a partner and a learner, and the client becomes a problem solver, a goal definer and the person responsible for his own healthcare and management. The professional is seen, not fixed within the walls of an institution, but as extending the rehabilitation process into the client's environment, enabling negotiation of community interactions and resolution of environmental barriers.

ACKNOWLEDGEMENT

Parts of this chapter are based upon Whalley Hammell (1994a; 1994b) for which permission has been granted.

REFERENCES

Banja, J.D. (1990) Rehabilitation and empowerment, *Archives of Physical Medicine and Rehabilitation*, **71**, pp. 614–5.

Brown, J.F. (1992) Another ethical issue without a resolution. . .to some. *SCI Psychosocial Process*, **5**(2), 42–3.

CAOT (1991) *Occupational Therapy Guidelines for Client Centred Practice*, Canadian Association of Occupational Therapists and Health Services Directorate, Health Services Promotion Branch, Health and Welfare Canada, Toronto, Ont., pp. vii, 17, 38, 74, 99, 110.

Cook, D.W. (1981) A multivariate analysis of motivational attributes among spinal cord injured rehabilitation clients. *International Journal of Rehabilitation Research*, **4**(1), 5–15.

Cyr, L.B. (1989) Sequelae of spinal cord injury after discharge from the initial rehabilitation program. *Rehabilitation Nursing*, **14**(6), 326–9.

Feaver, S. and Creek, J. (1993) Models for practice in occupational therapy: part 2, What use are they? *British Journal of Occupational Therapy*, **56**(2), 59–62.

Illich, I., Zola, I.K., McKnight, J. *et al.* (1977) *Disabling Professions*, Marian Boyars, London, p. 11.

Johnston, M., Gilbert, P., Partridge, C. and Collins, J. (1992) Changing perceived control in patients with physical disabilities: an intervention study with patients receiving rehabilitation. *British Journal of Clinical Psychology*, **31**(1) 89–94.

Jordan, S.A., Wellborn, W.R., Kovnik, J. and Saltzstein, R. (1991) Understanding and treating motivational difficulties in ventilator dependent SCI patients. *Paraplegia*, **29**(7), 431–42.

Kanellos, M.C. (1985) Enhancing vocational outcomes of spinal cord injured persons: the occupational therapist's role. *American Journal of Occupational Therapy*, **39**(11), 726–33.

Law, M. (1993) Evaluating activities of daily living: directions for the future. *Canadian Journal of Occupational Therapy*, **47**(3), 233–7.

Law, M., Baptiste, S., Carswell-Opzoomer, A. *et al.* (1991) *Canadian Occupational Performance Measure*, Canadian Association of Occupational Therapists, Toronto, Ont.

Mahon-Darby, J., Ketchik-Renshaw B., Richmond, T.S. and Gates, E.M. (1988) Powerlessness in cervical spinal cord injury patients. *Dimensions of Critical Care Nursing*, **7**(6), 346–55.

Maslow, A.H. (1970) *Motivation and Personality*, Harper and Row, New York, NY, pp. 15–23.

Oliver, M., Zarb, G., Silver, J. *et al.* (1988) *Walking into Darkness: the Experience of Spinal Cord Injury*, Macmillan, Basingstoke.

Ozer, M.N. (1988) *The Management of Persons with Spinal Cord Injury*, Demos, New York, NY, pp. 107–13.

Peloquin, S.M. (1990) The patient–therapist relationship in occupational therapy: understanding visions and images. *American Journal of Occupational Therapy*, **44**, 13–21.

Pollock, N. (1993) Client centered assessment. *American Journal of Occupational Therapy*, **47**(4), 298–301.

Rotter, J.B. (1966) Generalised expectancies for internal versus external control of reinforcement. *Psychology Monograph*, **80**, 1–28.

Seligman, M. (1975) *Helplessness: on Depression, Development and Death*, W H Freeman, San Francisco, CA, pp. xvii.

Sim, J. (1990) Physical disability, stigma and rehabilitation. *Physiotherapy Canada*, **42**(5), 232–8.

Somers, M.F. (1992) *Spinal Cord Injury Functional Rehabilitation*, Appleton and Lange, East Norwalk, CT, pp. 77–9.

Steele, D.J. Blackwell, B., Gutman, M.C. and Jackson, T.C. (1987) The activated patient: dogma, dream or desideratum? Beyond advocacy: a review of the active patient concept. *Patient Education and Counseling*, **10**, 3–23.

Steinglass, P., Temple, S., Lisman, S.A. and Reiss, D. (1982) Coping with spinal cord injury. The family perspective. *General Hospital Psychiatry*, **4**, 259–64.

Taylor, D.P. (1974) Treatment goals for quadriplegic and paraplegic patients. *American Journal of Occupational Therapy*, **28**(1), 22–9.

Trieschmann, R.B. (1986) The psychosocial adjustment to spinal cord injury, in *Management of Spinal Cord Injuries*, (eds R.F. Bloch and M. Basbaum), Williams and Wilkins, Baltimore, MD, p. 314.

Trieschmann, R.B. (1988) *Spinal Cord Injuries. Psychological, Social and Vocational Rehabilitation*, 2nd edn, Demos, New York, NY, pp. viii, 37, 39, 114, 285.

Tucker, S.J. (1984) Patient–staff interaction with the spinal cord patient, in *Rehabilitation Psychology* (ed. D.W. Krueger), Aspen, Rockville, MD, p. 262.

Whalley Hammell, K.R. (1994a) Establishing objectives in occupational therapy practice. I. *British Journal of Occupational Therapy*, **57**(1), 9–14.

Whalley Hammell, K.R. (1994b) Establishing objectives in occupational therapy practice. II. *British Journal of Occupational Therapy*, **57**(2), 45–8.

Whiteneck, G.G., Charlifue, S.W., Gerhart, K.A. *et al.* (1992) *Guide for Use of the CHART: Craig Handicap Assessment and Reporting Technique*, Craig Hospital, Englewood, CO.

Willems, E.P. (1972) The interface of hospital environment and patient behaviour. *Archives of Physical Medicine and Rehabilitation*, **53**, 115–22.

Yerxa, E.J. and Baum, S. (1986) Engagement in daily occupations and life satisfaction among people with spinal cord injuries. *Occupational Therapy Journal of Research*, **6**(5), 271–83.

FURTHER READING

Caplan, B. and Shechter, J. (1993) Reflections on the 'depressed', 'unrealistic', 'inappropriate', 'manipulative', 'unmotivated', 'noncompliant', 'denying', 'maladjusted', 'regressed', etc patient. *Archives of Physical Medicine and Rehabilitation*, **74**, 1123–4.

CAOT (1991) *Occupational Therapy Guidelines for Client Centred Practice*, Canadian Association of Occupational Therapists and Health Services Directorate, Health Services Promotion Branch, Health and Welfare Canada, Toronto, Ont.

Curtis, K.A. (1985) Physical therapist role satisfaction in the treatment of the spinal cord injured person. *Physical Therapy*, **5**(2), 197–200.

Davis, A., Davis, S., Moss, N. *et al.* (1992) First steps towards an interdisciplinary approach to rehabilitation. *Clinical Rehabilitation*, **6**, 237–44.

McGrath, J.R. and Davis, A.M. (1992) Rehabilitation: where are we going and how do we get there? *Clinical Rehabilitation*, **6**, 225–35.

Trieschmann, R.B. (1988) *Spinal Cord Injuries. Psychological, Social and Vocational Rehabilitation*, 2nd edn, Demos, New York, NY.

2

Education as the key to rehabilitation

Education is the acquisition of the art of the utilisation of knowledge. This is an art very difficult to impart.

(Whitehead, 1929)

INTRODUCTION

Rehabilitation has been defined as the process of learning to live with a disability in the context of one's own environment (Trieschmann, 1986). If this premise is held to be true, then the principles of learning must become the concern of everyone involved in the rehabilitation process.

Research has suggested that all disciplines represented on the rehabilitation team devote a portion of their professional effort to the education of their patients. Indeed, it is proposed that a rehabilitation hospital actually serves as an educational facility as well as a medical facility. Study has further indicated that nurses in a rehabilitation facility direct more effort towards teaching patients than any other single category of activity (Bleiberg and Merbitz, 1983). It is therefore important to examine how rehabilitation personnel are teaching, as the typical education programmes which these staff have themselves undergone have not included training about how to teach. It is suggested that rehabilitation medicine would benefit from a more systematic focus upon patient education, with emphasis upon methods of skill acquisition and relevant teaching practices. As a means of outcome measurement flowing from this approach, there should be quantification of objective learning measures, not a checklist of the topics it is believed have been taught.

Research study in the United States indicated that people with spinal cord injuries had the highest rate of rehospitalization of any diagnostic group (Zook *et al.*, 1980). Further studies have found that repeat hospitalizations are especially common in the first four years after injury and then diminish (Young *et al.*, 1982). This would seem to indicate that learning about living with the disability has an impact upon reducing the incidence of complications; but also that such learning has not successfully occurred during formal rehabilitation. Rehospitalization is a major barrier to independent living; it is costly not only in financial terms but also in the detrimental impact upon the lifestyle of the individual and the opportunity cost that this represents.

Trieschmann (1986) proposes that the learning experience is a dynamic process which starts at the time of injury and continues for the remainder of the person's life. It would therefore be reasonable to conclude that a primary mandate of the rehabilitation team is of assisting the patient to learn successfully how to learn, how to solve problems creatively and how to use experience as a positive learning process.

This chapter will discuss learning theory and the role of education in the rehabilitation process.

LEARNING PROCESS

Learning has been described as being the key to successful rehabilitation. It may also be proposed that a primary goal in the education of people with spinal cord injuries is to increase independence. (**Independence** is used to mean thinking for oneself, being self-governing – it does not relate solely to the performance of physical skills.) The link between learning and independence is crucial in the rehabilitation process.

Education is about imparting the confidence to pose a question and about imparting the responsibility to find the answer. For patient education to be successful, it must involve more than the provision of information. The education process must be an interactive effort which enables the individual to assume responsibilities and achieve independence (McVeigh, 1989).

THEORIES OF LEARNING

It has been suggested that man's power to change himself, that is, to learn, may be his most impressive attribute, but what is learning?

Learning may be described as the process of changing behaviour in a positive direction. It is the discovery of the personal meaning and relevance of ideas. It is defined as a consequence of experience, an evolutionary process. Importantly, it is also a co-operative and collaborative process. These could equally be stated as definitions of the process of rehabilitation.

Bruner (1960) defined the act of learning as having three parts:

1. The **acquisition** of new information;
2. The **transformation** of the information, manipulating it, dealing with it in a way that enables the learner to progress beyond it;
3. **Evaluation**, that is, checking whether the way in which the new information has been transformed and manipulated is adequate to the task and appropriate to the needs of the individual.

The process of being educated must appear to the learner to have some eventual value for him. The learning experience must have meaning and relevance. It must therefore evidently be concerned with the individual's own perception of his learning needs.

Unfortunately, there has been a tendency to label as 'poorly adjusted' any individual who questions the values of his learning experiences. It has been suggested that a learner who is labelled 'poorly adjusted' may not actually fit this label but may be rebelling against a learning experience which he perceives as having a lack of meaning and value for him (Pine and Boy, 1977).

To build knowledge successfully, new information and ideas must be related to an existing cognitive base. Basic concepts should be thoroughly understood and new ideas should be presented in relation to this previous knowledge.

Many writers advocate facilitation of learning centred upon problem identification and problem solving. This **problem-based learning** is the learning that results from the process of working towards the understanding or resolution of a problem

(Barrows and Tamblyn, 1980). Such learning will not only facilitate community re-integration but may influence survival itself. The principles of adult education require that the learner is an active participant in an interactive process, not the passive recipient of an educational programme that has been designed by others on his behalf. The high incidence of preventable complications of spinal cord injury would seem to indicate that the traditional presentation of information is not achieving its goals, hence these learning programmes must be re-evaluated.

In answer to the question: 'What is learning?', the theorists point to a process entailing problem solving, personal change, a personal experience that is unique to the learner and to the personal relevance of ideas. These concepts speak of action and involvement on the part of the learner in which a client-centred, problem-based approach to information would appear to be more appropriate to the acquisition of knowledge than a teacher-centred, subject-based approach. In the latter method, the client is a passive recipient of information and does not learn to learn. Perhaps the traditional methods by which healthcare professionals ('the experts') seek to pass along to their patients that information which they feel must be learned are therefore inappropriate. There is a sense in which 'we tried to teach them, but they didn't learn' (McVeigh, 1989).

HOW DO PEOPLE 'LEARN BEST'?

It has been proposed that people learn best when they are helped to define their own problems, decide on a course of action and importantly, evaluate the consequences of their decisions (Coles, 1989).

Educators have also emphasized the importance of enhancing the learning process by strengthening the link between the actual learning experience and the reflection that follows it. Schon (1983) urges the healthcare professional to encourage a reflective dialogue or conversation with a client to place knowledge into the framework and context of the individual's life and experiences. 'Learning is facilitated in an atmosphere in which evaluation is a co-operative process with emphasis on self-evaluation' (Pine and Boy, 1977).

Experiential learning is a process that requires the full involvement of the learner. What is being learned and how it is being learned are of personal relevance. Through this process, power, or locus of control (Rotter, 1966, see Chapter 1) are shifted from the teacher to the learner. The learner learns to reflect upon his own experience as a basis for assessment of his learning needs, his resources and his objectives. In this way, current learning is related to the past, the present and the future (Woolfe, 1987).

In summary, the learner must be personally involved in the learning process, be encouraged and able to reflect, to integrate his observations and to use this information in a problem-solving way.

The therapist needs to be aware that people have different styles of learning just as they have different types of personality. The approach to learning must therefore be both individualized and flexible.

Traditional presentation of information requires the individual to memorize that information considered to be important by the teacher. Focus tends to be upon disconnected facts or pieces of information. Although many pieces of information might be gleaned, these would be unrelated to experience, would lack personal meaning and relevance and importantly, they cannot be connected or linked to other pieces of information to solve problems. A more personal learning plan will assist individuals in drawing together the information they have assimilated, in asking questions and in centring their learning in their own reality and experience.

Some learners will appreciate the provision of visual aids or written material, or personal demonstration. Unfortunately, many centres have relied solely upon written manuals of information for their clients, irrespective of reading abilities, language preferences, cognitive levels or preferred learning style.

APPLICATION OF LEARNING THEORY IN REHABILITATION

The concept of patient education may be considered in the application of three key words: 'active', 'process' and 'change'. In this context, **active** reflects the need for the patient's full involvement, **process** signals a continuing series of actions or events that aim to help the patient learn how to maintain or improve his current health status. **Change** refers to the acquiring of new knowledge, new skills, new values or beliefs and, importantly, new behaviour (Nursing 87, 1987).

Criticism has been levelled at traditional health education which places the greatest emphasis upon teaching input rather than either process or outcome. An example is found in the literature of a two-day workshop, for people with spinal cord injuries and their families, which had 32 defined learning objectives (defined by the staff) and a schedule for the order in which each topic was to be presented, which was also decided by the staff (Nelson and Kelley, 1983). It is difficult for the learner to be an active participant in the learning process when he is unable to assess his own learning needs and objectives, or to learn new skills and information at the appropriate time.

In addition to determining the patient's preferred style of learning, it is important to time the presentation of information and skills. The patient is more likely to be actively involved in learning when the material being presented is most immediately applicable and relevant.

Educators have emphasized the need to get a patient actively involved in identifying his own learning needs and goals. Active participation and involvement in goal setting are essential to ensuring that the priorities and lifestyle of the patient are considered. These issues have been examined in Chapter 1. They are a key component of the process of enabling a regaining of independence and of encouraging personal control and responsibility. Schon (1983) describes a **reflective contract**, in which the patient joins with the professional in making sense of a situation, achieving in the process a sense of increased involvement and control.

Traditionally, care givers have sought to protect the patient or client from real or potential harm, by taking control over what is learned, when it is learned and how it is learned. However, in an environment in which the patient is active in defining his own problems and identifying his own goals, he must also be permitted to test out his own ideas, to be creative and to take risks (Nursing 87, 1987).

COMPLIANCE AND CONTROL

This raises an important issue concerning power and control. The healthcare team has tended to view patient education as a means to ensure 'compliance' and of preparing the patient to fit into a predetermined role. In Chapter 1 this issue of power and control has already been examined in relation to the rehabilitation process. This is equally relevant to the process of education within the context of rehabilitation and of learning to live with an acquired disability in the context of one's own environment – both physical and sociocultural.

Early education philosophers such as Dewey (1913) and Whitehead (1929) viewed education not in terms of ensuring compliance with a predetermined role but as enabling people to govern their own destinies; not to prepare people to comply but to equip them with the problem-solving skills to enable them to gain greater control over their lives. Many educators even consider the word 'compliance' to be repugnant, with its inherent implications of subservience, dependence and unquestioning obedience to authority (D'Onofrio, 1980).

If we accept the premise that the person who has sustained a spinal cord injury is going to have to seize responsibility for his own health, decisions and actions, then we must ensure that this same person has as much opportunity as possible for input and involvement during the learning process.

LEARNING AND EMPOWERMENT

Perhaps it would be pertinent to examine again the relationship between empowerment and rehabilitation. Banja (1990) proposes that it is the notion of **empowerment** that is the conceptual cornerstone of rehabilitation. It is empowerment that enables a patient to take control of his life, to be responsible for managing his physical condition and to make choices concerning his values and options. These are parallel to the factors that produce an optimal learning process and it is no coincidence that a problem-based learning approach both facilitates and results from empowerment. Health education that is philosophically grounded in the model of client–professional partnership produces not only an efficacious method of learning and transferring knowledge but is also a process by which the learner gains confidence in his ability to solve further problems based on the application and utilization of the knowledge that he has gained.

The ultimate goal of rehabilitation is to enable a regaining of independence. This implies more than independence in purely self-care skills (see Introduction). It is proposed that if people are unable to make their own decisions or solve problems without assistance, they are dependent. Hence problem-solving ability is one of the keys to independence for people with disabilities.

PROBLEM-SOLVING AND LEARNING

It has already been proposed that people are best able to learn when they have defined their own problems, examined their options, decided upon a course of action that is consistent with their values and goals and, finally, re-evaluated their experience and the outcome of their action (Figure 2.1). With reference to the education of people with disabilities, it would appear that solving problems is not only compatible with rehabilitation but it is a prerequisite to the latter's success.

Empowerment is a key issue, as is the concept of choice and control. Education provides the link between the theory and the reality, the process and the change.

Frieden and Cole (1984) describe the problem-solving process as using the following steps.

1. Identification and analysis of a problem – care in identifying and defining the problem will reduce the potential for ineffective solutions.
2. Developing alternative solutions – reflecting upon past experiences and thinking creatively about the possible outcomes of different courses of action.
3. Comparing alternatives and selecting an optimal solution – the individual needs to be able to anticipate possible consequences of his actions. This process may be facilitated by reflecting upon past experience and the consequences of previous decisions made in similar circumstances. Additionally, discussion with a peer group of people who are living with spinal cord injuries may help to identify possible options and alternative solutions.
4. Implementing the decision – this involves a deliberate course of action to initiate change. Risks are involved in implementing a course of action; and anticipation of likely sequelae is an essential component at this stage.

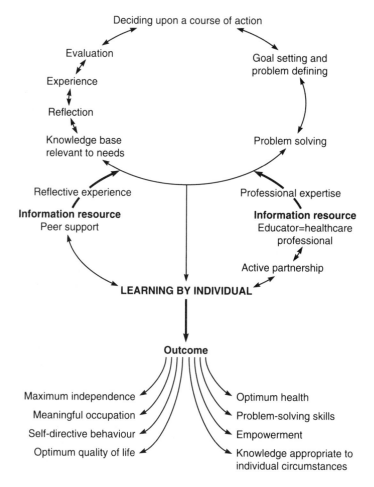

Deciding upon a course of action

Evaluation

Experience

Reflection

Knowledge base
relevant to needs

Goal setting and
problem defining

Problem solving

Reflective experience

Information resource
Peer support

Professional expertise

Information resource
Educator=healthcare
professional

Active partnership

LEARNING BY INDIVIDUAL

Outcome

Maximum independence

Meaningful occupation

Self-directive behaviour

Optimum quality of life

Optimum health

Problem-solving skills

Empowerment

Knowledge appropriate to
individual circumstances

Figure 2.1 The process of patient learning.

5. Evaluating experience and improving the solution, if appropriate – this crucial stage in the problem-solving process is
frequently ignored as attention is focused upon new issues.
Growth is derived, however, by learning from one's mis-
takes, to profit from experience. An empowered patient will
be better equipped to make use of reflection and experiential
learning if he has not been protected from the consequences
of his actions by his healthcare providers.

Reed and Sanderson (1992), in their occupational therapy text, closely link therapy with teaching, and solving problems with defining problems. They outline the role that the therapist plays in teaching an individual to examine a problem by carefully defining the situation, outlining a variety of possible options and selecting what appears to be the most satisfactory and potentially successful solution. If necessary, the solution may be modified or an alternative option tried to achieve optimal results. They emphasize that the advantage of the problem-solving method in therapy is that the individual can solve future problems based on this learning approach.

PEER LEARNING

In a recent research project, the author visited people with spinal cord injuries who were living in their own homes in England (Hammell, 1991). Concern was frequently expressed that the therapists in the spinal units had no knowledge or awareness of what it really means to live with a disability in the community. Frustration was directed at a generic rehabilitation process that aims to teach certain predetermined skills and is out of context with the specific and unique environment of the client, his values or lifestyle. After discharge these people were able to identify what additional skills they needed to acquire, yet this was the time when formal rehabilitation had ended and they had no one to ask for specific advice. This indicates a double flaw in the traditional in-patient rehabilitation process. Firstly, the client may not acquire the skills he needs to function in his own sociocultural and physical environment and, secondly, the rehabilitation team are blissfully ignorant of any additional problems they could have assisted their clients to overcome. Hence, no changes are made to the rehabilitation agenda, or to the assessment and goal-planning processes.

It has been suggested that people learn best from others who are in a similar situation. This would certainly seem to be the case for people with spinal cord injuries. Living life from a wheelchair is an experience shared by few healthcare professionals. Although some students have spent a day in a wheelchair, this serves primarily as a novelty experience and they are unlikely to have allowed their assumed disability to prevent them from reaching a toilet or lecture room, for example. Similarly, although the mechanics of a tenodesis grip can be taught by a therapist, the subtle adjustments of grip that are involved in daily living could usefully be shared by someone who uses a tenodesis grip in every activity. Anyone who has learned to ride a horse will doubtless have appreciated being taught by someone who has experienced the complexities of the required movements and responses themselves. Our clients may feel the same way. Only a person with a spinal cord injury knows what it is like to have a spinal cord injury and only carers know what it is like to provide full support for someone who is physically dependent. Gardner *et al.* (1985) suggest that the rehabilitation staff on a spinal unit may know all about spinal cord injury yet will still fail to appreciate its reality.

Clearly, rehabilitation professionals have a wealth of knowledge, experience and insight to share with their clients. They may see possibilities where a client sees none and they may have learned from others with spinal cord injuries. However, involvement of peers in a learning process provides the added dimension of experience upon which to base some reflection. This will be of benefit not only to the newly injured individual but also to the therapist who can learn from someone who has already learned to live with a disability.

BARRIERS TO LEARNING

Members of the rehabilitation team must be aware of potential barriers to learning. In the early stage of spinal cord injury management the patient may be unable to participate actively in the decision-making process, due partly to shock, severe pain and medications. This is a time when the medical model, which seeks to define and address purely physiological issues, may be appropriate. The initial phase of treatment may be regarded as a crisis in the individual's life and represents a sudden and devastating transition from independence to dependence. Once this acute phase is resolved, the patient may begin to participate actively in his care and in making decisions and choices.

The rehabilitation process requires the acquisition of new knowledge and skills. This requires the ability to concentrate, understand and process information. The information must also be retained, retrieved, integrated and used in a meaningful way. Researchers have examined the neuropsychological deficits that may be present in people with acute spinal cord injuries. They have found that concentration and initial learning ability appeared to be partially impaired, in comparison to control subjects. Severe impairments were apparent in the ability to adapt to new situations. The researchers identified other neuropsychological problems that could interfere with rehabilitation following a spinal cord injury, including poor attention span, impaired memory function and altered problem-solving ability (Roth *et al.*, 1989). These findings have major implications for the implementation of a learning experience as well as for the whole rehabilitation process for people with spinal cord injuries. Rehabilitation is an intensive process with much learning expected in the early stages. Indeed, even in many developed countries, financial restraints have served to limit the entire formal rehabilitation process to just a few weeks.

It is important to recognize the presence and nature of any neuropsychological deficits, as these may compromise the achievement of an optimal outcome from the rehabilitation process (see also Chapter 4 regarding concomitant head injuries). Such cognitive problems will present serious impediments to learning and should not be misinterpreted by the rehabilitation team as being symptoms of denial or depression (see Chapter 7). However, as research studies have indicated a prevalence of major depressive episodes among people with acute spinal cord injuries to range from 10% to 30%, learning during the early weeks of rehabilitation may be further compromised (Davidoff *et al.*, 1990).

After full consideration of the physiological, psychological, sociocultural and environmental factors that may prevent optimal learning, the therapist may be able to identify when meaningful learning can begin by the nature of the questions asked by the patient.

It is important that the rehabilitation team clearly understands what their patient believes they are saying. When a nurse, for example, speaks of the danger of forming a pressure sore, does the patient understand by 'sore' a small blister or a raw patch of skin, or does he visualize a gaping wound with life-threatening potential? (Basta, 1991).

In summary, the therapist can assist the learning process by awareness of potential barriers to learning, by adjustment of role from 'authoritative' to 'partnership' and by seeking co-operation from peers to provide reflective experiences for the patient.

LEARNING NEEDS AND MASLOW'S HIERARCHY

The person who has sustained an injury to the spinal cord must learn an impressive amount of new information. Survival depends to a very real extent upon correct management. The person with a very high lesion (and thus no use of hands or arms) must not only learn new information but be able to relay it effectively to a care giver. The success of his future life depends upon his ability to direct effectively other people in his care and hence to become a teacher himself (McVeigh, 1989).

The left-hand column of Table 2.1 illustrates some of the many complex issues that a person with a spinal cord injury must face in seeking an independent and fulfilling lifestyle within the parameters of his physical condition. These have been ranked according to Maslow's hierarchy of physiological and psychological needs (Maslow, 1970). This may provide a useful frame of reference for the patient and therapist in establishing collaborative priorities of learning needs. In the right-hand column are some suggested learning responses that could usefully be related to the identified needs.

Lawes (1985) presented the results of an international study of educational practices in spinal injury units. He divided into three areas the topics in which the various units stated that they needed educational programmes. These were:

- anatomy and physiology, e.g. bladder and bowel management, pressure sore prevention, spasticity;
- social areas, e.g. social skills, sexuality, sports and leisure, activities of daily living;
- resources, e.g. aids and equipment, community resources, financial management, benefits, employment and housing.

This is a comprehensive assessment of learning needs, reflecting many of the topics listed in the model (after Maslow) in Table 2.1.

Once again it must be reinforced that the provision of information to clients must not be based solely on what the healthcare providers decide that the client should know and when he should know it. The timing and nature of the topic

Table 2.1 Relating learning needs to Maslow's hierarchy. (Adapted from Starck, 1980; Nursing 87, 1987)

Basic physiologic issues

Paralysis	Cause and prognosis
Respiratory problems (life threatening)	Breathing exercises
	Assisted coughing
Urinary tract dysfunction	Fluid intake regimens
	Urinary tract management
Autonomic hyperreflexia (life threatening)	Prevention and diagnosis
Muscle spasticity	Prevention of contractures
Bowel incontinence	Dietary needs, care routines
Loss of sensation	Need for turning and positioning to prevent soft tissue damage
Altered temperature regulation	Summer/winter implications
Infections (life threatening)	Early detection and appropriate use of medications

Security issues

Altered mobility, uncertainty regarding long-term care provision, problems with transportation, financial uncertainty and insecurity, increased susceptibility to physical hazards	Safe use of mobility equipment, management of stress, problem identification, evaluation of options, awareness of local resources, identifying goals and investigating alternatives, peer learning and modelling

Love and belongingness issues

Barriers to involvement in social and religious activities, role reversals within family, changes in social persona, limitations in touching, alterations in sexual expression	Maintenance of important family and social relationships, learning from peers how to be expressive sexually and to function effectively in diverse social situations

Self-esteem

Frustrations from environmental barriers – architectural and social/attitudinal, altered body image, alteration of roles, dissatisfaction with lack of involvement in meaningful occupation, discomfort in asking for help	Adjustment to role changes, seeking information from knowledgeable others – peers and professionals, developing planning skills, developing assertiveness, actively working to reduce environmental barriers, reflection and experiential learning, engagement in meaningful occupations

Self-actualization

Altered lifestyle, lack of spontaneity, barriers to career fulfilment, dissatisfaction with the amount of control, choice and responsibility. Barriers to participation, in intellectual, political, cultural, social and religious arenas, changes in roles, barriers to life goal fulfilment, powerlessness	Engagement in meaningful occupation, integration of disability, learning process can allow patient 'activation' enabling identification of new goals and interests, the learning process should also facilitate the seizing of responsibility. Initiative and independence in decision-making and problem-solving skills. Identification of factors that contribute to life satisfaction and quality of life.

must be decided in collaboration between educator and client. If the client is preoccupied with a rampant urinary tract infection, for example, he is likely to be more concerned about the prevention of future such episodes than to discover how to transfer to and from the floor.

Learning needs may be expressed in terms of a hierarchy of importance and this may be a useful reminder to consider topics other than the 'low-level', physiological issues. It has been suggested that rehabilitation services in the past focused upon physiological restoration followed by maximum physical function and discharge. Consideration of all facets of the functioning adult in a model such as Maslow's serves as a useful reminder that there is more to learn about living with a disability than transfers, skin care and getting dressed.

SETTING GOALS

Chapter 1 included a study of client-centred goal setting in a rehabilitation programme. This approach is further advocated when establishing goals and devising a learning plan in a collaborative educational environment. Implicit in this approach is the belief that this provides the client with practice in solving problems and making decisions. These are the skills that will be needed in establishing future goals and in making realistic plans. The teaching process should concentrate on collaborative problem solving rather than on the provision of solutions.

This is a challenging agenda for the therapist who has received a training which places emphasis upon setting goals for clients and not in co-operation with clients. Taylor (1974) found little correlation between the goals of therapists and those of their spinal cord injured clients. Such discrepancies will present serious problems in an educational context if the therapist is not presenting information that the client desires but what it is perceived that he needs. This is a situation in which the client receives the mixed message that he should become independent (making responsible plans and decisions) yet act dependently (co-operating, complying and accepting the goals set by others) (Tucker, 1980).

When teaching people with spinal cord injuries about their injury and its sequelae, the focus must be upon the information required to solve problems that may occur in carrying out the required regimens. By encouraging participation, the client will learn to approach problems with the regimen by thinking through possible solutions and to cope when such problems occur (McVeigh, 1989).

The person with high-lesion quadriplegia must become not only a learner but also a teacher if his needs are to be fulfilled. This will only occur if the individual has learned to become fully responsible for his own care. Rehabilitation should not result in a person who is dependent not only for physical care but also dependent on others for making decisions and solving problems related to the disability.

FAMILY INVOLVEMENT IN THE LEARNING PROCESS

Spinal cord injury poses great adaptation demands both on the injured person and on those who live with him. There has, however, been a lack of systematic studies of the partners and families of severely injured people which is only recently being addressed. This may reflect the tendency of rehabilitation workers to focus upon the adaptation and learning process solely of the individual who has been injured, despite the frequent acknowledgement that spouses and close support people play a major role in the rehabilitation process. Family education has rarely been addressed despite the recognition that family support is one of the most important factors in successful rehabilitation outcome and that, at discharge, the spouse frequently becomes responsible for the continuation of the partner's rehabilitation process and, sometimes, for the provision of continuing care (Peters *et al.*, 1990).

If the client and his family are waiting for a 'miracle cure', they may initially show little interest in an education programme that enables them to learn about life with a spinal cord injury. However, if the staff can emphasize that maintenance of the body in an optimal condition is important in case of any future functional return, this may help to focus their attention and interest (Zejdlik, 1992).

The process of education should be open to include any significant people whom the client would like to involve. The choice should be the client's. Staff members who are accustomed to making decisions on behalf of their clients may feel, for example, that the mother of a 17-year-old with paraplegia should learn about his care. To the young man himself, who may have already left home and will certainly have been physically independent of his mother for many years, this could be an unnecessary, unwelcome and embarrassing intrusion. Conversely, someone with a new spinal cord injury may wish to involve his partner or spouse in learning about his disability and how best to minimize its impact. It may therefore be appropriate for the client to time such events as range of motion exercises or catheterizations to coincide with the time his partner is able to visit.

If rehabilitation is assumed to be the process of learning to live with a disability in one's own environment then it would appear to be essential to include members of that close personal environment in a shared learning experience. Unfortunately, the reality has frequently been quite different and exclusion has been more common than inclusion.

SUMMARY

People with spinal cord injuries need to learn a great amount of information to maintain their health status. Many will also need to learn how to relay their care needs clearly and effectively to others. Principles of adult education require that a learner is an active participant in an interactive process, not a passive recipient of a programme designed for him. The high incidence of preventable complications of spinal cord injury indicates that the current presentation of information is not achieving its goals.

It is proposed that the outcomes of a successful learning process will include self-determination, effective coping skills, participant satisfaction and, ultimately, enhanced quality of life (see Figure 2.1).

A newly disabled person must learn to trust in his abilities, form a new relationship with his environment and live creatively. He cannot afford to be a conformist. Education in a rehabilitation context should enable the individual to learn how to learn, to use experience as a constant modifier of new knowledge and to solve problems creatively.

REFERENCES

Banja, J.D. (1990) Rehabilitation and empowerment (commentary). *Archives of Physical Medicine and Rehabilitation*, **71**, 614–5.

Barrows, H.S. and Tamblyn, R.M. (1980) *Problem Based Learning*, Springer, New York, NY, p. 1.

Basta, S.M. (1991) Pressure sore prevention education with the spinal cord injured. *Rehabilitation Nursing*, **16**(1), 6–8.

Bleiberg, J. and Merbitz, C. (1983) Learning goals during initial rehabilitation hospitalization. *Archives of Physical Medicine and Rehabilitation*, **64**, 448–51.

Bruner, J.S. (1960) *The Process of Education*, Harvard University, Cambridge, MA, pp. 48–9.

Coles, C. (1989) Self assessment and medical audit: an educational approach. *British Medical Journal*, **299**, 807–8.

Davidoff, G., Roth, E., Thomas, P. *et al.* (1990) Depression among acute spinal cord injury patients: a study utilizing the Zung Self-rating Depression Scale. *Rehabilitation Psychology*, **35**(3), 171–9.

Dewey, J. (1913) *Interest and Effort in Education*, Southern Illinois University, Carbondale and Edwardsville, IL.

D'Onofrio, C.N. (1980) Patient compliance and patient education: some fundamental issues, in *Patient Education: an Enquiry into the State of the Art* (ed. W.D. Squyres), Springer, New York, NY, pp. 271–2.

Frieden, L. and Cole, J.A. (1984) Creative problem solving, in *Rehabilitation Psychology* (ed. D.W. Krueger), Aspen, Rockville, MD, pp. 69–79.

Gardner, B.P., Theocleous, F., Watt, J.W.H. and Krishnan, K.R. (1985) Ventilation or dignified death for patients with high tetraplegia. *British Medical Journal*, **291**, 1620–2.

Hammell, K.R.W. (1991) *An Investigation into the Availability and Adequacy of Social Relationships Following Head Injury and Spinal Cord Injury: a Study of Injured Men and their Partners*, MSc thesis (Rehabilitation Studies), University of Southampton, Southampton.

Lawes, C.J. (1985) Patient education in practice: an international survey of spinal injury units. *International Journal of Rehabilitation Research*, **8**(3), 321–9.

Maslow, A.H. (1970) *Motivation and Personality*, Harper and Row, New York, NY, pp. 15–23.

McVeigh, K. (1989) Reflections on the process of education for the patient with high quadriplegia, in *The Management of High Quadriplegia. Vol. 1. Comprehensive Neurologic Rehabilitation* (eds G.G. Whiteneck, C. Adler, R.E. Carter *et al.*), Demos, New York, NY, pp. 263–270.

Nelson, A.L. and Kelley, B. (1983) Patient and family workshops. *Rehabilitation Nursing*, **8**(6), 13–16.

Nursing 87, (1987) Understanding basic concepts, in *Patient Teaching*, Nursing 87, Springhouse Corp., Springhouse, PA, pp. 1, 14, 60–61.

Peters, L.C., Stambrook, M., Moore, A.D. and Esses, L. (1990) Psychosocial sequelae of closed head injury: effects on the marital relationship. *Brain Injury*, **4**(1), 39–47.

Pine, G.J. and Boy, A.V. (1977) *Learner-centered Teaching. A Humanistic View*, Love, Denver, CO, pp. 112–13, 124.

Reed, K.L. and Sanderson, S.N. (1992) *Concepts of Occupational Therapy*, 3rd edn, Williams and Wilkins, Baltimore, MD, pp. 134, 170.

Roth, E., Davidoff, G., Thomas, P. *et al.* (1989) A controlled study of neuropsychological deficits in acute spinal cord injury patients. *Paraplegia* **27**, 480–9.

Rotter, J.B. (1966) Generalised expectancies for internal versus external control of reinforcement. *Psychology Monograph*, **80**, 1–28.

Schon, D.A. (1983) *The Reflective Practitioner – How Professionals Think in Action*, Jossey-Bass, San Francisco, CA.

Starck, P. L. (1980) Maslow's needs and the spinal cord injured client. *Rehabilitation Nursing*, Sept/Oct, 17–20.

Taylor, D.P. (1974) Treatment goals for quadriplegic and paraplegic patients. *American Journal of Occupational Therapy*, **28**(1), 22–9.

Trieschmann, R.B. (1986) The psychosocial adjustment to spinal cord injury, in *Management of Spinal Cord Injuries*, (eds R.F. Bloch and M. Basbaum), Williams and Wilkins, Baltimore, MD, pp. 303–4.

Tucker, S.J. (1980) The psychology of spinal cord injury: patient–staff interaction. *Rehabilitation Literature*, **41**(5–6), 114–22.

Whitehead, A.N. (1929) *The Aims of Education*, Macmillan, New York, p. 6.

Woolfe, R. (1987) Experiential learning in workshops, in *Running Workshops*, (Coping with Crisis Research Group), Open University, Croom Helm, Beckenham, pp. 1–15.

Young, J.S., Burns, P.E. and Witt, G.A. (1982) Medical charges incurred by the spinal cord injured during the first six years following injury. *SCI Digest*, **4**(2), 19–34.

Zejdlik, C.P. (1992) Individual and family health education, in *Management of Spinal Cord Injuries* (ed. C.P. Zejdlik), Jones and Bartlett, Boston, MA, p. 206.

Zook, C.J., Savickis, S.F. and Moore, F.D. (1980) Repeated hospitalization for the same disease: a multiplier of National Health Costs. *Milbank Memorial Fund Quarterly*, **58**(3), 454–71.

3

Spinal cord injury: aetiology, incidence and impairments

When meditating over a disease, I never think of finding a remedy for it, but, instead, a means of preventing it.

(*Louis Pasteur, 1884*)

HISTORICAL PERSPECTIVE

The catastrophic nature of spinal cord injury was described by an Egyptian physician as early as 2500 BC. (Grundy and Swain, 1993), yet spinal cord injury remained a sentence of death until as recently as the 1940s. During the First World War, 80% of people who sustained a spinal cord injury died within two weeks (Stover and Fine, 1986). It was the introduction of sulfanilamides and antibiotics in the 1940s that changed the rates of survival and provided Western countries with the challenge of caring for thousands of men who had sustained spinal cord injuries during the Second World War.

Sir Ludwig Guttmann, in Britain, recognized that survivors of spinal cord injury required more than nursing care. Extensive rehabilitation services were also required to enable these men to achieve the highest quality of life, even if this was thought to be fairly short. Through the pioneering work of Guttmann, and others in the USA, increased understanding was gained concerning spinal cord injury. The development of efficient management led to a reduction in mortality and increased numbers of incomplete lesions although, by the 1960s, mortality associated with quadriplegia was still 35% (Grundy and Swain, 1993).

There was a gradual change in the pattern of survival from low-lesion paraplegia in the 1950s, high-lesion paraplegia in the 1960s and low-lesion quadriplegia in the 1970s. These changes coincided with advances in the development of limited antibiotics, full spectrum antibiotics, improved respiratory care and cardiopulmonary resuscitation (CPR), (Menter, 1989). Finally, in the 1980s, people with spinal cord injuries at or above C4, resulting in high-lesion quadriplegia, have also been surviving in significant numbers. Expert medical services provided at the scene of the accident and, in North America, the training in CPR of large numbers of the general public, have assisted in saving lives. Improved diagnosis, equipment and training in hospitals has enabled long-term survival.

Superior knowledge concerning the management of spinal cord injury now exists, which serves both to minimize disabilities and complications while being more cost effective. The next decades should see greater access to specialized care for more people with acute injuries and improvements in rehabilitation services. It is possible to enable all people with spinal cord lesions to achieve productive, fulfilling and quality lifestyles. Quantity of life has been assured. Quality of life must become our larger goal.

INCIDENCE AND PREVALENCE

Spinal cord injury is not a notifiable condition, hence figures for annual incidence are inaccurate and vary according to the source. Estimates in the USA indicate that there are about 8000–10 000 new traumatic spinal cord injuries per year with almost a quarter of a million people who are living with spinal cord injuries (DeVivo *et al.*, 1980). The incidence of non-traumatic spinal cord injury is difficult to determine but is estimated to be at least equal to that of traumatic injury.

In the UK, it is estimated that there are between 900 and 1000 new injuries per year and about 40 000 people living with spinal cord injuries.

In the USA (where a database enables more accurate analysis of injury patterns), the median age at injury is 25 and the mode, that is, the most frequent age at injury, is 19 years. A total of 61% of spinal cord injuries in the USA are sustained between 16 and 30 years of age (Stover and Fine, 1986). Hence spinal cord injury predominantly affects young people who are poised to achieve their life goals and become economically independent. Spinal cord injury occurs more frequently among males than among females. The ratio of males to females is usually estimated to be 82:18% in the developed world. This figure is also imprecise, as only the USA has a spinal cord injury database. Ratios will differ according to aetiology and country.

AETIOLOGY OF TRAUMATIC INJURY

The aetiology of spinal cord injuries in the UK is illustrated in Figure 3.1. Industrial legislation, seat belt legislation and sports regulations have done little to alter the aetiology or incidence of this injury. Spinal cord injuries due to diving have been described as an 'epidemic'. Prevalence of the injury is increasing exponentially, as it is in other countries. Among the over-75 age group in the USA, about 60% of spinal cord injuries are the result of falls (Stover and Fine, 1986).

The nationwide USA figures mask individual idiosyncracies. In cities such as Los Angeles, Miami, Chicago and Washington DC, the number of spinal cord injuries caused by acts of violence is double or triple that of 10 years ago. Acts of violence are reportedly the primary cause of spinal cord injuries in southeast Michigan, or 42.7% of the total (Weingarden and Graham, 1992). Gunshot wounds have recently become the prime cause of spinal cord injuries admitted to the Rancho Los Amigos Medical Center near Los Angeles. It is reported that over 35% of the 300 spinal cord injuries admitted in 1990 were caused by gunshot wounds (Zeeb, 1991).

Stover and Fine (1986) further indicate that spinal cord injuries, nationwide, occur in cycles, with the lowest number in February, rising to the greatest number in July and decreasing steadily again until February. Similarly, injuries reach a peak on weekends.

Of critical importance is the distribution of neurological injuries according to aetiology. Stover and Fine indicate that, from their national statistics, fully 91.8% of spinal injuries caused by sporting activities result in quadriplegia (44.7% complete and 47.1% incomplete injuries). Falls account for 16.9% complete quadriplegias (47.8% quadriplegias) whereas acts of violence have a distribution of 42.4% complete paraplegias and 16.1%

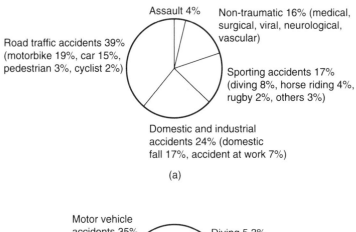

Assault 4%   Non-traumatic 16% (medical, surgical, viral, neurological, vascular)

Road traffic accidents 39% (motorbike 19%, car 15%, pedestrian 3%, cyclist 2%)

Sporting accidents 17% (diving 8%, horse riding 4%, rugby 2%, others 3%)

Domestic and industrial accidents 24% (domestic fall 17%, accident at work 7%)

(a)

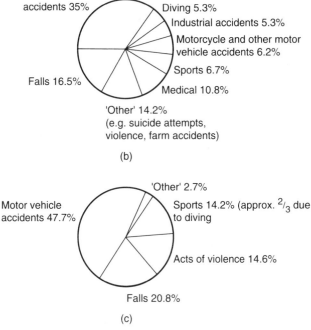

Motor vehicle accidents 35%

Diving 5.3%

Industrial accidents 5.3%

Motorcycle and other motor vehicle accidents 6.2%

Sports 6.7%

Falls 16.5%

Medical 10.8%

'Other' 14.2% (e.g. suicide attempts, violence, farm accidents)

(b)

'Other' 2.7%

Motor vehicle accidents 47.7%

Sports 14.2% (approx. $\frac{2}{3}$ due to diving

Acts of violence 14.6%

Falls 20.8%

(c)

Figure 3.1 Causes of spinal cord injury. (a) UK in 1992 (Spinal Injuries Association, 1992); (b) Canada in 1992 (Canadian Paraplegic Association, 1993); (c) USA 1973–1985 (Stover and Fine, 1986).

complete quadriplegias (14.4% incomplete quadriplegias). In motor vehicle accidents, 23.2% result in complete quadriplegias, 30.8% incomplete quadriplegias and 28.4% complete paraplegias.

In other countries, different patterns of aetiology emerge. In Denmark, it is reported that the proportion of traumatic spinal cord injuries due to suicide attempts rose from 3.5% (1965 to 1974) to 13% (1985–1987) (Biering-Sørensen *et al.*, 1992). In Armenia, over 200 people sustained spinal cord injuries during the 1988 earthquake. The subsequent mission by the League of Red Cross and Red Crescent societies led to the establishment of the first spinal cord injury rehabilitation unit in what was still the Soviet Union. In Soweto, the largest urban, black township in South Africa, the inter-related factors of poverty, apartheid, oppression and violence lead to most cord injuries (64%) being caused by acts of violence. A total of 42% of people sustained their injuries due to stabbings, whereas 22% were shot by the police (Cock, 1989a; Cock, 1989b).

In Singapore, 24% of spinal cord injuries occurring between 1973 and 1984 were sustained due to falls from incompleted high-rise buildings and unsafe (primarily bamboo) scaffolding (Tan and Balachandran, 1987). In Madras, India, 66% of patients with spinal cord injury sustained their trauma by falling either from a height or into unprotected wells (Shanmugasundaram, 1988).

In countries such as Lebanon, Nicaragua, Zimbabwe and Cambodia, wars have created tens of thousands of people with traumatic disabilities, including many spinal cord injuries. However, it is estimated that most people with spinal cord injuries in developing countries die within two years of their injuries due to a lack of adequate treatment facilities (New Internationalist, 1992). Hence, the whole concept of 'rehabilitation' will remain largely the prerogative of the developed world until issues surrounding acute care management, prevention of complications, poverty, powerlessness, disadvantage and stigma are addressed in developing nations.

PREVENTION OF TRAUMATIC INJURY

Spinal cord injury is a condition of comparatively low incidence but of great cost to the individual and to society. Cure is not possible, hence considerable attention must be directed towards preventing its occurrence.

In the USA, comprehensive databases exist to compile information about each spinal cord injury. From this information, trends can be identified and preventive measures, education or legislation can be directed accordingly. Wigglesworth (1992) advocates the formation of an Australian Spinal Injuries Registry to identify the causes of spinal cord injury and hence appropriate intervention measures. In those countries where such a recording system does not exist, it is difficult to determine the primary targets for intervention – or even the number of people sustaining the injury. More than just the cause of injury is important, as there is a relationship between the cause of injury and the anatomic location of injury. For example, motor vehicle accidents which result in spinal cord damage show a 54% proportion of quadriplegias. The incidence of quadriplegia following a sports related spinal injury is a startling 91.8% (Stover and Fine, 1986).

Parsons and Lammertse (1991) outline three strategies to prevent injuries:

- persuading people to alter risky behaviour through education, for example, not diving in natural environments;
- requiring that people change their behaviour through legislation, such as the mandatory use of seat belts;
- providing automatic protection by product and environment design, such as air bags and safety elements in vehicle design.

Motor vehicle accidents

Automobile accidents are a major cause of spinal cord injury. Analysis of these accidents in North America has found them to be most common on rural, high-speed roads, in the dark and on a weekend. Frequently the accident is a single-vehicle rollover but may involve a head-on collision. There is an association with alcohol use, driving with undue care and unsafe speed (Wing and Cain, 1992). An Australian study indicated that 38 out of the 44 motor vehicle accidents that resulted in spinal cord injuries involved a single-vehicle rollover accident (that is, over 86%)

(Wigglesworth, 1992). The highest rate of severe cervical injury is caused by rollover accidents but severe neck injuries also occur in frontal or side impact crashes. Of those who sustain the more serious neck injuries, 97% are not wearing seat belts. It is important to note that positive changes in car design such as seat belt provision, air bags, interior padding and energy absorbing steering wheels, which help to reduce the incidence and severity of spinal cord and other severe injuries have required legislation to enforce standards. Kraus *et al.* (1982) showed that following the introduction of USA federal standards of vehicle design, the rates of spinal cord injuries from car crashes in the USA declined.

Diving

Diving injuries form a significant proportion of all spinal cord injuries. Many are fatal and survivors are significantly more likely to have quadriplegia than paraplegia. It is apparent that relatively little impact is required to cause spinal cord injuries when diving and few people have noticeable bruising or abrasions to the head. Those involved with prevention of spinal cord injuries from diving recommend that inexperienced divers need a deeper and larger area in which to dive than do experienced divers, thorough education in technique and thorough attention to water depths, their entry angle and arm positions. As the natural environment (where approximately 50% of Canadian dive-related spinal cord injuries occur) cannot be thoroughly judged, it is recommended that people do not dive in lakes, rivers or oceans. It is further proposed that the only safe way to use a waterslide is sitting up (Wing and Cain, 1992).

Sports and recreation

Spinal cord injuries resulting from accidents in sports and recreation appear to be increasing in Canada and this trend may parallel other developed countries where these activities are growing.

Examination of the statistics has shown the considerable disproportion of quadriplegias caused by sporting accidents. Survival rates are considered to be high following these injuries, as the incidence of multiple trauma is rare. Hence, sports-related injuries constitute a considerable burden on society in medical costs and even greater personal costs to the individual who sustains the injury.

In the USA, football has been a major cause of spinal cord injury but the incidence is declining because of changes in rules and tactics. Similarly, in South Africa, the UK and Ireland, where rugby has contributed to significant numbers of spinal cord injuries, rule changes and educational programmes have been initiated.

In Canada, the emergence of ice hockey as a major cause of spinal cord injury (in particular, high cervical injury) has caused the Committee on Prevention of Spinal Injuries Due to Hockey to recommend stricter rule enforcement, especially those against checking from behind; neck muscle conditioning for players and research on equipment design and injury mechanisms. Study suggests that non-professional players are especially at risk of injury due to lack of muscle conditioning; or lack of awareness of how to sustain an impact and of the implications of collisions into the boards (Tator and Edmonds, 1984).

Spinal cord injuries are caused by a variety of sporting activities, for example, boxing, snow-mobiling, horse riding, trampolining, toboganning, bicycling, gymnastics and hang gliding, and in each activity the mechanism of injury is unique. It is proposed that the medical profession should be a leader in data collection regarding epidemiology and should be adaptable in promoting appropriate prevention strategies.

Work injuries

Industries attempt to improve financial returns by minimal safety standards and little attempt to reduce accidents or work related injuries. Government legislation in the form of occupational safety and health regulations is maintained under public pressure and demands for worker protection (Wing and Cain, 1992). In countries where such pressure has not been mobilized, industries have little incentive to provide a high level of safety, as this entails considerable cost and effort. Work injuries continue to contribute significantly to the worldwide cause of traumatic spinal cord injuries.

IMPAIRMENT

Levels of injury

Injury to the spinal cord may produce damage that results in complete or incomplete impairment of function. A **complete** lesion is one where motor and sensory function is absent below the level of injury. A complete lesion may be caused by a complete severance of the spinal cord, by nerve fibre breakage due to stretching of the cord or due to ischaemia of the cord resulting from interruptions of the total blood supply.

An **incomplete** lesion will enable certain degrees of motor and/or sensory function below the level of injury to remain intact. There are recognized patterns of incomplete cord injuries.

Central cord syndrome

This lesion occurs almost exclusively in the cervical region and is typically due to a hyperextension injury, often from fairly minor trauma. Classically there is flaccid weakness of the arms (lower motor neurone) and spastic, although relatively strong leg function (upper motor neurone). There is generally sacral sensory sparing and partial bladder and bowel function. Prognosis for neurological and functional improvement is good, although hand function characteristically remains poor.

Brown-Séquard syndrome

The signs of this syndrome are of a hemisection of the spinal cord and it is commonly the result of a stab wound. On the side of the injury (ipsilateral) there is reduced or absent motor power but relatively normal pain and temperature sensation. Because the spinothalamic tract crosses to the opposite side of the cord, the contralateral or uninjured side has good motor power but loss of sensitivity to pinprick and temperature (ASIA, 1992; Grundy and Swain, 1993).

Anterior cord syndrome

This syndrome is the result of a combination of direct trauma and ischaemia of the corticospinal and spinothalamic tracts. The lesion produces a variable loss of motor function and reduced sensitivity to pain and temperature. Proprioception is preserved (ASIA, 1992; Grundy and Swain, 1993).

Conus medullaris syndrome/cauda equina lesions

These injuries involve damage to the conus medullaris (sacral cord) or the spinal nerves forming the cauda equina. This usually results in an areflexic (flaccid) bladder and bowel, loss of motor function to the legs with sparing of sensory function (ASIA, 1992).

Upper motor neurone and lower motor neurone lesions

A spinal cord injury may produce damage to upper motor neurones, lower motor neurones or to a combination of both upper and lower motor neurones.

Upper motor neurones originate in the brain and are located within the spinal cord. An upper motor neurone lesion produces spasticity of limbs below the level of lesion, increased muscle tone and spasticity of bowel and bladder functioning. The reflex arcs are intact but no longer under central control. An upper motor neurone injury will be located at or above T12. The spinal cord ends at L1 as the conus medullaris. Below this is the cauda equina.

Lower motor neurones originate within the spinal cord where they receive nerve impulses from the upper motor neurones. The lower motor neurones travel outside the central nervous system to provide motor impulses to a specific muscle group and to receive sensory information from the body to transmit back to the upper motor neurone in the spinal cord. Lower motor neurones may be damaged at the level of the upper motor neurone lesion but are more commonly identified when occurring at or below T12. Patients exhibit flaccid paralysis of the legs, decreased muscle tone at rest, loss of reflexes and atonicity of bladder and bowel. Men will experience an inability to achieve reflex erections. (Burke and Murray, 1975; Zejdlik, 1992)

Assessment of impairment

Systematic examination of the dermatomes (sensory) and myotomes (motor) will enable evaluation of the cord segments affected by the spinal cord injury. From this assessment, the neurological level can be determined. Medical texts from different countries may give differing interpretations of the level of an injury. The **skeletal level** refers to the location of the greatest vertebral damage, detected by radiographic examination. For example, radiographs may show a fracture/dislocation of C6 on C7. Neurological damage may occur above and below the level of bony injury. Confusion may occur, as both the vertebrae and the spinal nerves are numbered, and these numbers do not entirely correspond. The **neurological level** is described as the most caudal segment (the lowest) of the spinal cord with normal sensory and motor function on both sides of the body (ASIA, 1992). This classification has been adopted by the American Spinal Injury Association (ASIA) and is the definition assumed in the current work. Following the example above, of the C6/C7 skeletal level of injury, the patient may have absent elbow flexors but sensation to pinprick on top of the acromioclavicular joint, indicating a neurological level of C4. This latter designation is of the greater relevance in terms of functional expectations and rehabilitation goals.

Motor examination

The ASIA requires a motor examination which entails testing a key muscle (one on the right and one on the left side of the body) in 10 paired myotomes. Testing must be done on both sides, as damage to the cord may not be symmetrical and some sparing may be evident on one side of the body. A **myotome** refers to the collection of muscle fibres innervated by a single spinal segment. Individuals may vary slightly in their innervation of various muscles – many muscles being innervated by more than one nerve segment. For example, the triceps is innervated by the C6, C7 and C8 roots. If C6 is the last, normally functioning root after a spinal cord injury, one person may have a third of his triceps spared and another may have sparing of half, and hence more function. The 10 muscles in the ASIA test were chosen not only because of their ease of testing but also because of their consistency for being innervated by the segments indicated (ASIA, 1992; Figure 3.2).

MOTOR

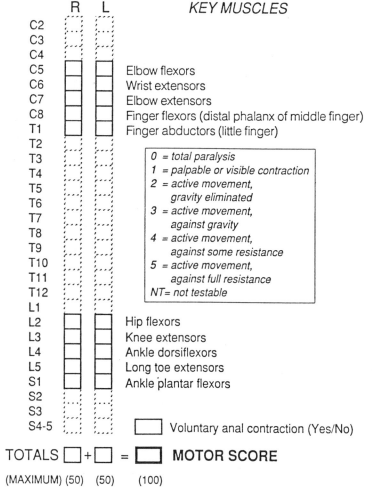

KEY MUSCLES

	R	L	
C2			
C3			
C4			
C5			Elbow flexors
C6			Wrist extensors
C7			Elbow extensors
C8			Finger flexors (distal phalanx of middle finger)
T1			Finger abductors (little finger)

0 = total paralysis
1 = palpable or visible contraction
2 = active movement,
    gravity eliminated
3 = active movement,
    against gravity
4 = active movement,
    against some resistance
5 = active movement,
    against full resistance
NT= not testable

L2			Hip flexors
L3			Knee extensors
L4			Ankle dorsiflexors
L5			Long toe extensors
S1			Ankle plantar flexors

☐ Voluntary anal contraction (Yes/No)

TOTALS ☐ + ☐ = ☐ **MOTOR SCORE**

(MAXIMUM) (50) (50) (100)

Figure 3.2 Motor classification of spinal cord injury. (From ASIA, 1992.)

Sensory examination

The ASIA neurological examination requires sensory assessment through testing 28 dermatomes on the right and left sides

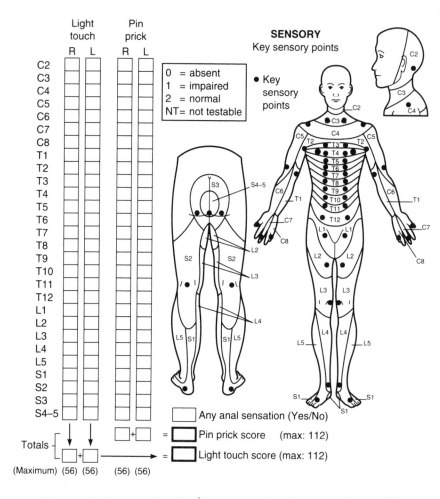

Figure 3.3 Sensory classification of spinal cord injury. (From ASIA, 1992.)

of the body. **Dermatome** refers to an area of skin innervated by sensory axons from one spinal root (ASIA, 1992). These key points are indicated in Figure 3.3. At each of these points, sensitivity to pinprick and light touch is examined. Appreciation of these sensations is scored separately at each point, based on the scale outlined in the Figure.

Neurological extent of injury

The scheme for classifying the neurological extent of spinal cord injury was developed by Frankel and colleagues (1969) and is widely used. The American Spinal Injuries Association Impairment Scale (1992), modified from the Frankel scale, to grade degree of impairment, is as follows.

A = Complete. No sensory or motor function is preserved.

B = Incomplete. Sensory but not motor function is preserved below the neurological level.

C = Incomplete. Motor function is preserved below the neurological level. The majority of key muscles below the neurological level have a muscle grade less than 3.

D = Incomplete. Motor function is preserved below the neurological level. The majority of key muscles below the neurological level have a muscle grade greater than or equal to 3.

E = Normal. Sensory and motor function is normal. (Reflexes may be abnormal).

Functional expectations

The motor and sensory examinations outlined above will provide the means of assessing the neurological status of the patient. This will serve as a guide for the expected functional potential of the individual. However, it is impossible to state unequivocally what a person with a particular level of spinal cord injury will attain in terms of actual functional ability. From a rehabilitation perspective, the designated neurological level of spinal cord lesion will serve as an **indicator** of potential function. It cannot be viewed as completely predictive of actual functional achievements.

Levels of injury and their incidence

Spinal cord injured survivors are not only becoming more numerous but they are also surviving more serious levels of injury in increasing numbers. Cervical cord injury is now the most common level of injury admitted to trauma units in the developed world, accounting for more than 50% of all spinal cord injuries (Stover and Fine, 1986). Hence, more people are surviving with quadriplegia than with paraplegia. In the USA, the proportion of complete lesions has decreased over the past decades. This is not the picture, however, in the developing world. In Turkey, for example, poor emergency care, delayed evacuation and inadequate primary treatment and acute care mitigate against survival for quadriplegics, 91.9% of spinal cord injured survivors being paraplegic. Only 10% of lesions are incomplete (Dincer *et al.*, 1992).

Aetiology of non-traumatic injury

Parsons and Lammertse (1991) estimate the incidence of non-traumatic spinal cord injury to be approximately equal to that of traumatic injuries. In the UK, the Spinal Injuries Association estimates 16% of spinal cord injuries to be non-traumatic (SIA, 1992) and in Canada, the Canadian Paraplegic Association estimates 10.8% of lesions to occur from medical causes (CPA, 1993). These figures are likely to be low, as most records will not list 'spinal cord lesion' as a primary diagnosis.

The aetiology of such injuries may be developmental or acquired. Burke and Murray (1975) outline the following non-traumatic aetiologies.

Developmental aetiologies include:

- spina bifida
- scoliosis
- spondylolisthesis
- familial paralysis.

Acquired aetiologies may be:

- infective
  - bacterial abscess
  - tubercular spine
  - viral, e.g. poliomyelitis, transverse myelitis
- degenerative
  - spondylosis
  - intervertebral disc herniation
- neoplastic
  - benign or malignant (cancer is a more common cause of cord dysfunction than trauma (Staas *et al.*, 1988)).
- vascular, e.g.
  - dissecting aneurysm

    –spontaneous anterior artery thrombosis
    –embolism
- metabolic
- neurological
    –multiple sclerosis
    –amyotrophic lateral sclerosis (motor neurone disease)
- iatrogenic
    –radiation
    –surgical intervention
    –spinal injection
    –vaccination
- psychological.

Spinal cord injury: impairments

Spinal cord injury is a complex form of serious trauma. It causes loss of motor, sensory and autonomic function leading to disruption of almost every system of the body.

(Bélanger, 1992)

Approximately 37% of people who sustain spinal cord injuries in the developed world die before hospitalization. Most of these deaths are associated with multiple and massive trauma (Staas *et al.*, 1988).

A comparatively small percentage of all spinal fractures and dislocations result in injury to the spinal cord. The spine is especially vulnerable to injury at the two points where a highly mobile segment of the spine meets a comparatively immobile segment, i.e. at C6/C7 and T12/L1.

The spinal cord is only rarely lacerated or completely transected by the trauma to the spinal column. More usually, the physical trauma initiates a destructive process within the spinal cord. Staas describes this process as consisting of haemorrhage, vascular wall necrosis, central haematoma and oedema. Grundy and Swain (1993) indicate that, as radiographic images of the spine represent a final position of the vertebrae and do not indicate the forces generated in the injury, they are not a reliable guide to the severity of cord damage.

A complete spinal cord injury will result in absent sensory and motor function below the level of lesion. In addition, virtually every system of the body will be impacted by the

injury. The severity of the impact will depend upon the level of
lesion but may include impairments such as:

- bladder dysfunction
- bowel dysfunction
- respiratory dysfunction – normal breathing function
  depends upon the action of the diaphragm (innervated from
  C2 to C4), the intercostals (innervated from T2 to T12), the
  abdominal muscles (innervated from T6 to L1)
- impairment of sexual function
- cardiac impairments – bradycardia is common following
  cervical lesions because of vagal tone arising from the intact
  parasympathetic system
- orthostatic hypotension (especially cervical lesions)
- poikilothermia – inability to regulate body heat and assumption of the temperature of the environment. Lesions above
  T8. Paralysis of sweating and vasomotor control of the skin,
  and the inability to shiver. Increased potential of hypothermia, the higher the lesion above T8.
- metabolic disturbances
- reflex sweating (cervical lesions)
- gastrointestinal complications – atony, loss of motility
- hypotension, decreased vascular tone (above T5)
- pain
- autonomic hyperreflexia (lesions above T6) (see Chapter 4)
- skin (affected by impaired circulation, loss of sensation)
  subject to pressure sores and trauma
- oedema (Burke and Murray, 1975; Staas *et al.*, 1988; Ozer,
  1988).

Autonomic nervous system

The autonomic nervous system is governed by the hypothala-
mus. Neurones descending through the spinal cord form three
groups:

- cranial outflow (brain stem)
- thoracolumbar outflow (T1 to L1)
- sacral outflow (S2 to S4).

The thoracolumbar outflow gives rise to the sympathetic
division of the autonomic nervous system. This sympathetic

system prepares the body for stress responses. The parasympathetic division arises from the craniosacral outflows. This system controls normal body functioning, initiating digestion or contracting the bladder to initiate voiding. These are more specific responses than those of the generalized sympathetic system (Zejdlik, 1992).

A spinal cord injury, particularly a cervical injury, will produce autonomic system dysfunction. The normal balance of the sympathetic and parasympathetic divisions is upset, and this inhibits the maintenance of a stable internal environment. Autonomic system impairments produce disabilities that are often severe. Some are unique to spinal cord injury. Impairments of upper and mid thoracic sympathetic outflow have a major impact. Vagal nerve activity is unopposed. The individual with a cervical or high thoracic lesion will be unable to regulate pulse rate, blood pressure and temperature in response to changes in position or environmental temperature. Inability to maintain cardiac output may produce syncope, especially in the early stages after injury (Ozer, 1988).

EMERGENCY MANAGEMENT

Although the effect of the initial trauma is irreversible, emergency management and acute care will determine the patient's progress **for life**.

Emergency care for all victims of trauma will focus primarily upon the maintenance of adequate ventilation and circulation. In addition, the major objective of emergency care is to stabilize the spine, preventing all active and passive movements, maintaining the normal curvature and protecting the spinal cord from further neurological damage. Excellent emergency care is evidenced by increasing proportions of patients who have incomplete rather than complete lesions.

Airway

Management of the airway in acute spinal cord injury can be a very complex problem. CPR will require a modified jaw thrust manoeuvre rather than neck hyperextension (Zejdlik, 1992). Bélanger (1992) warns that individuals who have cervical or high thoracic injuries, with disruption of the sympathetic outflow tracts, may suffer severe bradycardia or cardiac arrest during intubation because of unopposed vagal stimulation, hence each episode of suctioning must therefore be as brief as possible.

Breathing

Respiratory function may be mildly to severely compromised, depending upon the neurological level of injury. Individuals who experience respiratory dysfunction will exhibit rapid, shallow respirations, laboured abdominal breathing and will increase their use of the accessory muscles of respiration.

Circulation

Spinal cord injuries above T6 may produce neurogenic shock. This is the body's response to the sudden loss of sympathetic control and is characterized by hypotension, bradycardia and hypothermia. Thermal reflector blankets may be necessary in winter to prevent hypothermia in poikilothermic individuals (primarily those with cervical injuries, Grundy and Swain, 1993).

Paralytic ileus

This is not uncommon following spinal cord injury, hence a nasogastric tube is usually inserted in all individuals with acute cord injuries (Bélanger, 1992).

Urinary tract

Spinal shock and interruption of the autonomic nervous system leads to bladder atonicity. Individuals with a suspected or confirmed spinal cord injury will therefore have an indwelling foley catheter inserted to prevent overdistention of the bladder.

Skin care

Loss of vasomotor skin tone and sensation leads to the risk of pressure sores, even in the earliest hours after cord lesion. The patient should not be lying on debris such as glass or gravel, should have objects removed from his pockets and should not be left lying on a spine board longer than is absolutely necessary (Zejdlik, 1992; Bélanger, 1992; Grundy and Swain, 1993). Bélanger (1992) and Zejdlik (1992) provide a thorough and comprehensive protocol for excellent emergency management of the acute spinal cord injured patient.

SPECIALIZED SPINAL INJURY UNITS

Clinicians and researchers throughout the world are in agreement upon the need for quick and immediate transportation of the acutely injured patient to a spinal centre, using air transportation if distances are great. Donovan and Bedbrook (1982) recommend that the individual with an acute spinal cord injury should remain at an emergency care facility only long enough for life saving and emergency measures, for insertion of a nasogastric tube and placement of an indwelling catheter connected to a closed urinary drainage system.

Research studies have found that people who have early admission to a specialized spinal unit suffer less complications, have shorter lengths of stay, reduced costs and more successful outcomes from medical care and rehabilitation processes. However, although in Switzerland and Australia, virtually every individual with an acute spinal cord injury is admitted to a specialized unit, in the UK, less than half the people who sustain spinal cord injuries will receive specialized care. There are too few spinal units and those that exist are not evenly distributed to provide adequate or equal coverage for the whole country. Patients who are not treated at a spinal unit may be the victims of 'inappropriate treatment. . .given because doctors often failed to understand the pathophysiology of the injury' (Carvell and Grundy, 1989).

Despite the recognition of catastrophic medical complications, increased disability and increased costs, in the USA, 50–70% of people with spinal cord injuries are still denied access to a specialized unit and expert care (Zejdlik, 1992).

Inappropriate and inadequate treatment during emergency, acute care and rehabilitation can lead to an increase both in the severity of the impairment and the resulting disability.

REFERENCES

American Spinal Injury Association (1992) *Standards for Neurological and Functional Classification of Spinal Cord Injury* (Revised), American Spinal Injury Association, Chicago, IL.

Bélanger, L.M.A. (1992) *Emergency Management and Transfer of the Individual with a Suspected Spinal Cord Injury*, University Hospital, Shaughnessy Site, Vancouver, BC, pp. 4, 7, 17–18.

Biering-Sørensen, F., Pedersen, W. and Giørtz-Müller, P. (1992) Spinal cord injury due to suicide attempts. *Paraplegia*, **30**(2), 139–44.

Burke, D.C. and Murray, D.D. (1975) *Handbook of Spinal Cord Medicine*, Macmillan, Basingstoke.

Canadian Paraplegic Association, (1993) Annual Report, *Caliper*, **XLVIII**, 4.

Carvell, J. and Grundy, D. (1989) Patients with spinal injuries. Early transfer to a specialised centre is vital. *British Medical Journal*, **299**, 1353–4.

Cock, J. (1989a) Hidden consequences of state violence: spinal cord injuries in Soweto, South Africa. *Social Science and Medicine*, **29**(10), 1147–55.

Cock, J. (1989b) Life 'inside the shell': a needs survey of spinal cord injured wheelchair users in a black South African township. *Disability, Handicap and Society*, **4**(1), 3–20.

DeVivo, M.J., Fine, P.R., Maetz, M. and Stover, S.L. (1980) Prevalence of spinal cord injury: a re-estimation employing life table techniques. *Archives of Neurology*, **37**, 707–8.

Dincer, F., Oflazer, A., Beyazova, M. *et al.* (1992) Traumatic spinal cord injuries in Turkey. *Paraplegia* **30**(9), 641–6.

Donovan, W.H. and Bedbrook, G. (1982) Comprehensive management of spinal cord injury. *Clinical Symposia*, CIBA **34**(2), 4.

Frankel, H.L., Hancock, D.O., Hyslop, G. *et al.* (1969) The value of postural reduction in the initial management of closed injuries of the spine with paraplegia and tetraplegia. *Paraplegia*, **7**(1), 179–92.

Grundy, D. and Swain, A. (1993) *ABC of Spinal Cord Injury*, 2nd edn, British Medical Journal, London, pp. 1, 4, 6, 13.

Kraus, J.F., Frantin, C.E. and Riggins, R.S. (1982) Neurologic outcome and vehicle crash factors in motor vehicle related spinal cord injuries. *Neuroepidemiology*, **1**, 223–38.

Menter, R. (1989) Introduction to high quadriplegia care, in *The Management of High Quadriplegia*, (eds G.G. Whiteneck, C. Adler, R.E. Carter *et al.*), Demos, New York, NY, p. 1.

New Internationalist (1992) Disabled lives: difference and defiance. *The New Internationalist*, July, p. 233.

Ozer, M.N. (1988) *The Management of Persons with Spinal Cord Injury*, Demos, New York, NY, pp. 30–56.

Parsons, K.C. and Lammertse, D.P. (1991) Rehabilitation in spinal cord disorders: 1. Epidemiology, prevention and system of care of spinal cord disorders. *Archives of Physical Medicine and Rehabilitation*, **72**, S293–4.

Pasteur, L., (1884) Address to the Fraternal Association of former students of the École Centrale des Arts et Manufactures, Paris, 15 May 1884, in *Medical Quotations*, (eds J. Daintith and A. Isaacs, 1989), Collins, London.

Shanmugasundaram, T.K. (1988) The care of SCI patients in developing nations – can we stem the rot? *Paraplegia*, **26**, 10, 11.

Spinal Injuries Association (1992) *Annual Review*, Spinal Injuries Association, London.

Staas, W.E., Formal, C.S., Gershkoff, A.M. *et al.* (1988) Rehabilitation of the spinal cord-injured patient, in *Rehabilitation Medicine: Principles and Practice*, (ed. J.A. DeLisa), J.B. Lippincott, Philadelphia, PA, pp. 635–59.

Stover, S.L. and Fine, P.R. (1986) *Spinal Cord Injury: the Facts and Figures*, University of Alabama, Birmingham, AL, pp. 2, 14, 15, 21, 24, 27, 34, 35.

Tan, E.S. and Balachandran, N. (1987) The causes, pattern and effects of spinal injury in Singapore. *Clinical Rehabilitation*, **1**, 101–6.

Tator, C.H. and Edmonds, V.E. (1984) National survey of spinal injuries in hockey players. *Canadian Medical Association Journal*, **130**, 875–80.

Weingarden, S.I. and Graham, P. (1992) Young spinal cord injured patients in nursing homes: rehospitalization issues and outcomes. *Paraplegia*, **30**(12), 828–33.

Wigglesworth, E.C. (1992) Motor vehicle crashes and spinal cord injury. *Paraplegia*, **30**(8), 543–9.

Wing P.C. and Cain, K. (1992) Spinal cord injury prevention, in *Management of Spinal Cord Injuries*, 2nd edn, (ed. C.P. Zejdlik) Jones and Bartlett, Boston, MA, pp. 31–49.

Zeeb, K. (1991) Bullet wounds and spinal cord injury. *Spinal Network Extra*, Summer, 22–3.

Zejdlik, C.P. (1992) *Management of Spinal Cord Injuries*, 2nd edn, Jones and Bartlett, Boston, MA, pp. 7, 60–1, 69–71, 87–103.

4

Acute care and reduction of disability

It is sometimes said that a patient with a spinal cord injury is too ill to be moved to a major center. Actually, these individuals are too sick to be safely managed in small hospitals or in large hospitals where fragmentation of services and specialty groups prevent the overall view of their complex problems . . . over and above the humane factor, favorable prognosis as to the life expectancy and stability of neuromuscular disability justifies a considerable investment of time, money and effort required to rehabilitate the patient with a spinal cord injury.

(Schweigel and Peerless, 1971)

Reduction of disability

An **impairment** is defined as an abnormality or loss of function (WHO, 1980). The impairments that may result from a spinal cord injury were delineated in Chapter 3 and may include motor or sensory loss or dysfunction, autonomic system dysfunction, loss of voluntary control over bowel and bladder and impairments of respiratory function. The impairments that are the sequelae of a spinal cord injury cannot be cured. However, correct and creative management of impairments will prevent many of them from leading to significant disabilities or to lifestyle handicaps.

The World Health Organisation (1980) defines **disability** as a restriction or inability to perform an activity due to the impairment, and a **handicap** as the limitation of life roles or lifestyle that may result from impairment and disability. The loss of voluntary bladder control, for example, need not equate with incontinence, embarrassment and a subsequent reduction in outings and activities. Proper management can allow the individual with a spinal cord injury to empty the bladder at appropriate times and hence prevent the creation of a handicapping condition.

This chapter outlines some of the ways in which the sequelae of spinal cord lesion impairments can be minimized, disabilities reduced, complications avoided and hence how potential lifestyle handicaps can be diminished. Therapists will need to be familiar with this information, as much has relevance to treatment interventions.

ACUTE CARE

Spinal shock

'Spinal shock' is a state that immediately follows a traumatic spinal cord injury. Although its physiological basis is not entirely clear, it is attributed to the sudden loss of the influence of the supraspinal tracts. The effects become more profound with higher levels of cord lesions.

Spinal shock is characterized by generalised flaccidity below the level of the lesion and the disappearance of reflex activity. This is a transient condition, lasting from a few hours to several weeks and may be evident in the presence of both temporary or permanent neurological losses.

The features characteristic of spinal shock are:

- hypotension and decreased cardiac output;
- bradycardia (due to the unopposed effects of the parasympathetic nervous system);
- hypothermia (due to the body's inability to conserve heat);
- priaprism (especially with cervical lesions);
- ventilatory impairment (particularly with cervical lesions). This is one of the most serious complications, with high risk of morbidity and mortality;
- bladder flaccidity, leading to urine retention with overflow voiding. Emergency management entails placement of an indwelling catheter, replaced by regular intermittent catheterisations to prevent overdistention and chronic bladder wall atonicity;
- paralysis of peristalsis (especially with higher lesions);
- risk of pressure sores, due to loss of vasomotor tone and

reduction of tissue perfusion. Regular turning is essential, positioning should prevent gravitational oedema and high-quality pressure stockings should be worn. Passive range of motion exercises and ankle-pumping exercises are especially important during this stage.

The end of the period of spinal shock is indicated by a return of reflex activity in the spinal cord, in the presence of an upper motor neurone lesion. Flaccidity persists if the lesion is at the sacral level (Burke and Murray, 1975; Ozer, 1988; Zejdlik, 1992; Grundy and Swain, 1993).

Acute care

Much controversy exists in the medical community concerning the philosophy of management for the acute traumatic spinal cord injured patient. 'The question of operative intervention and stabilization versus conservative management without surgery remains unsettled despite the mountain of published literature' (Brooks and Ohry, 1992).

Successful acute care management is dependent upon excellent positioning and extraordinary attention to regular and correct turning. The methods for positioning, turning and lifting acutely injured patients are clearly described and illustrated by Grundy and Swain (1993). The primary aim of positioning is to support the injured spine in a good healing position. Secondarily, the aim is to maintain limbs and joints in a functional position, hence reducing the incidence of spasticity and preventing contractures and deformity. Regular turning by four people every two hours is essential to relieve pressure and prevent the formation of sores. The Egerton turning and tilting bed may be used, particularly for paraplegic patients. The Stryker frame, in which the patient is 'sandwiched' between anterior and posterior sections and turned between supine and prone positions using a circular turning mechanism, may also be used (Grundy and Swain, 1993).

In the acute phase of management, the patient will be carefully observed and monitored for two common and potentially fatal complications: paralytic ileus and acute peptic ulceration. Patients with cervical injuries, particularly complete cervical lesions, are at the highest risk of gastrointestinal complications due to severe autonomic nervous system dysfunction (Zejdlik, 1992; Grundy and Swain, 1993).

Psychological care

Spinal cord injury represents serious trauma, potentially life threatening and disrupting almost every body system. Early, crisis-oriented care will be focused upon efforts to ensure patient survival, prevent neurological deterioration, stabilize the spine and maintain optimal physiological functioning. The body cannot, however, be treated in isolation from the person, and thorough consideration to psychological components of care are essential.

Most patients who are not unconscious will be aware that something is seriously wrong with them. Initial concerns may centre upon fear of death. In many individuals, initial awareness of the consequences of the injury may be dulled and they may be unable to absorb all the implications. Some clinicians attribute this to **denial** – a psychopathological reaction but, in reality, it may be a response to the impacts of acute care management (see Chapter 7). The patient may suffer the combined effects of anaesthesia, pain, sleep deprivation, medications and total immobilization. Disorientation may result from constant artificial lighting and electric monitors that contribute to auditory disturbance. Under such conditions it is difficult to assimilate new information. Further, it is normal to sustain some hope for recovery and, as it is not usually possible to predict accurately the prognosis while the patient is still in spinal shock, maintenance of hope should not be discouraged.

Information should be provided repeatedly, full explanations of procedures should be given and sensitive psychological support must be a care priority for every member of staff.

Sensory deprivation

Acute spinal cord injury results in both sensory deprivation (absolute reduction of sensory input) and perceptual deprivation (distortion of the patterns of sensory stimulation rather than reduction in amount). Sensory deprivation is shown to lead to perceptual changes, intellectual and cognitive impairments, psychomotor effects and an inability to tolerate the

present situation. Sensory deprivation is due to absent proprioceptive and motor feedback below the level of lesion. Enforced
immobility removes kinaesthetic feedback and produces visual
restrictions. Perceptual deprivation may be auditory – due to
monotonous, continuous sounds and an inability to control
noise level. Olfactory stimulation may be reduced due to nasal
congestion (due to the physiology of spinal shock). Gustatory
stimulation may also be disrupted while no food is being given
by mouth (Krishnan *et al.*, 1992).

Krishnan and colleagues further report that spinal cord
injured patients complain of noises that do not exist, strange
and vivid visual experiences and uncomfortable or painful
limb positions. Abnormal sensory perceptions precede acute
behavioural disturbances. These behavioural disturbances are
experienced with greater frequency with high level lesions.

More importantly, Krishnan's group contend that a recognition of the role and reduction of sensory input in behavioural
disturbance makes it possible to pre-empt such occurrences.
They found that a major factor in the occurrence of behavioural
disturbances was the absence or low frequency of support from
family or others important to the patient. All staff have a role in
encouraging and facilitating visits from these influential people,
involving them in care and ensuring they have accommodation
close to the unit.

Psychological reactions to traumatic spinal cord injury must
be seen not purely in the context of the physical injury but in
relation to interactions with the hospital environment and with
social supports (Trieschmann, 1988; Krishnan *et al.*, 1992).

Family involvement

During the course of past clinical experience, the author has
been interested in the process of adjustment to a traumatic
disability. In particular, there was an interest into what factors
the disabled person perceived as being important in mitigating
the severity of the life changes and facilitating positive adaptation. The response has been unanimous – that the support
of close friends and family was the most important factor in
enabling adaptation to drastically changed circumstances.
However, there has frequently been an additional comment,
that rehabilitation professionals – who see themselves as being

important to the process of adjustment to a traumatic disability – need to learn more about what is of prime importance to the individuals themselves: that is, the support of friends and family (Hammell, 1991).

Although many researchers have acknowledged the considerable impact of family support upon positive rehabilitation outcomes, little has been written concerning the impact of the injury upon the family or what actions can be taken by the treatment team to include the family in the treatment and rehabilitation process, to maximize their coping skills and eventual adaptation (Trieschmann, 1988).

It is suggested that it is often harder for family members to adapt to a traumatic spinal cord injury than it is for the injured person himself (Oliver, 1981).

The crisis that arises from the traumatic injury produces a sense of uncontrollability and helplessness among family members. There is disruption of routine and uncertainty about the future. Severe emotional stress results from a situation that is clearly serious, is potentially life threatening and may be the most severe crisis the family has ever experienced. Such emotions may be compounded by a feeling of anger at the injured person for contributing to, or not avoiding the accident that caused the injury; and subsequent guilt for sustaining such thoughts at a time when the individual is so vulnerable (Trieschmann, 1988).

Practical problems may be a further concern. Travel to and from the hospital, sudden loss or reduction of income, dealing with lawyers and insurance companies and coping with child care may compound the stress the family experiences. Krishnan *et al.* (1992) proposes that relatives should be encouraged to spend as much time as possible with the patient to maintain maximum involvement with him. However, they recommend a balance between attendance at the unit and maintaining as normal a lifestyle as possible. They suggest developing a visiting rota so that responsibility for support is shared and there is high quality as well as quantity of interaction.

In addition to encouraging family visiting, enhancing communication and involving the family in planning and making decisions, it is important for staff to understand that the crisis impacts upon a pre-existing structure of relationships. Not all marriages are positive and fulfilling, not all parents enjoy a good rapport with their children. Spinal cord injury 'does not change the nature of a particular relationship as much as it may magnify and intensify both its flaws and strengths' (Woodbury and Redd, 1987).

There is an inter-relationship between the needs of the patient and those of his family and friends. The more understanding that healthcare workers have of what they are experiencing, the more likely they are to be able to help both them and the client. Family involvement is essential in the process of rehabilitation and should be included from the beginning of treatment. It is proposed that ignoring the importance of family members during spinal cord injury management is akin to treating the patient without assessing all his body systems, or to treating the patient in a vacuum. However, reality has frequently been quite different.

Typically, family members have found that rigid ward practices and administration seem to be designed to exclude the family rather than involve them (Tucker, 1980; Oliver *et al.*, 1988). Indeed, nursing staff exclude family members from involvement in care tasks on the ward that they may be expected to perform themselves, following the patient's discharge. 'All the attention [at the spinal unit] is on helping the spinal cord injured person to cope. There is nothing for the partner or friends. At that stage, you are told you can ask questions – but you don't even know what questions to ask' (wife of a man with a spinal cord injury, quoted in Hammell, 1991).

Expanding the approach to treatment from a purely medical view to a psychosocial vision incorporates the responsibility to attend to the psychological and social needs not only of the patient but of his support system – who are themselves facing a crisis event. The response to disability of the important people in the patient's life may dictate his own response and outcome. The healthcare team must communicate to the family that their involvement is valued. The family and the patient face a shared future and must likewise share in the rehabilitation process – starting in acute care.

Concomitant head injury

Trauma which is of the severity required to cause damage to

the spinal column and cord may also produce a traumatic head injury. The most common causes of head and spinal cord injuries (motor vehicle accidents and falls) have similar mechanisms of injury. The injury to the brain can range from mild to severe. Even though most concomitant head injuries are mild the sequelae can still have substantial impact upon rehabilitation: impaired problem-solving skills, poor abstract reasoning, attention and concentration deficits, fatigue, reduced speed of information processing, memory impairment, diminished capacity for new learning, poor judgement and social inappropriateness (Roth *et al.*, 1989; Davidoff *et al.*, 1992; Hildebrand and Weintraub, 1992).

Estimates of incidence vary according to the criteria used in assessment. Contrary to expectation, no significant correlations have been found between the occurrence of traumatic brain injury and either the level or completeness of cord injury. Consultation with an expert head injury team will ensure appropriate treatment of the sequelae of moderate or severe head injuries. As learning and adaptation are the main elements in a rehabilitation programme following traumatic spinal cord injury, it is important to identify those patients who exhibit evidence of mild head injuries. Deficits of attention, concentration, memory and judgement pose considerable obstacles to active participation in an interactive rehabilitation programme and the requisite learning of new skills. Hence early vocational evaluation or discharge may be contraindicated and intellectual functioning potential may not be evident until later in the rehabilitation programme. Thorough assessment will prevent head injuries from remaining undetected and their sequelae unevaluated.

However, skilled neuropsychological assessment is essential, as test performance can be adversely affected by many of the sequelae of an acute traumatic spinal cord injury and its management – for example, pain, depression, fatigue, poor motivation for tests, medications, functional impairments, sensory deprivation, sleep deprivation or the effects of general anaesthesia (Trieschmann, 1988; Davidoff *et al.*, 1992). The psychologist can suggest compensation strategies to the rehabilitation team to overcome the inherent problems encountered in treating those individuals who experience cognitive deficits.

Environmental control

The deleterious effects of acute care management upon a person with a spinal cord injury have been noted. Early treatment may reinforce a sense of helplessness, powerlessness and lack of control (see Chapter 1). Sensory deprivation and loss of the ability 'to do' may reduce motivation and the ability to engage in purposeful activity.

The medical philosophy of 'doing no harm' is appropriate in the early management of spinal cord injury: every effort must be made to enable the individual to engage in activity and to experience early interaction with his environment. Successful rehabilitation will be dependent upon an active, involved individual, not one who has learned helplessness and passivity.

Technological devices exist to provide early control over the environment, stimulation and purposeful activity. It is important to note that these devices constitute a small portion of the cost of other services provided in acute care and, as they make a positive contribution to the wellbeing of the client, should be as much a part of the treatment milieu as monitors and respirators. Environmental control units are thoroughly examined in Chapter 6.

Splinting the hand

There is a consensus among spinal cord injury clinicians that static splinting is essential for persons with cervical lesions and further, that this intervention must begin immediately upon admission to hospital, and certainly within 48 hours. (Krajnik and Bridle, 1992; Zejdlik, 1992).

The purposes and aims of splinting the quadriplegic hand are as follows.

1. To maintain a hand that looks 'normal' and free of deformities, preserving the anatomical alignment, functional position of the fingers, the normal arches of the hand and the thumb web space.
2. To maintain a hand that is pleasant to hold.
3. To provide a tenodesis grip for those with lesions at C6 or C7.
4. To maintain full, passive range of motion.

5. To retain future possibilities for tendon transplants or dynamic hand splinting.

Left untreated, interruption of vasoconstriction below the level of lesion will produce oedema, and the subsequent collagen deposits will be transformed into fibrous tissue, adhering to the ligaments and joint capsules resulting in lost elasticity and contractures (Krajnik and Bridle, 1992). Prevention of contractures involves elevation of the limb, passive range of motion and splinting. Muscle imbalance puts patients at risk of developing 'claw hand' deformities, especially with lesions at C7 and C8. Splinting the quadriplegic hand prevents deformity of the intrinsic minus hand, prevents overstretching of muscles (particularly wrist extensors), protects and stabilizes flail joints and maintains joint integrity and functional position (Krajnik and Bridle, 1992).

The occupational therapist will form a splint (**orthosis**) from thermal plastic, based upon evaluation of the individual client. For the highest lesions, splinting is concerned with hygiene and maintenance of appearance (see Chapter 6). For lower cervical lesions, splinting provides functional position of the hand and wrist in preparation for a natural tenodesis function, to maintain hand function in the event of motor function return, for cosmesis and hygiene. The opponens splint is most usually applied (Figure 4.1). This maintains the thumb in opposition to the first two fingers, maintains the web space and allows for full finger flexion. If the wrist extensors are weak (C4/C5) a long opponens is necessary to prevent stretching of the extensor tendons (see Figure 6.1, Chapter 6). The short opponens is fabricated if the patient has active wrist extensors (Krajnik and Bridle, 1992; Zejdlik, 1992). A utensil slot can be added to either opponens splint to allow early self-feeding or for other functional activities.

The person with C6 or C7 quadriplegia will be dependent for hand functional activities upon a **tenodesis** action. Tenodesis is the natural flexion of the fingers that occurs when the wrist is extended. In the absence of active finger movement, tenodesis provides a grip and the ability to pick up things. Contractures of the hand are encouraged in this instance but the web space between the thumb and first fingers must be maintained to allow for grasp with the thumb in adduction (Zejdlik, 1992).

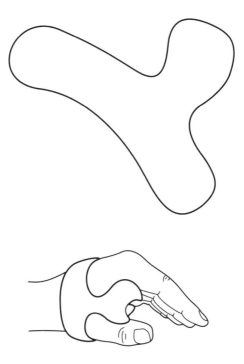

Figure 4.1 Short opponens splint and pattern. Indications: active wrist extensors; training tenodesis action; intrinsic minus hand. Maintain: adequate web space; palmar arch; thumb in abduction, directly under second metacarpophalangeal joint; ensure metacarpophalangeal flexion is not impeded (Rehabilitation Institute of Chicago, 1985; Malik, 1979).

Grasp is released by relaxing the wrist. Splinting for these people aims to allow for functional contracture of the quadriplegic hand (see Ford and Duckworth, 1987 and Curtain, 1993).

The long opponens splint allows for maintenance of the flaccid wrist in neutral or up to 30° of dorsiflexion, the thumb is rotated at the carpometacarpal joint and abducted. The metacarpophalangeal (MCP) joints will be allowed to flex. The addition of a bar may hold the MCP joints in flexion.

Splints should be worn continually when the patient is in bed, removed only for washing, checking for red pressure spots and for performing passive range of motion exercises (see below).

Full and clear explanation must be provided to the patient regarding the philosophy of splinting. This should include the hazards of contractures (impaired hygiene, cosmesis and reduced functional potential) and, if applicable, the benefits to the individual of a hand that is trained to perform most activities associated with daily living – self-care, productive occupations and leisure activities. Prevention is easier than correction. Potential recovery of hand function with incomplete spinal cord lesions makes preservation of the architecture of the hand even more important.

Range of motion

The pathophysiology that leads to the development of contractures was briefly outlined with regard to splinting the hand. Contractures develop quickly in the presence of immobility, muscle imbalance or muscle paralysis. Prevention involves performing range of motion exercises, hand splinting and positioning (Krajnik and Bridle, 1992).

Passive movements of paralysed limbs should be commenced within the first days following admission. Manoeuvring each joint through its full range of motion will help to:

* prevent joint deformities
* maintain joint mobility
* stimulate circulation
* prevent muscle shortening
* prevent contractures
* prevent joint pain caused by contractures.

Severe contractures can lead to:

* skin maceration, fungal infection, skin ulceration
* problems with adequate body positioning, leading to increased risk of pressure sores
* uneven pressure distribution in sitting, leading to the formation of pressure sores
* inability to propel a wheelchair
* reduced ability to transfer independently
* reduced capacity for self-care activities.

Maintenance of range of motion is especially relevant if the injury to the cord is incomplete and motor return is possible.

Any impairment in the range of motion at a joint will hamper self-care activities of daily living, for example, dressing, transferring or positioning. Limitations in the range of motion of the neck may prevent the individual with a high lesion from using a mouthstick and may limit the choices for controlling both a powered wheelchair and an environmental control unit.

Bromley (1991) recommends that passive movements are given to the patient twice daily during the period of spinal shock and daily thereafter until the patient is able to maintain full mobility through his own activities. Ozer (1988) reiterates the importance of maintaining full range of motion during the phase of spinal shock. Assisted, active movements are given to all the muscles that remain innervated, from the first day after injury, avoiding any neck movement if there is a cervical lesion.

Some further qualifications exist. Shoulder range-of-motion exercises are not given if this may compromise the alignment of the healing spine, for example, while the patient is lying on a Stryker frame, hence excellent positioning is especially important (see below). Absence of sensation produces a vulnerable joint. Great care therefore should be taken to avoid overstretching soft tissues, as this may lead to joint capsule fibrosis and resulting deformity. Movements should be smooth, slow and rhythmic (Bromley, 1991).

It is especially important to ensure that the finger flexors of people with C6 quadriplegia are allowed to tighten into partial flexion. An effective tenodesis grip is dependent upon tight finger flexors when the wrist is moved into extension. During range of motion exercises the fingers must be flexed while the wrist is extended. When the fingers are extended, the wrist must be flexed. In this instance, range of motion is performed to maintain freedom of the joint capsules rather than to stretch the intrinsic muscles. Intrinsic stretching will reduce hand function through ineffective tenodesis.

Every member of the treatment team must be aware of the importance of range-of-motion exercises and ensure that the patient receives 10 minutes of proximal-to-distal movements of each limb on a daily basis while in acute care (Bromley, 1991). Correction of deformity is highly undesirable and must be avoided.

Shoulder pain in acute traumatic quadriplegia

Shoulder pain in acute quadriplegia is a prime example of a needless disability and potentially preventable, severely handicapping condition which may result from poor initial management of the cord lesion impairment. Shoulder pain has been a documented problem among acutely injured patients with cervical lesions (Waring and Maynard, 1991).

Waring and Maynard (1991) studied acutely injured quadriplegic patients retrospectively and found that 75% had shoulder pain documented in their records. Forty per cent of these people had onset of pain within three days after injury and 52% within the first two weeks. Pain was frequently bilateral and associated with loss of normal shoulder range of motion. Silfverskiold and Waters (1991) reported that 78% of their quadriplegic patients had shoulder pain, severe enough to create functional disability, within the first six months after injury. Once this problem has been allowed to develop, it is extremely difficult to treat.

Persistent shoulder pain results in severe functional impairment, is a barrier to participation in a rehabilitation programme, and limits performance of self-care activities, wheelchair propulsion and participation in occupational and recreational activities.

Factors that contribute to shoulder pain in acute quadriplegia include:

- weakness of shoulder girdle muscles (especially lesions above C6) which limits active joint movement, leading to muscle shortening;
- muscle imbalance due to paralysis, spasticity, inflammation or trauma, leading to loss of muscle integrity to maintain the humeral head depressed and in the glenoid fossa;
- pain from nerve root injury. Cervical dermatomes, which provide sensory innervation to the shoulder joint and tissues, cross the shoulder joint;
- referred pain, especially from cervical spine fractures and/or dislocations and accompanying trapezius muscle pain;
- direct trauma due to poor positioning, turning procedures and transfers (Waring and Maynard, 1991).

Shoulder pain in acute cervical injuries is a separate issue from the common, chronic, overuse syndromes to be discussed in Chapter 5. The relationship between pain during acute care and the development of chronic problems has not been researched.

It has been proposed that rotator cuff imbalance in quadriplegic patients may produce abnormal glenohumeral motion during active or passive range of motion exercises. This may result in subluxation, synovial and capsular inflammation due to joint stress and tendonitis. Inflammation produces pain, increases spasticity and further reduces range of motion (Silfverskiold and Waters, 1991). The importance of performing smooth, slow movements cannot be overemphasised. If passive or active abduction of the arms is not performed, the pectoralis and latissimus dorsi muscles will shorten and future attempts to abduct the shoulder will meet resistance and produce pain (Scott and Donovan, 1981).

Waring and Maynard (1991) recommend early and consistent shoulder range-of-motion exercises as a means of preventing acute shoulder pain. They report that delay in initiation of these exercises was found to be a significant risk factor for shoulder pain.

However, shoulder pain has been found to develop in the presence of diligent, twice-daily, passive range-of-motion exercises (Scott and Donovan, 1981). Scott and Donovan report that care in positioning the arms effectively prevents shoulder pain.

The correct positioning of the arms of patients with acute, traumatic quadriplegia, to prevent shoulder pain, contractures and adhesive capsulitis is shown in Figure 4.2.

Heterotopic ossification

Heterotopic ossification (HO) is the formation of bone in abnormal locations, usually periarticular soft tissues. This is a frequent complication following spinal cord injury, the incidence being higher amongst those with complete neurological injuries.

The cause is unknown, although local trauma such as from vigorous stretching (particularly overstretching during the period of spinal shock) is suspected as a contributory factor. Risk factors are unclear but appear to be cumulative and include age, completeness of lesion, presence of pressure sores and spasticity. The hip joint is most commonly affected, with the knee, shoulder and elbow being involved less frequently. HO always occurs below the level of neurological lesion.

HO usually presents with localized redness, joint swelling or stiffness, induration and possible referred pain. Heterotopic ossification may substantially limit range of motion and hence

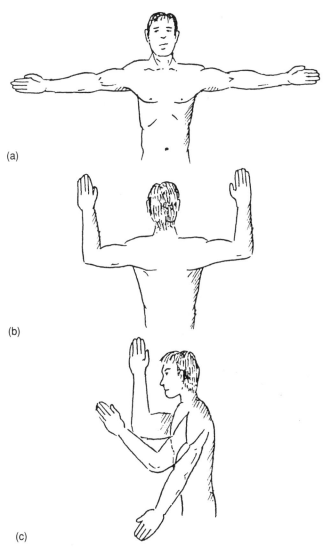

(a)

(b)

(c)

Figure 4.2 Arm positioning for patients with quadriplegia. (a) Supine lying: shoulder abducted to 90°, elbows in full extension; (b) prone lying: shoulder abducted to 90°, elbow flexed to 90°; and (c) side lying: lower arm, 90° shoulder flexion, 90° elbow flexion, top arm, full extension. The underlying shoulder may be protected from pressure by pulling it gently forward (to prevent direct load on the humeral head and acromion process) and/or by using an axillary pillow. The hands and arms must always be supported (S.J. Tuck, after Zejdlik, 1992).

adversely affect mobility, self-care, functional independence and engagement in productive activity. This problem most commonly develops 1–4 months after injury, although lesions may develop as late as one year after injury.

Early research discouraged the use of range-of-motion exercises but later studies have discounted this theory, finding no increase in the formation of bone deposition with exercise. Treatment protocols now involve regular, gentle range-of-motion exercises and extreme diligence in reducing the increased susceptibility to pressure sores (Formal, 1992; Zejdlik, 1992; Grundy and Swain, 1993).

Managing spasticity

Spasticity typically occurs below the level of neurological lesion among people who have upper motor neurone lesions. It is not seen until after spinal shock has subsided and may give the patient and his family the mistaken impression that voluntary muscle activity is returning.

Spasticity is characterised by hypertonicity, hyperactive stretch reflexes and clonus. Burke and Murray (1975) report that virtually all patients with cervical lesions have spasms, 75% of those with thoracic lesions and under 60% of those with lumbar lesions.

Spasticity is produced or increased by many internal or external stimuli, including:

- changes in position
- cutaneous stimulation
- tight clothing
- bladder or kidney stones
- urinary tract infection
- catheter blockage
- faecal impaction
- pressure sores
- anal fissure
- ingrowing toenail
- fracture
- burns
- infection
- emotional stress (Grundy and Swain, 1993).

Any unusual increase in spasticity should be investigated as a possible manifestation of pathology. Individuals vary in the degree of spasticity that they experience and the impact this has upon their activities. People who experience mild or moderate spasticity may learn to trigger this effect at certain times to enhance their performance of specific activities, for example, transferring or turning in bed. Conversely, those who experience strong spasticity may suffer serious impediments to independent functioning; people with incomplete lesions may experience spasticity that overrides voluntary muscle control to prevent walking. Others may experience spasms strong enough to throw them out of the wheelchair. Hence, 'the problem must be defined in terms of the disabilities that spasms create in the context of the person's own life' (Ozer, 1988).

Spasticity may have some considerable benefits. It:

- confers protection against pressure sore formation
- maintains muscle bulk
- decreases osteoporosis
- improves venous return.

Severe spasticity clearly has some disadvantages.

- Severe spasticity and imbalance of opposing muscle groups predisposes to the development of contractures.
- It interferes with sitting balance, transfers, control of powered chair and functional activities.
- It may create sleep disturbance (both for the person with the spinal cord injury and/or his or her partner).
- It may cause skin breakdown. Repetitive clonus may lead to friction and shearing. Flexion or extension spasms of the legs may cause trauma by hitting hard objects, heel loops, etc.

Spasticity is a common impairment following spinal cord injury, but may be prevented from becoming a disabling condition, handicapping the individual in his pursuit of a fulfilling and productive lifestyle.

Spasticity is decreased by proper positioning and passive range of motion exercises. However, daily activity provides effective passive range to critical joints for many individuals, therefore many people do not require formal, daily range-of-motion exercises to maintain adequate control of spasticity and to avoid contractures. Severely handicapping spasticity may be treated with medications; however, these may have severe side effects and withdrawal symptoms, and should be carefully tailored to meet the individual needs of the client (Ozer, 1988).

Preventing contractures

Contractures are produced by the effects of immobilization, spasticity or imbalance between opposing muscle groups. Therapists will be involved in the prevention of contractures and conservative treatment in the form of gradual stretching of affected muscles. Serial splinting may be necessitated but great care is required to prevent the formation of pressure sores on anesthetic areas.

Once a contracture occurs, spasticity is increased and deformities will be inevitable. Contractures interfere with skin integrity, prevent optimal positioning, interfere with personal hygiene, impair cosmesis, interfere with independent self-care activities and produce significant degrees of pain.

Yarkony *et al.* (1985) compared the incidence of contractures between a spinal cord centre and general hospital acute care: 'Patients treated in the general hospitals had a statistically significant increase of contractures compared to spinal centre patients'. Contractures allowed to develop at the general hospital were commonly of the hips, knees and ankles.

Passive stretching of spastic muscles and regular standing (if possible) are helpful in relieving spasticity and preventing contractures. Range of motion is performed as frequently as the clinical situation indicates.

Contractures commonly occur due to flexor spasticity in antigravity muscles and are common in the hip flexors, knee flexors and ankle plantar flexors.

Care of the quadriplegic shoulder and hand have already been examined. Flexion contractures of the elbows preclude independent push-ups for pressure relief and transfers. Hip flexion contractures are detrimental to optimal positioning, independent transfers and dressing. Additionally, hip flexion contractures may exert excessive pressure on bony prominances.

Hip and knee flexion contractures can be avoided by regular prone lying (once the patient is medically stable). Stable, long sitting for dressing requires substantial hamstring stretching and 110° of hip flexion. Prevention of ankle plantar flexion deformities requires diligent passive range of motion, in association with correct wheelchair footplate positioning to provide optimal ankle alignment. A footboard may be used when lying supine. Feet should be positioned at the end of the mattress in prone lying and not forced into plantar flexion. High-top runners may help to preserve good position of the ankles.

Positioning

In the acute stages of treatment, or at other times when the spinal cord injured person must spend significant periods of time in bed, assiduous attention to positioning will help to reduce spasticity and the formation of contractures and deformity.

Positioning is appropriate below the level of neurological lesion. Optimal positioning of the quadriplegic arms has already been examined. Bromley (1991) outlines the following positions for the lower limbs in supine and side lying.

Supine:

- hips extended, slightly abducted
- knees extended (**no** pillows under knees)
- ankles dorsiflexed (use of splints may produce pressure sores)
- toes extended.

Side lying:

- hips 20° of flexion, with two pillows between the knees
- knees flexed enough to allow stability
- ankles dorsiflexed
- toes extended.

DISABILITY REDUCTION: ACUTE AND LONG-TERM MANAGEMENT

Dependent oedema

Dependent, or gravitational oedema is characterized by bilateral, pitting oedema in dependent body parts which is relieved by changing position. The problem is aggravated by spinal shock (Zejdlik, 1992).

Dependent oedema may be problematic due to poor vasomotor control and the loss of assistive muscle pumping action for venous return.

Management requires:

- constant support of the arms and hands of quadriplegic patients on pillows (in bed) and on arm troughs or wheelchair trays;
- support of the legs when seated, using wheelchair footrests;
- encouragement of frequent position changes;
- protection of the skin from trauma;
- performance of range-of-motion exercise to improve circulation, while taking care not to force oedematous joints, thereby causing additional trauma;
- regular and frequent elevation of the legs;
- venous circulation is aided by wearing high-quality, anti-embolitic stockings. These should be full length and must be checked frequently to ensure that they do not cause a tourniquet effect. Alternatively, tensor bandages may be wrapped spirally, from foot to thigh and secured with tape rather than pins to avoid the risk of skin damage (Zejdlik, 1992).

Dependent oedema is common when the patient is first resuming a sitting posture following bed rest. However, as time progresses, local vasomotor tone improves (particularly in the presence of upper motor neurone lesions and subsequent spasticity) and the problem will resolve for most individuals (Burke and Murray, 1975).

Prevention of deep vein thrombosis and pulmonary embolism

Deep vein thrombosis (DVT) and pulmonary embolism are reported to be the major post-injury complications among patients with spinal cord injuries, with an incidence reported to range from 49% to 72%. Pulmonary embolism is the leading cause of death among patients who survive the period immediately following the spinal cord trauma (Merli *et al.*, 1988).

Contributing factors to the development of DVT include venous system stasis due to loss of muscle pump action, hypercoagulability, possible local trauma, pressure of the calf muscles on the bed and prolonged immobilization (Burke and Murray, 1975; McCagg, 1986). Additional risks include obesity, smoking, poor nutritional status, associated hip or long-bone fractures, multiple trauma, or high, complete quadriplegia (Zejdlik, 1992).

Although there is a time-honoured tradition of daily leg circumference measurements, studies have shown that this is of no value in a spinal cord injured population (Swarczinski and Dijkers, 1991). However, all staff working with the patient should observe for signs of swelling, erythema or low-grade increase in temperature (McCagg, 1986). Diagnosis of a DVT precludes passive range of motion for both legs until anticoagulation therapy is successful (Bromley, 1991). The condition commonly occurs within the first two or three weeks after injury, and the study by Merli *et al.* (1988) suggests that external pneumatic compression with gradient elastic stockings may form part of an effective prophylactic regimen for this client group.

Zejdlik (1992) outlines a programme for effective management focused upon increasing peripheral blood flow, preventing blood pooling in the extremities and protecting venous walls from trauma or pressure. This incorporates:

- active and passive range-of-motion exercises;
- ankle-pumping exercises about five times on each foot after every turn;
- applying high-quality, custom-fit elastic stockings to exert a compression force;
- limb positioning to prevent oedema;
- regular, two-hourly turns and correct positioning (avoiding pressure behind the knee and never putting pillows under the knees in supine lying);
- laboratory technicians being warned against taking blood specimens from the legs, to avoid venous punctures;
- avoiding an increase in blood viscosity by not allowing the patient to become dehydrated.

Orthostatic hypotension

Orthostatic, or postural, hypotension refers to the dramatic plummet in blood pressure that occurs when a patient with a lesion above T5 moves from a horizontal to an upright position. Similar in pathology to postural oedema, orthostatic hypotension produces the most severe symptoms among those with cervical lesions. In people with quadriplegia, postural changes produce no significant sympathetic response to prevent venous pooling in dependent areas of the body, to increase the pumping action of the heart or peripheral vascular resistance. Decreased venous return and diminished cardiac output are exacerbated by bed rest.

Symptoms of orthostatic hypotension are most severe in the early stages after injury, being quickly reversed when the patient resumes a reclined position. It is suggested that regular and frequent changes of position can be important factors in stimulating a vasoconstrictor response and in restoring control (Ozer, 1988). Once the individual with quadriplegia resumes regular activity, adaptation to this condition occurs and it is no longer problematic in most instances, despite still being demonstrable by blood pressure recording.

This is generally a short-term problem, which is managed in the immediate post-acute period by the use of high-quality, pressure gradient stockings and abdominal binders. Abdominal binders should be fitted below the rib cage, between the waist and the gluteal fold (Zejdlik, 1992; Grundy and Swain, 1993). The aim is to reduce the pooling of blood in the abdomen and lower extremities.

It is essential that all rehabilitation staff are aware of this potential problem and its immediate remedy. The patient should be encouraged to alert the therapist to symptoms of dizziness, weakness and blurred vision before fainting or black-outs. Blood pressure may be increased by lowering the head of the bed or tilt table or by tilting the wheelchair backwards. The patient should be instructed to breathe deeply, the therapist can assist expiration by placing a hand firmly on the diaphragm to elicit a vasoconstriction reflex (Zejdlik, 1992).

The patient should be reassured that the problem will resolve with time and that the attendant member of staff will take immediate action to remedy orthostatic hypotension should its symptoms occur.

Autonomic hyperreflexia

Autonomic hyperreflexia (autonomic dysreflexia) is a life-threatening syndrome unique to people with spinal cord injuries above T6. **This is a severe, acute medical emergency which can lead to cerebral haemorrhage and death.** It is therefore essential that every care giver who interacts with people who have spinal cord lesions is aware of the signs and symptoms of autonomic hyperreflexia. It is imperative that swift and appropriate action is taken immediately to alleviate the symptoms and prevent morbidity and mortality.

Individuals with spinal cord lesions above T6 are unable to preserve autonomic homeostasis by an interaction of sympathetic and parasympathetic activity. Although an intact nervous system produces a sympathetic response to a variety of stimuli, in those with cord lesions above T6 (and especially cervical lesions), there is massive and unregulated reflex sympathetic activity below the lesion level.

Signs and symptoms of autonomic hyperreflexia may include a combination of:

- severe hypertension
- pounding headache
- shivering and chill
- facial flush/blotchiness above the level of lesion
- bradycardia (or tachycardia)
- profuse sweating above and below the level of lesion
- piloerection ('goose bumps')
- dilated pupils
- pallor
- nasal congestion (Guttmann's sign)
- increased spasticity
- blurred vision
- anxiety

and less commonly:

- nausea
- confusion
- lethargy
- periods of unresponsiveness.

Rapid intervention should prevent the dangers that are inherent in autonomic crises and include loss of consciousness, atrial fibrillation, seizures, aphasia, retinal, subarachnoid or cerebral haemorrhage and death (Bloch, 1986; Colachis, 1992).

Autonomic hyperreflexia is usually caused by overdistention of the bladder or bowel but may be produced in response to various noxious visceral or other stimuli below the level of spinal cord injury. Stimuli reported to trigger hyperreflexia include:

- bladder distention (possibly due to blocked catheter), bladder irrigation, bladder calculi or infection
- defecation, rectal distention, digital stimulation, enemas
- cutaneous stimulation
- fractures, heterotopic ossification
- range-of-motion exercises, passive stretching of the hip, sudden position changes, such as on tilt table
- ejaculation
- labour
- surgery, cystoscopy, catheterisation
- pressure sores
- ingrowing toenails
- constricting clothing, leg bag straps, pressure stockings (Bloch, 1986; Braddom and Rocco, 1991).

An episode of autonomic hyperreflexia not associated with the usual causes can be an important sign of visceral pathology, for example, pulmonary embolism or abdominal emergency.

Autonomic hyperreflexia may occur at any time after the period of spinal shock and is significantly more common among those with cervical lesions than high thoracic lesions.

Treatment

Treatment consists of removing the precipitating cause.

The patient's head should be elevated to 45° if possible to counteract the hypertension with orthostatic hypotension. Clothing should be loosened. The source of nerve stimuli is sought, catheter and drainage tubes checked, rectum checked for bowel impaction, and skin and toe nails inspected. Blood pressure should be monitored. Catheterisation may be indicated. If symptoms are not relieved, immediate medical assistance should be sought (Braddom and Rocco, 1991; Grundy and Swain, 1993).

The patient should be fully cognizant with the prevention,

symptoms and amelioration of autonomic hyperreflexia, as staff in community hospitals are rarely knowledgeable about handling this emergency. Braddom and Rocco (1991) recommend carrying an information card in case of emergency. The well-informed and educated individual is more likely to prevent and survive autonomic hyperreflexia.

Regulating body temperature

Individuals with spinal cord injuries are susceptible to both heat prostration and hypothermia due to major impairments in the body's ability to modify heat production and loss.

Thermoregulation is impaired because of the following factors.

- Shivering does not occur below the level of a complete spinal cord injury. Those with lesions above T4 are unable to increase their metabolism because of the limited amount of available musculature (Ozer, 1988).
- Vasoconstriction is absent.
- Sweating is reduced below the level of injury in paraplegia and is almost absent in quadriplegia.
- The systemic response to intense localized cold stress is reduced in quadriplegia (Bloch, 1986).

The degree of dysfunction is directly proportional to the body area that experiences loss of thermoregulatory mechanisms (Zejdlik, 1992). People with quadriplegia exhibit an excessive rise in core temperature and a decreased ability to withstand hot and humid environments. Individuals with quadriplegia and high thoracic lesions are poikilothermic – being unable to regulate body heat effectively and tending to assume the temperature of the environment. Improvement in vasomotor control and increased tolerance to heat occurs over time, even among people with quadriplegia (Ozer, 1988).

Individuals with quadriplegia are considered to be at high risk of developing accidental hypothermia. To conserve body heat, the individual with quadriplegia should take care to wear warm clothing when going outside in cool temperatures, however briefly. Sheepskin-lined boots, long underwear and layers of natural fibre clothing may be necessary in especially cold environments such as in Canada. Duvets or warm bed covers are essential – hot water bottles or electric blankets are unsuitable because of the potential for burn damage to desensitized skin.

In some instances, profuse sweating may occur above the level of injury. The client must be kept dry to prevent chills hence bed linen or clothes may need to be changed frequently.

To dissipate body heat, the individual should avoid going outside in extremely high temperatures. Air conditioning, fans and spray bottles may all help to maintain a comfortable body temperature and should be used where possible.

An elevated temperature that is not a response to a high environmental temperature will need to be thoroughly investigated and treated (Zejdlik, 1992).

Bloch (1986) indicates that, despite major changes in the ability of people with spinal cord injuries to modify heat production and loss, clinically significant disturbances of body temperature are uncommon. This is presumably due to the appropriate application of the preventive measures indicated above.

Respiratory care

A conscientious, comprehensive and consistent approach to respiratory care plays a significant role in maintaining optimal health in the person with an acute spinal cord lesion, in preventing complications and ensuring long-term respiratory health. The respiratory therapist or physiotherapist will perform a detailed and thorough assessment of the client, following which, the principles of a maintenance programme for bronchial hygiene are:

- promotion of ventilation and gas exchange;
- promotion of airway humidification;
- preventing secretion retention by promotion of mobilization and expectoration;
- increasing muscular strength and endurance;
- prevention of pulmonary complications;
- improvement in force of cough (Bromley, 1991; Zejdlik, 1992).

Regular turning and positioning

The regular turning regimen which is essential in preventing the formation of pressure sores is also important in preventing stasis of secretions in dependent areas of the lungs. Even minor changes of position will prevent accumulation of secretions. Prone lying and postural drainage are advocated if they do not compromise early spine stability and if they are tolerated by the client (Bromley, 1991). Good posture is important in sitting, to prevent restriction in movement of the diaphragm. If the individual is unable to maintain good postural alignment, use of the Obus or Jay back supports may be beneficial. People who have higher lesions with paralysis of the abdominal muscles and rib cage may initially have problems in breathing when sitting upright.

Goldman and associates (1986) report that the abdominal wall in people with quadriplegia is twice as compliant as in normal subjects. In erect postures, the abdominal contents fall forwards unopposed and the diaphragm flattens, hence impairing the only respiratory muscle that is available to the quadriplegic in expanding the rib cage. Abdominal binders decrease the compliance of the abdominal wall, increasing intra-abdominal pressure and pushing the diaphragm into a position of greater mechanical advantage hence decreasing the effort required to breathe.

When normal subjects lie down, vital capacity decreases by 7.5%. When people with quadriplegia who have been tilted head up, lie down, vital capacity increases by about 45%. If the abdomen is supported by a binder the difference is reduced to 28%. Goldman found a significant increase in vital capacity in the sitting position when abdominal binders were applied. Abdominal binders have a dual impact in reducing the effects of postural hypotension.

Care should be taken to ensure that the abdominal support is not positioned over the rib cage, as this would serve to restrict chest expansion and be counterproductive (Zejdlik, 1992).

The abdominal support is not usually required on a long-term basis but may be gradually discontinued as the client adjusts to the respiratory demands required in sitting. However, improvements in respiratory function have been demonstrated amongst people with chronic quadriplegia, when using an abdominal binder (Scott *et al.*, 1993).

Assisted cough

Those individuals who have little or no abdominal muscle paralysis will be able to cough effectively to clear lung secretions; however, for people who have high thoracic or low cervical lesions, coughing may be achieved by leaning well forward in the chair and pressing the chest against one arm, to compensate for absent abdominal musculature.

People with lesions of C5 and above will require assistance from another person. With the client lying supine, the helper spreads both hands across the lower rib cage and upper abdomen of the client and thrusts inwards and upwards in co-ordination with the client's efforts to cough (see Brownlee and Williams, 1987; Bromley, 1991). Great care must be taken with this procedure in the acute stages of treatment, before fracture sites have healed and when abdominal complications may be present. This manoeuvre may be performed while the client is seated, if this is necessary.

Good bronchial hygiene will require continued attention to assisted coughing throughout life.

Breathing exercises

People with spinal cord injuries who wish to participate in active and competitive sports will require an aggressive programme of breathing exercises.

However, it is important for all people with spinal cord injuries to build up respiratory muscle strength, improving ventilation to all parts of the lung by slow, relaxed deep breathing exercises. Although early exercises concentrate on diaphragmatic breathing, some therapists recommend progression by using weights to provide resisted exercise for the diaphragm. Weights should be positioned on the upper abdomen, not on the ribs.

Those clients who have innervated intercostal musculature may perform breathing exercises while the therapists provide localized pressure against the chest wall. Absent proprioceptive feedback may be compensated for by using mirrors (Brownlee and Williams, 1987). The aims of resisted exercises are to improve strength and endurance and postpone fatigue. Use of neck accessory muscles in respiration to assist a weak diaphragm in high-lesion quadriplegia is discouraged. Attention is given instead to strengthening the diaphragm. Future use of a mouthstick for functional activities will be severely hampered if the individual is using his neck muscles to assist respiration. Mobility may also be impaired if the individual is unable to drive a powered chair with his head or chin.

Routine respiratory care should be initiated at the earliest phase of treatment. People with spinal cord injuries are at risk of developing hypoxia, atelectasis and pneumonia, pulmonary oedema, pulmonary emboli and pneumothorax (Zejdlik, 1992). Smoking is actively discouraged, as any further compromise of lung function will be seriously detrimental to the health and activity level of the individual.

Attention to respiratory hygiene must also be a lifelong process. Respiratory complications now constitute the leading cause of death among people with spinal cord lesions both during the acute phase and also during later years, especially among people with quadriplegia. Most respiratory deaths are attributed to pneumonia. Hence considerable effort must be taken to promote optimal respiratory hygiene and function (refer to Clough *et al.*, 1986).

Urinary tract management

Despite advances in urological management, urinary tract complications remain a major cause of morbidity and mortality for people with spinal cord lesions. Successful and diligent management of the urinary tract is of the utmost importance in a comprehensive lifetime care programme.

The term **neurogenic bladder** refers to a group of symptoms that arises from neurological rather than urological pathology. The neurological pathology may result in the loss of voluntary control of voiding, altered bladder tone and of its ability to contract, altered ability of the bladder to empty, altered bladder capacity and ability to store urine and an altered degree of resistance of the sphincters controlling flow from the bladder (Zejdlik, 1992). The nature of neurogenic bladder dysfunction will vary according to the presence of an upper or lower motor neurone lesion.

There are four primary aims in the urinary tract management programme:

1. To achieve a reliable method of bladder management which is socially acceptable to the client and those close to him; and which is compatible with his lifestyle.
2. To maintain a low-pressure system and to prevent bladder overdistention. High residuals, obstruction, infection or infrequent draining can produce overdistention of the bladder and subsequent damage to the kidneys.
3. To ensure the bladder fills adequately and achieves as complete emptying as possible.
4. To prevent and control infection (Zejdlik, 1992).

Intermittent catheterisation

An indwelling catheter is inserted within the emergency period immediately following a spinal cord injury and this may allow for accurate, early measurement of urine output and prevent detrusor overdistention. However, use of an indwelling catheter for over a week is invariably associated with infection, hence intermittent catheterisation is instituted as early as possible in most centres as the treatment of choice for acute spinal cord injuries (Zejdlik, 1992; Grundy and Swain, 1993). Intermittent catheterisation is performed regularly (every few hours), using a strictly sterile technique.

Self-intermittent catheterisations

Once the spinal cord injured patient is able to sit up, it is possible to start self-intermittent catheterisations. Individuals who catheterise themselves may use a clean method rather than sterile technique, although many sources recommend a sterile procedure while in hospital because of the high risk of contamination (Herschorn and Gerridzen, 1986; Zejdlik, 1992). People with high lesions may choose to continue sterile intermittent catheterisation, directing a care attendant in this procedure.

Both men and women may choose intermittent catheterisation on a long-term basis. The benefits include freedom from an external collecting device or from an indwelling catheter (with its inherent high risks of infections and calculi), enhanced sexual relations and improved personal hygiene – most particularly for women (Zejdlik, 1992). It is also the method of choice among most people who have a lower motor neurone lesion. Although this technique demands some manual dexterity, Ford and Duckworth (1987) clearly outline methods of self-catheterisation for those with minimal hand function.

Indwelling catheter

Long-term indwelling urethral catheterisation is often the method of choice for urinary drainage by women (particularly with quadriplegia), older people and those with poor or absent hand function. Unfortunately, infection is inevitable, there is a tendency to develop bladder calculi and trauma may be sustained to the urethra and bladder neck. Nonetheless, these complications can be minimised by assiduous attention to fluid intake, maintenance of an acidic urine and appropriate use of medications. Despite the potential problems, an indwelling catheter can provide the method of choice for those who have encountered incontinence or who are unable to perform independent catheterisations (Zejdlik, 1992; Grundy and Swain, 1993).

External collection systems

For some individuals, the inability to predict or control voiding may necessitate some means of protection from incontinence.

Several different types of condom drainage are available for men, using condoms that are self-adhesive and rolled into place, have adhesive strips or adhesive applicators. A connecting tube attaches to a leg bag. Scrupulous attention to personal cleanliness and hygiene are as essential with this method of management as with every other, to prevent infection and serious, permanent damage to the urinary tract. Further attention to skin condition is indicated, as prolonged exposure to adhesives and moisture may promote skin breakdown.

Unfortunately, no satisfactory method of external urine collection has yet been designed for women, hence the use of absorbent padding is indicated, if this is acceptable to the client.

Some people may achieve varying degrees of successful

urinary management by Valsalva manoeuvre (bearing down), by tapping or manual expression (Credé) to induce a contraction (Grundy and Swain, 1993). Sacral anterior root stimulators (radio-linked implants) are an alternative method of achieving continence for some people (Brindley *et al.*, 1986).

Complications

Autonomic hyperreflexia is a potentially fatal hazard among those with high lesions (above T6) and is typically triggered by bladder overdistention, blocked catheter, calculi, urinary tract infection or overfilled drainage bags (see pp. 96–99). The patient and all his care givers should be aware of the symptoms and immediate management of autonomic hyperreflexia.

Urinary tract infections remain a significant threat to people with spinal cord injuries with a high incidence of morbidity, re-admission to hospital and life-threatening complications. For long-term prevention of urinary tract infection, Grundy and Swain (1993) recommend a high fluid intake (if possible) and ensuring effective bladder emptying.

The management of the urinary tract provides a clear example of an impairment that is a sequelae of spinal cord injury but which may be prevented from becoming a significantly disabling, or handicapping condition by appropriate choice of drainage method and by assiduous attention to the long-term prevention of potential complications.

Any infection or complication of urinary tract management will delay and prolong the initial process of rehabilitation and will be a significant barrier to the achievement of a quality lifestyle in the community. (See also the National Institute on Disability and Rehabilitation Research consensus statement on urinary tract management (NIDRR, 1992)).

Bowel management

A bowel management programme may be started once the period of spinal shock has ended. During spinal shock the bowel is flaccid and requires regular, gentle manual evacuation to prevent distention.

The great majority of people with spinal cord injuries are able to control evacuation, with unintentional evacuations occurring rarely – if at all.

The individual who has an upper motor neurone lesion is able to make use of the local reflex activity which remains intact. Digital stimulation, (using one gloved finger, plenty of lubricant and gentle, circular motions), may be sufficient to trigger reflex emptying of the bowel. Additionally, a Dulcolax suppository inserted past the sphincter and placed against the bowel wall may produce reflex evacuation. Most individuals will be able to sit on a padded toilet seat for this procedure, allowing gravity to assist elimination, ensuring privacy and preventing pressure sore formation. A footstool may be used to assist balance and prevent excessive pressure on the thighs. People who have high lesions will require the assistance of an attendant and may prefer to lie on one side in bed, with the knees and hips flexed. Use of dry edge underpads will ensure that bed linen is not soiled and will facilitate thorough clean up.

Individuals with poor hand function may be able to use simple aids to enable independent suppository insertion.

The timing and frequency of bowel evacuation should be chosen to suit the individual's previous habit and his lifestyle.

Successful long-term bowel management will depend upon a nutritious, high-fibre diet and generous fluid intake. If problems develop it may be beneficial to keep a record of diet, fluid intake, exercise and bowel routines to identify any emerging patterns.

Laxatives are not recommended, most particularly their long-term use is discouraged. Use of enemas is also contraindicated. The dilation of the lower bowel produced by enemas causes a loss of bowel tone – the opposite of the desired effect (Zejdlik, 1992).

Management of the bowel is more difficult in lower motor neurone lesions because of the lost reflexes and flaccid sphincters (usually lesions at T12 and below). Daily planned evacuations are recommended, using the strong abdominal muscles to perform a Valsalva manoeuvre, manual evacuation and possible use of a strong stimulant suppository (Zejdlik, 1992). (See also Ford and Duckworth, 1987; Zejdlik, 1992).

Pressure sore prevention

Pressure sores interfere with every aspect of the physically disabled patient's life, from active participation in a rehabili-

tation program to returning to the community as a productive
and creative person.   (Donovan *et al.*, 1988)

A pressure sore is formed as a result of ischaemia caused by
unrelieved pressure, particularly over a bony prominence.
People with spinal cord injuries are at particular risk from unrelieved pressure due to loss of sensation, loss of voluntary movement and impaired circulation caused by loss of vasomotor
control (Bromley, 1991).

Pressure sores contribute a major cause of re-admission to
hospital despite being wholly preventable. It is almost unbeliev-
able that, in the late 20th century, pressure sores are frequently
allowed to develop while a patient is in acute care in a hospital
and wholly reliant upon conscientious nursing care for maintenance of his skin integrity. McGregor (1992) emphasizes that such
negligence represents a very serious breakdown in care and
should be a very rare occurrence.

The incidence of pressure sores has been found to be especially high among those patients who experience delay in transfer to a specialist spinal unit (or are treated solely at a general
hospital), significantly contributing to longer hospitalization
and greatly increased costs. McGregor (1992) states: 'Resent-
ment is likely if it is inferred that the cause of the pressure sore
lies in a failure in the system of care – but this is usually always
the fact of the matter'.

> Of all the preventable complications to which the spinal cord
> injured patient is vulnerable, this is the costliest. If a pressure
> sore severe enough to require even one plastic surgical pro-
> cedure develops it increases the total cost of the patient's care
> fivefold. . . . Yet in the correct environment it does not occur.
>   (Donovan *et al.*, 1984)

The most common sites of pressure sores are over the ischial
tuberosities, greater trochanter and sacrum. The scapulae and
elbows are also at risk for people with quadriplegia. The sore
may affect not only the skin but subcutaneous fat, muscle
and bone.

Pressure sores contribute a huge economic burden to the
healthcare system and to society, are associated with a high
mortality rate in addition to placing severe handicap upon the

individual, curtailing his activities and reducing his opportunities for socialization, recreation, productivity and quality of life.

Prevention of pressure sores relies upon a few basic principles which should be initiated at the earliest stage of care and thereafter continued by the individual throughout his life.

1. While in bed, the spinal cord injured person must be turned, or turn himself regularly. This will be every two hours during the stage of spinal shock and every three hours thereafter, day and night (Bromley, 1991).

2. Each individual will need to shift his weight every 15 minutes when first sitting in a wheelchair. Once skin tolerance increases, he will need to determine his desired frequency of push-up lifts or weight shifts while seated. An attendant may perform this task for people with high lesions, or an automatic tilt feature on a powered wheelchair may allow independent weight shift (see Chapter 6).

3. Scrupulous cleanliness is essential, with no urine or faecal matter allowed to remain in contact with the skin.

4. Pillows may be positioned between the legs while in bed to prevent contact between the knees and ankles.

5. The skin should be protected from friction shearing forces, for example, from poor lifting techniques, or from sitting in bed with the head elevated and subsequent excessive shearing force over the sacrum.

6. The skin must be checked twice daily, using a mirror, to identify any change in colour, bruising, induration, blistering, infected hair follicles, pimples or other signs of pressure irritation.

7. If a red mark on the skin is detected, which does not fade within 30 minutes, the individual should avoid all pressure on the area until the redness and induration disappears.

8. A rash on the skin, caused by allergy from drugs, medications, soaps, food or other irritants should be treated as though it was a pressure sore.

9. Pressure is concentrated in deeper tissue close to the bone, hence a small ulcer on the skin may overlie a much larger, deep area of tissue destruction.

10. Ischaemia will be increased by a raised temperature. Particular attention must be paid during times of fever and during extremely high environmental temperatures. Some

    wheelchair cushions will contribute to raised skin tempera-
    ture in certain individuals.

11.   Skin should be prevented from burning due to heat
       exposure. Protection is necessary in direct sunlight. The
       individual should also be cautious about sitting too close to
       a fire, to hot pipes or radiators.
12.   Hot plates or drinks should not be carried directly on the
       lap.
13.   Hot water bottles or electric blankets should not be used.
14.   Sharp objects should be kept away from anesthetic areas of
       the body. Items should therefore not be carried in back
       pockets.
15.   Feet and legs should be protected from bumping into
       objects and causing local skin trauma.
16.   Smoking is significantly and positively correlated with the
       formation of pressure sores.

Studies indicate that the formation of pressure sores among
people with spinal cord injuries living in the community are
caused, not purely by mechanical factors, but by psychosocial
variables. Anderson and Andberg (1979) determined that a high
degree of satisfaction with life was correlated with a low incidence of pressure sore formation. Heilporn (1991) describes a
syndrome of passivity, helplessness and failure to assume
responsibility for healthcare among people with repeat hospitalizations for recurring pressure sores.

These studies indicate again the need to expand the process of
rehabilitation from a mechanical, medical model to one that
respects the need of each individual for purposeful activity and
further, to the requirement of enabling patients to become active
in their own care management, in making decisions and in
solving problems. Quality of life and satisfaction with life are to
be viewed as more than psychosocial outcome measures but as
crucial factors in determining health and preventing needless
complications.

Some spinal units are addressing the needs of people with
spinal cord injuries living in the community by establishing
community-based support services with particular emphasis on
reducing the incidence of pressure sores. Such a programme in
Scotland has enabled close liaison between people who have
spinal cord injuries and their community nurses. There has been

a subsequent and marked reduction in the number of individuals requiring hospitalization and/or plastic surgery due to sores (McGregor, 1992). At Odstock Hospital in England, a pressure clinic was established as the central part of the educational programme for the prevention of pressure sores. The clinic acts as an information source not only for former patients but also offers training for general hospital and community healthcare workers. A community liaison nurse visits former patients at home to provide advice. Results show a reduction of over 50% both in the incidence of pressure sores and in the re-admission rate due to sores (Dover *et al.*, 1992).

SURVIVAL AND MORTALITY

> The outlook for most persons who sustain spinal cord injuries has improved considerably in the last two decades.
>
> (DeVivo *et al.*, 1992a)

A series of Canadian studies traced all patients with spinal cord injuries discharged from Toronto's Lyndhurst Hospital between 1945 and 1980. The most recent report noted a marked decrease in deaths due to renal disease (formerly the primary cause of mortality) but a marked increase in deaths due to suicide, liver disease and alcohol abuse (Geisler *et al.*, 1983).

In the USA, DeVivo and associates have examined survival and mortality following spinal cord injury (1989; 1992a; 1992b). They report that, although mortality rates for many people with spinal cord injuries have declined dramatically in the past few decades, many cause-specific mortality rates remain substantially above normal. The prognosis for older people who sustain neurologically complete quadriplegias remains very poor. DeVivo reports that mortality due to renal failure has been steadily declining. The leading known cause of death among people with quadriplegia and those over 55 was found to be pneumonia, with unintentional injuries and suicide being the primary cause for people with paraplegia and those under 55 years of age (1989).

A recent British study represents the largest investigation conducted to date of people who have lived for more than 20 years since sustaining spinal cord injury (Whiteneck *et al.*, 1992; Whiteneck, 1993). Findings indicate that the extent of neurological impairment appears to be related to survival and to causes of death. Renal disorders contributed to the highest mortality among people with paraplegia whereas respiratory disorders were the primary causes of death for those with quadriplegia. The study additionally found that, with increasing time since injury, causes of morbidity and mortality more closely mirror those of the general ageing population, although occurring at younger ages than would be expected among the normal population. Primary causes of death for all the subjects with spinal cord injuries were:

- renal failure 19.6% (22.8% in those with paraplegia, 15.8% in quadriplegia)
- respiratory system disease 13.8% (11.2% in paraplegia, 19.3% in quadriplegia)
- neoplasms 11.0%
- heart disease 19.1% (myocardial infarction 10.5%, other heart disease 8.6%
- accidents and injuries 6.1%.

(Other causes each constituted less than 5% of total mortality) (Whiteneck, 1993).

Research has suggested that mortality after spinal cord injury is correlated with lower levels of social and vocational activities and lower life satisfaction (Krause and Crewe, 1987; Krause, 1991; Krause and Kjorsvig, 1992). This is of prime importance to the rehabilitation team, as it suggests that a comprehensive psychosocial approach to rehabilitation, including identification of meaningful productive activity, fulfilling leisure pursuits and social re-integration may not only enhance rehabilitation outcomes but may also influence survival itself. In comparison to the spinal cord injured survivors, those who had died had reported three highly significant differences in perceived problems, namely depression, loneliness and boredom (Krause and Kjorsvig, 1992).

> The relationship between poor psychological, social and vocational adjustment with mortality reaffirms the need to address these issues as part of a comprehensive rehabilitation programme. (Krause, 1991)

It may thus be emphasized that those variables loosely termed 'quality of life' and only recently considered in assessment of rehabilitation outcome may actually be instrumental in ensuring survival. Krause proposes that quality of life and length of life are closely related following spinal cord injury.

This finding poses a clear challenge to the development of comprehensive, personally meaningful rehabilitation programmes and post-discharge services. Many of the factors that influence survival are firmly within the mandate of the rehabilitation professions. Self-destructive behaviour, substance abuse, suicide, social isolation, depression, loneliness and boredom must thus be of considerable concern to the rehabilitation team. Mortality following spinal cord injury is seen to be more than a medical issue. Hence attention to engagement in meaningful occupations, to socialization and community re-integration during a rehabilitation programme are to be considered more than optional extras – the 'icing on the cake'. Rather they may be relevant to survival itself (Krause and Crewe, 1987).

REFERENCES

Anderson, T.P. and Andberg, M.M. (1979) Psychosocial factors associated with pressure sores. *Archives of Physical Medicine and Rehabilitation*, **60,** 341–6.

Bloch, R.F. (1986) Autonomic dysfunction, in *Management of Spinal Cord Injuries* (eds R.F. Bloch and M. Basbaum), Williams and Wilkins, Baltimore, MD, pp. 149–63.

Braddom, R.L. and Rocco, J.F. (1991) Autonomic dysreflexia: a survey of current treatment. *American Journal of Physical Medicine and Rehabilitation*, **70,** 234–41.

Brindley, G.S., Polkey, C.E., Rushton, D.N. and Cardozo,L. (1986) Sacral anterior root stimulators for bladder control in paraplegia: the first 50 cases. *Journal of Neurology, Neurosurgery and Psychiatry*, **49,** 1104–14.

Bromley, I. (1991) *Tetraplegia and Paraplegia – a Guide for Physiotherapists*, 4th edn, Churchill Livingstone, Edinburgh, pp. 6, 18–20, 27–30, 37, 39.

Brooks, M.E. and Ohry, A. (1992) Conservative versus surgical treatment of the cervical and thoracolumbar spine in spinal trauma. *Paraplegia* **30**(1), 46–9.

Brownlee, S. and Williams, S. (1987) Physiotherapy in the respiratory care of patients with high spinal injury. *Physiotherapy*, **73**(3), 148–52.

Burke, D.C. and Murray, D.D. (1975) *Handbook of Spinal Cord Medicine*, Macmillan, Basingstoke, pp. 27–9, 36–8, 67.

Clough, P., Lindenhaur, D., Hayes, J. and Zekarny, B. (1986) Guidelines for routine respiratory care of patients with spinal cord injury. *Physical Therapy*, **66**(9), 1395–402.

Colachis, S.C. (1992) Autonomic hyperreflexia with spinal cord injury. *Journal of the American Paraplegia Society*, **15**(3), 171–86.

Curtin, M. (1993) The management of the C6 quadriplegic patient's hand. *British Journal of Occupational Therapy* **56(12)**, 455.

Davidoff, G.N., Roth, E.J. and Richards, J.S. (1992) Cognitive deficits in spinal cord injury: epidemiology and outcome. *Archives of Physical Medicine and Rehabilitation*, **73**, 275–84.

DeVivo, M.J., Kartus, P.L., Stover, S.L. *et al.* (1989) Cause of death for patients with spinal cord injuries. *Archives of Internal Medicine*, **149**(8), 1761–6.

DeVivo, M.J., Rutt, R.D., Black, K.J. *et al.* (1992a) Trends in spinal cord injury demographics and treatment outcomes between 1973 and 1986. *Archives of Physical Medicine and Rehabilitation*, **73**, 424–30.

DeVivo, M.J., Stover, S.L. and Black, K.J. (1992b) Prognostic factors for 12-year survival after spinal cord injury. *Archives of Physical Medicine and Rehabilitation*, **73**, 156–62.

Donovan, W.H., Carter, R.E., Bedbrook, G.M. *et al.* (1984) Incidence of medical complications in spinal cord injury: patients in specialised compared with non-specialised centres. *Paraplegia*, **22**, 282–90.

Donovan, W.H., Garber, S.L., Hamilton, S.M. *et al.* (1988) Pressure ulcers, in *Rehabilitation Medicine: Principles and Practice*, (ed. J.A. DeLisa), J.B. Lippincott, Philadelphia, PA, pp. 476–91.

Dover, H., Pickard, W., Swain, I. and Grundy, D. (1992) The effectiveness of a pressure clinic in preventing pressure sores. *Paraplegia*, **30**(4), 267–71.

Ford, J. and Duckworth, B. (1987) *Physical Management for the Quadriplegic Patient* 2nd edn, F.A. Davis, Philadelphia, PA.

Formal, C. (1992) Metabolic and neurologic changes after spinal cord injury. *Physical Medicine and Rehabilitation Clinics of North America*, **3**(4), 783–95.

Geisler, W.O., Jousse, A.T., Wynne-Jones, M. and Breithaupt, D. (1983) Survival in traumatic spinal cord injury. *Paraplegia*, **21**, 364–73.

Goldman, J.M., Rose, L.S., Williams, S.J. *et al.* (1986) The effect of abdominal binders on breathing in tetraplegic patients. *Thorax*, **41**(12), 940–5.

Grundy, D. and Swain, A. (1993) *ABC of Spinal Cord Injury*, 2nd edn, British Medical Journal, London, pp. 6, 16–17, 19, 22–5, 27–8, 32–3.

Hammell, K.R.W. (1991) *An Investigation into the Availability and Adequacy of Social Relationships Following Head Injury and Spinal Cord Injury: a Study of Injured Men and their Partners*, MSc thesis (Rehabilitation Studies), University of Southampton, Southampton.

Heilporn, A. (1991) Psychological factors in the causation of pressure sores: case reports. *Paraplegia* **29**, 137–9.

Herschorn, S. and Gerridzen, R.G. (1986) The management of the neurogenic bladder, in *Management of Spinal Cord Injuries* (eds R.F. Bloch and M. Basbaum), Williams and Wilkins, Baltimore, MD, pp. 117–33.

Hildebrand, K.H. and Weintraub, A.H. (1992) The combination injury: spinal cord injury with concomitant traumatic brain injury, in *Management of Spinal Cord Injury*, 2nd edn, (C.P. Zejdlik), Jones and Bartlett, Boston, MA, pp. 571–81.

Krajnik, S.R. and Bridle, M.J. (1992) Hand splinting in quadriplegia: current practice. *American Journal of Occupational Therapy*, **46**(2), 149–56.

Krause, J. and Crewe, N. (1987) Prediction of long term survival among persons with spinal cord injury: an 11 year prospective study. *Rehabilitation Psychology* **32**, 205–13.

Krause, J. S. (1991) Survival following spinal cord injury: a fifteen year prospective study. *Rehabilitation Psychology*, **36**(2), 89–98.

Krause, J.S. and Kjorsvig, J.M. (1992) Mortality after spinal cord injury: a four year prospective study. *Archives of Physical Medicine and Rehabilitation* **73**, 558–63.

Krishnan, K.R., Glass, C.A., Turner, S.M. *et al.* (1992) Perceptual deprivation in the acute phase of spinal injury rehabilitation. *Journal of the American Paraplegia Society*, **15**(2), 60–5.

Malik, M.H. (1979) *Manual on Static Hand Splinting*, Harmarville Rehabilitation Center, Pittsburgh, PA.

McCagg, C. (1986) Postoperative management and acute rehabilitation of patients with spinal cord injuries. *Orthopedic Clinics of North America*, **17**(1), 171–82.

McGregor, J.C. (1992) Pressure sores: a personal comment. *Paraplegia*, **30**(2), 116–7.

Merli, G.J., Herbison, G.J., Ditunno, J.F. *et al.* (1988) Deep vein thrombosis: prophylaxis in acute spinal cord injured patients. *Archives of Physical Medicine and Rehabilitation*, **69**, 661–4.

NIDRR (1992) National Institute on Disability and Rehabilitation Research. Consensus statement, January 27–29, 1992. The prevention and management of urinary tract infections among people with spinal cord injuries. *Journal of the American Paraplegia Society*, **15**(3), 194–204.

Oliver, M. (1981) Disability, adjustment and family life – some theoretical considerations, in *Handicap in a Social World*, (eds A. Brechin, P. Liddiard and J. Swain), Open University and Hodder and Stoughton, London, p. 55.

Oliver, M., Zarb, G., Silver, J. *et al.* (1988) *Walking into Darkness: the Experience of Spinal Cord Injury*, The Macmillan Press, Basingstoke.

Ozer, M.N., (1988) *The management of persons with spinal cord injury*, Demos Publications, New York.

Roth, E., Davidoff, G., Thomas, P., Doljanac, R., Dijkers, M., Berent, S., Morris, J., Yarkony, G., (1989) A controlled study of neuropsychological deficits in acute spinal cord injury patients, *Paraplegia*, **27**, 480–9.

Schweigel, J., Peerless, S., (1971) A proposal for a spinal cord injury unit at Shaughnessy Hospital, Preliminary research review for Canadian Paraplegic Association, Vancouver, B.C., In *Management of spinal cord injuries*, 2nd edition, (C.P. Zejdlik, 2–4), Jones and Bartlett, Boston.

Scott, J.A., Donovan, W.H., (1981) Prevention of shoulder pain and contracture in the acute tetraplegia patient, *Paraplegia*, **19**, 313–19.

Scott, M.D., Frost, F., Supinski, G., Gonzalez, M., (1993) The effect of body position and abdominal binders in chronic tetraplegic subjects more than fifteen years post injury, *Journal of the American Paraplegia Society*, (abstract), **16**(2) 117.

Silfverskiold, J., Waters, R.L., (1991) Shoulder pain and functional disability in spinal cord injury patients, *Clinical Orthopaedics*, **272**, 141–5.

Swarczinski, C., Dijkers, M., (1991) The value of serial leg measurements for monitoring deep vein thrombosis in spinal cord injury, *Journal of Neuroscience Nursing*, **23**(5) 306–14.

Trieschmann, R.B., (1988) *Spinal cord injuries. Psychological, social and vocational rehabilitation*, 2nd edition, Demos Publications, New York.

Tucker, S.J., (1980) The psychology of spinal cord injury: patient–staff interaction, *Rehabilitation Literature*, **41**(5–6) 114–22.

Waring, W.P., Maynard, F.M., (1991) Shoulder pain in acute traumatic quadriplegia, *Paraplegia*, **29**, 37–41.

Whiteneck, G.G., (1993) Learning from recent empirical investigations, In *Aging with spinal cord injury*, (ed, G.G. Whiteneck), Demos Publications, New York.

Whiteneck, G.G., Charlifue, S.W., Frankel, H.L., Fraser, M.H., Gardner, B.P., Gerhart, K.A., Krishnan, K.R., Menter, R.R., Nuseibeh, I., Short, D.J., Silver, J.R., (1992) Mortality, morbidity and psychosocial outcomes of persons spinal cord injured more than 20 years ago, *Paraplegia*, **30**(9) 617–30.

WHO, (1980) *International classification of impairments, disabilities and handicaps: a manual of classification relating to the consequences of diseases*, World Health Organization, Geneva.

Woodbury, B., Redd, C., (1987) Psychosocial issues and approaches, In *Spinal cord injury. Concepts and management approaches*, (eds, L.A. Buchanan & D.A. Nawoczenski), Williams and Wilkins, Baltimore.

Yarkony, G.M., Bass, L.M., Keenan, V., Meyer, P.R., (1985) Contractures complicating spinal cord injury: incidence and comparison between spinal cord centre and general hospital acute care, *Paraplegia*, **23**, 265–71.

Zejdlik, C.P., (1992) *Management of spinal cord injuries*, 2nd edition, Jones and Bartlett Publishers, Boston.

5

Engagement in self-care activities

> Rehabilitation professionals' views of the real-life situation of people with disabilities may be biased by seeing only those with health problems, and then only in a hospital setting. They are likely to have less exposure to people who are living successfully in the community, yet these are the people with disabilities who have discovered means of coping that could benefit recently discharged individuals.
>
> (*Nosek, 1993*)

INTRODUCTION

For people who do not have a disability, physical health is rarely a goal in its own right. Rather, having a healthy body allows attainment of those things that are important in one's life – activities that make life worth living. The same is true for people with disabilities.

Ill health is a serious barrier to achievement of a fulfilling lifestyle, hence careful attention to healthcare management (as outlined in Chapter 4) is of considerable importance in enabling an individual who has sustained a spinal cord injury to achieve more personally meaningful goals. However, maintenance of the body in optimal health is not the primary goal of rehabilitation – but rather a means of achieving rehabilitation goals.

> Basic rehabilitation is a drag. It teaches you what you learned in the first four years of life – mobility, personal hygiene, avoidance of hazards, muscle development and other pretty unoriginal stuff. The best thing going for it is that not doing it is much worse than doing it. (Corbet, 1980)

Self-care activities are those tasks that are done routinely to maintain the individual's health and wellbeing in the environment. Self-care will include aspects of personal care, functional mobility and community management (Law *et al.*, 1991; CAOT, 1991). Each individual will have a personal and unique approach to self-care activities (as he will to all aspects of occupational performance) as a function of the social roles which must be fulfilled, the environment within which he will function (physical, social, economic and cultural) and his developmental stage (Law *et al.*, 1991).

Every individual must perform self-care activities, or have these activities performed on his behalf, to survive. An individual may try to perform alone all the occupations that are needed to function and survive, or some tasks may be shared with others. Satisfactory occupational performance may represent an individual's personal ability to achieve personal care tasks, including the use of adaptive equipment where necessary; or it may be interpreted as the ability to direct or manage others such as a personal care attendant who provides personal care on behalf of the client.

Mastery of self-care activities is only one aspect of a balanced and satisfying life. Self-care activities fulfil primarily physiological, security and to some extent, belonging needs (Maslow, 1970) and are hence only one aspect of a comprehensive and integrated rehabilitation process. These are the aspects that will be examined in this chapter.

Self-care activities are not only just one component of an integrated and balanced rehabilitation programme but also only one component of an integrated and balanced life. Engagement in occupations related to productivity, leisure and socialization (which fulfil needs for belonging, self-esteem and self-actualization) are of no less importance in a rehabilitation programme and these will be examined in Chapter 8.

FUNCTIONAL LEVELS

An understanding of functional levels and their implications is essential in enabling realistic and mutually agreed goals for achieving independence in self-care activities.

It is impossible to state unequivocally what a person with a particular level of spinal cord injury will attain in terms of actual functional ability. From a rehabilitation perspective, the designated neurological level of spinal cord lesion will serve as an indicator of potential function. It cannot be viewed as completely predictive of actual functional achievements.

Function may be affected by many variables, not limited to:

- level of injury
- body build, height, weight, proportion, strength, flexibility
- co-ordination
- kinetic awareness
- intellectual ability
- presence of other injuries
- physical and mental health
- individual differences in muscle innervation
- degree of spinal cord damage
- distribution of sparing, for example, central cord syndrome
- complications such as joint contractures or tendon shortening
- effects of spasticity (may be positive or negative)
- effect of body position on function
- family support
- age
- sex
- motivation
- previous employment and leisure activities
- previous fitness
- physical environment
- social environment
- cultural background and environment.

The emphasis on functional abilities which underlies many attitudes and practices concerning people with disabilities is disproportionate. While this dimension is undeniably important, it does not outweigh considerations of psychological strength or social opportunity in determining an individual's general level of independence.

(Nosek *et al.*, 1987)

IMPLICATIONS OF LEVEL OF INJURY
High-lesion quadriplegia
C1, C2:

- Partial innervation: sternocleidomastoid.
- Able to swallow, talk, chew and blow.
- No motor function below the chin.
- Complete lesions will require use of a respirator to enable breathing.
- Cough is absent.
- Vital capacity = 5–10% of normal (Zejdlik, 1992).
- Independent function of facial muscles enables use of mouthsticks and pneumatic wheelchairs and devices (see Chapter 6).
- Will require a reclining powered wheelchair.
- Patients with C1–C4 lesions will require fulltime attendant care services.

C3:

- Partial innervation: upper trapezius, diaphragm, levator scapulae.
- Motor function: neck control and movements, weak shoulder elevation.
- Breathing may necessitate a respirator.
- Reclining electric wheelchair with head or breath control (see Chapter 6).
- In lesions from C3 to C6, cough is non-functional.
- Vital capacity = 20% of normal (Zejdlik, 1992).

C4:

- Full innervation: diaphragm, trapezius.
- Partial innervation: deltoid.
- Motor function: good shoulder elevation (shrug), respiration (diaphragm). External rotation, protraction, retraction, depression weak.
- Independent respiration.
- Self-feeding possible with mobile arm supports
- Reclining electric wheelchair with head or breath control (see Chapter 6).

Quadriplegia

C5:

- Full innervation: deltoid, rotator cuff muscles, biceps.
- Partial innervation: rhomboids, internal/external rotators, brachialis, supinator.
- Motor function: good shoulder external rotation and protraction, **good elbow flexion**, supination. All other shoulder girdle movements weak.
- Some upper arm mobility.
- Potential for self-feeding and limited self-care activities (e.g. brushing teeth, rolling in bed, combing hair), using hand splints or specially adapted equipment.
- Electric wheelchair with hand control for functional mobility. Potential for lightweight, manual wheelchair with projection hand rims, on level ground.
- Fulltime care attendant probably required.

C6:

- Innervation: wrist extensors, trace triceps, latissimus dorsi, brachioradialis, pronator teres, pectoralis major.
- Motor function: good shoulder function, elbow flexion, **good wrist extension**, pronation. Weak elbow extension, wrist flexion; abduction, extension, flexion and opposition of thumb. Accessory muscles of breathing.
- Finger function absent. Tenodesis grip.
- The potential for independence in self care exists. Independent living will require considerable time and physical effort. Dependent upon all the variables previously delineated, it may be possible to achieve independence in a lightweight, manual wheelchair, transfers, feeding, hygiene, dressing, weight shifts and light household management, although this will only be realized by a few individuals.
- Driving is possible, using hand controls.
- May need part-time care attendant services and/or home helps.

C7:

- Innervation: triceps, wrist flexors, partial finger flexors, extensor digitorum, extensor digiti minimi.
- Motor function: shoulder function – all movements normal

or good; elbow – normal flexion, **good extension**; forearm – normal pronation, good supination; wrist – **good extension**, limited flexion; thumb – good abduction and extension, limited flexion and opposition; fingers – **good extension** and **good metacarpophalangeal flexion**, limited interphalangeal flexion.

- Independence is probable, despite impaired finger dexterity. Independent living will require considerable time and physical energy but is an option for most people at this level of lesion. Lightweight, manual wheelchair.
- The functioning of triceps is found to be a significant determinant for functional independence in self-care tasks. Those people who have triceps as their lowest functional muscle achieve a significantly greater amount of independence in self-care activities than those for whom wrist extensors are the lowest functioning muscle group (Welch *et al.*, 1986).
- In patients with lesions from C7 to T1, cough is non-functional.
- Vital capacity = 30–50% of normal (Zejdlik, 1992).

High-lesion paraplegia

C8:

- Fine hand control.

T1–T2:

- Poor balance (no abdominals).
- T2–T4, cough is weak.
- Vital capacity = 30–50% of normal (Zejdlik, 1992).

T3–T6:

- Increased respiratory function.
- Improved balance.
- Still requires assisted cough.

Paraplegia

T6–T12:

- Abdominals added. Good balance.
- Weak cough (to T10).

- Accessory muscles of respiration added.
- Vital capacity = 75–100% of normal (to T10) (Zejdlik 1992).
- In patients with lesions at T11 and below, cough is normal.
- Normal vital capacity (T11).

T12:

- Thoracic and back muscles added.

L1–L2:

- Hip flexion (aids caliper walking).

L3:

- Probable use of ankle-foot orthoses and sticks (canes).

L4:

- Hamstrings. Ankle foot orthoses.

L5:

- Good knee flexion.

S1, S2:

- Glutei – aid in standing balance.

S2, S3, S4:
- Bladder and bowel control. Sexual function.

CENTRAL CORD SYNDROME

Central cord syndrome is the most common type of incomplete traumatic quadriplegia, characterised by disproportionately more motor impairment of the arms than the legs. This syndrome generally has a good prognosis for neurological and functional improvement during rehabilitation.

Roth *et al.* (1990) found at least 70% of patients with central cord syndrome to be independent in drinking, feeding, dressing, grooming, bathing, bladder and bowel care at discharge. These individuals could also walk 50 m and climb stairs. Although age was one of the most important prognostic indicators, even older people achieved significant functional gains.

Hand function is identified as the last area to regain neurological recovery but long-term problems with pain and fatigue following central cord syndrome are also reported. It is therefore suggested that rehabilitation services for this group should include training in pain management, energy conservation techniques and intervention to alleviate environmental barriers at home and in the workplace.

SELF-CARE SKILLS

This section outlines areas of occupational performance that relate to self-care. It is a guide to some of the options and techniques that may be used by the person with a spinal cord injury and his therapists. This is not an exhaustive list, nor is it intended to be a 'how to' manual, as detailed procedural information is already available in other works.

Particularly recommended are:

- Ford and Duckworth (1987) regarding personal care/ functional mobility (quadriplegia).
- Hill (1986) regarding personal care, community management.
- Somers (1992) especially recommended concerning functional mobility.
- Nixon (1985) regarding functional mobility.
- Bromley (1991) regarding functional mobility.

The clinical skills of the therapist and the resourcefulness of the client may achieve far more creative means of achieving satisfaction with performance of self-care activities.

PERSONAL CARE

C1–C4

All aspects that relate to personal care must be performed on behalf of the person who has a high-lesion spinal cord injury. Many sources write that these people are 'dependent on an assistant' for personal care activities. Physical independence may indeed be implicit with this level of injury but all responsibility for personal care rests with the client himself.

At this level of lesion, the primary goal of intervention is to promote independent thought and restore a sense of control through self-governing behaviour. In the context of personal care, the rehabilitation process should enable the client to seize control over making decisions, solving problems and timing of procedures. The client who has a high-lesion quadriplegia will need to learn how to teach and direct a care giver in all personal care activities, taking responsibility for aspects such as remembering medications or wheelchair maintenance while not relinquishing control over what is worn, where personal items are stored or when skin checks are performed. Independence in personal care activities for the person with a high-lesion quadriplegia will consist of directing others to perform all functions on his behalf. Dependence will only be allowed to occur if the client has all decisions made and problems solved on his behalf. Such dependence is incompatible with the philosophy of rehabilitation (see also Chapter 6).

Pressure relief may be achieved by activating the tilt mechanism of a power wheel chair, if this feature is present.

C5

Acute care

- Self-feeding – in prone if on a Stryker frame, using angled utensil in universal cuff slot and a Futuro wrist splint, or long opponens splint with utensil slot.
- Hygiene and grooming – may brush teeth with brush in utensil cuff.

Long-term self-care

- Self-feeding – using long opponens or Futuro wrist splint, with universal cuff, plate guard, scooper dish, Dycem (non-slip plastic), angled cutlery, insulated cups, cup with a T-handle.
- Hygiene and grooming – may assist with dressing upper body. May use toothbrush in universal cuff, comb in cuff, electric razor with adapted holder. Fisher and Hunter (1992) describe an adapted make-up kit for women with C5 and C6 quadriplegia.

- Voiding – electric leg bag emptier (controlled by small on/off switch).
- Pressure relief – side-to-side leaning, leaning forwards.

C6

Acute care

Personal care management as C5, above.

Long-term self-care using a tenodesis grasp

- Self-feeding – large handle cups (thumb hooks through handle), adapted knife (Quad Quip cutlery, rocker knife or sharp cook's knife, folding, angled knife with serrated edge and built-up handle).
- Hygiene and grooming – shower chair (padded seat) or bath board, handheld shower head for shampooing, pump soaps, shampoos, toothpaste; long-handled brush, washing mitt, bath hoist, nail brush with suction cups, suction denture brush, make-up (see C5 above).
- Voiding – emptying leg bag (may have adapted valve release), inflatable or padded toilet seat, suppository inserter and/or adapted digital stimulator. May be able to perform self-catheterisations, apply condom and leg bag.
- Menstrual care – sanitary pads do not require good hand function.
- Dressing – loops on clothes. Will probably avoid clothes with buttons, or shirts which must be tucked into trousers. Dressing lower half in bed (if this is possible for the individual). Greater stability for dressing top half in a chair. Button hooks, Velcro fasteners, zipper pulls or rings. Long-handled shoe horn, shoes with Velcro or zip fasteners. Shoes may be worn up to one size larger to reduce pressure. Method chosen to dress will depend upon individual ability and choice. Women may choose to wear a stretch brassière that does not need to be fastened. Alternatively, back-fastening (done up at the front and turned) or front-fastening brassières may be manageable for some women, if it has a loop at the fastener edge to provide enhanced grip and leverage.

- Pressure relief – independent turning in bed. Independent weight shifts in chair, leaning from side to side, leaning forwards with side rotation, pushing up with elbows on armrests.
- Skin inspection – using a mirror (may have an adapted handle).

Much of the adapted equipment will be discarded as the client becomes more adept at using a functional grasp, hence clients may wish to borrow equipment in the early stages rather than spend considerable sums on items that will not have long-term use.

C7

Acute care

Personal care management as C5, above.

Long-term self-care

- Feeding – independent.
- Hygiene and grooming – independent. (Shower chair with padded seat, or bath board).
- Voiding – independent self-catheterisations, application of condom and leg bag. Suppository inserter and/or adapted digital stimulator. Inflatable or padded toilet seat.
- Menstrual care – may be able to insert tampon (adapted applicators are available).
- Dressing – independent. May use button hook.
- Pressure relief – independent weight shifts to relieve pressure.

Any of the equipment listed under C6 may also be useful for people with C7 lesions, especially in the early stages of rehabilitation.

Below C7

Independent in all personal care activities in a friendly environment.

C8–T6

Advisable to use inflatable or padded toilet seat and shower chair seat.

Tenodesis and dynamic splinting (C6/C7 quadriplegia)

The natural action of tenodesis was outlined in Chapter 4, i.e. when the wrist is extended, the fingers will flex. Encouragement of the tenodesis mechanics of the hand (by strengthening wrist extensors, maintaining web space and allowing finger flexors to shorten) enables someone with C6 quadriplegia to achieve considerable physical independence. People with C6 lesions have demonstrated the ability to transfer (using wrist extension), dress, (by hooking the flexed fingers through loops on clothing and footwear), hold cutlery and cups, drive and do light housekeeping tasks, all using a tenodesis grip.

Previous attempts to enhance the function of the C6 quadriplegic hand by dynamic splinting have met with limited results. An electrically powered prehension orthosis, for example, was designed to provide a grip for people with C5 lesions. This has generally proved incompatible with an active lifestyle, is prone to breakdown and does not enable participation in activities not possible by other means.

The flexor hinge splint provides the C6 hand with a strong grip but prohibits self-propulsion of a manual wheelchair. The Rehabilitation Institute of Chicago tenodesis splint may be used to enhance a weak prehension grip and has the advantage of being made to measure, on site by the occupational therapist and hence is easily adjustable. This is used primarily during tenodesis training.

Several studies have examined the use of dynamic splints following discharge and have reported contradictory findings.

Lee (1988) reported that 55% of people with C6 spinal cord lesions discarded their flexor hinge splints following discharge. The primary reason given was that subjects found they were able to achieve activities in other ways. Lee concludes that patients should be encouraged to maximize their use of the splints but this appears difficult to justify if they are able to perform activities to their satisfaction without having to rely upon orthotic intervention.

Similarly, Shepherd and Ruzicka (1991) report that 47% of those people with C6 lesions discarded their wrist-driven tenodesis splints after discharge. The common reason cited was the use of a natural tenodesis action of the hand to perform activities. However, Krajnik and Bridle (1992) found that 69% of people with C6 lesions continued to use their dynamic splints for at least some activities. Reports indicate that the activities for which dynamic splints are most useful are for writing, drawing and picking up heavy objects. Hence they may be indicated for students and for those whose employment or productive occupation necessitates certain fine movements of the hands.

A clearer understanding of the individual client's goals, interests, occupations and requirements for community living will provide the optimal protocol for provision of dynamic hand splints.

Upper limb reconstruction

The past two decades have seen a dramatic increase in the number of people with cervical cord lesions who survive the initial trauma and acute care to proceed through rehabilitation programmes.

There has been a subsequent increased interest in improving the function of the upper limb for people with quadriplegia below C5. In accordance with these goals an international group of surgeons are pursuing expertise in the reconstructive surgery of the quadriplegic arm and hand.

Active elbow extension may be restored using transfer of the posterior third of the deltoid muscle into the triceps tendon. Restoration of active finger flexion, thumb pinch and the functions of grasp and release have also been developed and documented, using transfers of extensor carpi radialis longus and brachioradialis (Lamb, 1992; Grundy and Swain, 1993).

Subjects are very carefully selected and surgery is not initiated until at least a year after injury. One of the drawbacks is the considerable period of limb immobilization following surgery. Patients are restricted from doing push ups, transfers, wheelchair mobility and heavy exercise for many weeks after tendon operations.

Patient selection will be dependent upon such aspects as age, occupation, choice of activities and goals, absence of spasticity, muscle grade, adequate hand sensation and a neurological level below C5. The patient is encouraged **not** to expect too much.

The absence of a standardized system for evaluation of upper limb function (with particular reference to the quadriplegic hand) has been problematic in relation to accurate documentation of outcome. Hence video recording before and after surgery has been suggested as probably the best way of assessing upper limb function for each individual (Lamb, 1992). This is also a useful means of showing prospective patients what can realistically be expected from surgical intervention of this nature.

Although it has been suggested that tendon transfers for people with quadriplegia represent small gains for big investments, Lamb (1992) indicates that: 'good results from surgery will depend very much upon the stimulation and encouragement which the patient receives after tendon transfers from an enthusiastic and skilful therapist'.

Surgeons working in this highly specialized field must build up considerable experience and expertise. Occupational therapists working as part of the surgical team must carefully research current knowledge in this area and likewise develop appropriate expertise. The rehabilitation period after surgery is crucial to the final outcome and the specialized, postoperative, occupational therapy management of the quadriplegic upper limb is documented by Trombly (1983), Ainsley *et al.* (1985), Johnstone *et al.* (1988) and Vanden Berghe *et al.* (1991).

Although surgical reconstruction of the quadriplegic upper limb does not restore 'normal' functioning, reports document successful outcomes and the very considerable role that skilful occupational therapy has to play in ensuring adequate education, correct post-surgical management and optimal performance of activities.

Wheelchair cushions

Pressure relief is a key aspect of personal care for the person who has a spinal cord injury. Selection and correct use of a wheelchair cushion is one of the single most important factors in the prevention of pressure sores. No one cushion is optimal for all people with spinal cord injuries. Selection will depend upon client needs and preferences, objective measurements and clinical judgements.

The aim is to select a cushion that will distribute pressure over the widest possible area. Weight distributed over a greater area will result in less propensity to skin breakdown and pressure sore formation. Choice of cushion will depend upon the individual's ability to relieve pressure, his muscle tone, sitting balance and stability and his degree of physical independence.

Many types of cushions are commercially available, including air-inflatable cushions, foam cushions and those filled with gel, foam or water. Three cushions will be outlined below: the ROHO, Jay and Ulti-mate. Although these have been used with great success by numbers of people with spinal cord injuries, this does not imply that other cushions are not appropriate or suitable for excellent pressure relief in certain individuals.

Cushions will need to be re-evaluated periodically not only to assess the condition and functioning of the cushion but also to determine whether it continues to meet the needs of the client. Changes in body build or activity level, for example, may necessitate a different choice of cushion.

The combined weight of the hands and arms constitute 10% of bodyweight, hence use of armrests will result in a significant reduction in seating force on the buttocks.

ROHO

The ROHO cushion consists of individual, interconnected air cells to allow distribution of bodyweight and to relieve peak pressures on the bony prominances. The high-profile cushion (10 cm high cells) is the design most commonly used by people with spinal cord injuries. Studies have found, in comparison with other cushions, that the high-profile ROHO cushion provides the greatest pressure reduction in the majority of subjects, carrying a larger percentage of total bodyweight and a more anterior centre of mass than other cushions. It has been found to produce the lowest incidence of skin breakdown per year. Nevertheless, this does not make it the cushion of choice for every individual's needs and lifestyle (Garber, 1985; Gilsdorf *et al.*, 1991; Garber and Dyerly, 1991; Tough and Chandler, 1992).

Individual cells may be tied off, if desired, or a customized cushion can be made to suit special situations. Dual manifolds may be used to adjust pressure distribution. The ROHO's inherent lack of stability is a problem for active individuals with paraplegia who may also find it difficult to transfer on and off the cushion. However, this is not usually a problem for those with high lesions and it is most commonly recommended for people with lesions above C6.

The ROHO Enhancer cushion increases lateral support and pelvic stability because of the dual manifold and three heights of air cells (5, 7.5 and 10 cm) arranged to ensure correct leg and pelvic position (Figure 5.1). Overinflation of the ROHO cushion will increase seated instability.

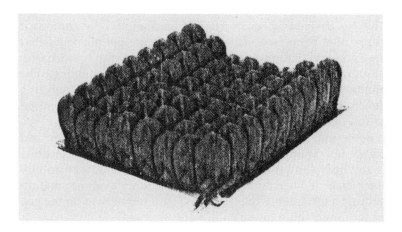

Figure 5.1   ROHO Enhancer.

The ROHO does not absorb moisture, is washable, does not promote perspiration in most individuals and allows for extended periods of sitting. It reduces shear forces and allows for some skin ventilation, as the air cells move with the user. Allergies to the ROHO's rubber have been reported and would preclude use of the cushion for these individuals. The ROHO cushion must be checked on a daily basis to ensure adequate inflation. Although the individual cell structure and material of the ROHO offer some support even when underinflated, overinflation is found to be less dangerous than underinflation. Care must be taken to ensure that internal air pressure is at an optimal level to provide the minimum of interface pressure.

Air pressures change at different altitudes so daily adjustments will need to be made if the individual is travelling between areas of differing height above sea level.

The ROHO may be damaged by smokers who drop hot ash or cigarette butts on to the rubber. Similarly, those who use narrow chairs without armrests may damage the cushion by allowing it to rub on the wheels of the chair.

Responsibility for cushion use, inflation and placement rests with the person with a spinal cord injury. He must direct others to perform these tasks if unable to do so himself.

Jay

The Jay cushion is constructed of an anatomically contoured supportive foam base, covered with Flolite gel-filled pouches and a cover. The moulded urethane foam base is washable, encourages pelvic stability and optimal leg positioning. The Flolite pad conforms to the shape of the individual, reducing effects of shear and friction. The Jay cushion may be customised to suit individual needs.

Some individuals report problems with transferring on and off the Jay cushion because of its contoured shape. The cushion is also heavy and some people find it hard to move it on and off their chair. If a narrow chair is used, the individual may end up sitting on the sides of the contoured base rather than on the gel, hence diminishing the cushion's effectiveness.

The Jay does not require daily adjustments although regular kneading of the Flolite pad is recommended to prevent gel from thickening at the edge of the pad. The Flolite pad requires periodic replacement and regular assessment to ensure that pooling of the gel is not decreasing coverage under bony prominances. Care should be taken to ensure that a bony or thin person does not 'bottom out'. An overfilled pad may be used in such instances.

Some individuals have reported allergies to the Flolite cushion and some people find perspiration to be a problem, caused by lack of skin ventilation. The vented 'air exchange' cover may help to alleviate problems associated with sweating. There have been reports of gel cushions freezing and creating sores from frostbite.

Jay also produce an 'active' cushion which is lighter, easier to move during transfers, has a softer, less contoured base and a smaller gel pad which does not extend under the thighs. It is suitable for some active individuals who can perform regular, independent weight shifts but does not provide the postural support required by many individuals with spinal cord injuries.

The Jay Protector consists of a small, lightweight Flolite pad in a waterproof cover, on a moulded foam base. This is suitable for short periods of sitting, for example in baths, in vehicles, during recreational activities or for sitting on the floor. The addition of a sling attachment allows the user to perform transfers with both arms while the cushion remains strapped in place. It should be emphasised that this does not replace a regular wheelchair cushion but provides short-term protection when the user leaves his wheelchair.

Jay also produce an excellent modular back support (Figure 5.2). Adjustable lumbar and lateral supports allow for control of posture and stability while a Flolite spinal insert provides pressure protection for bony protrusions. The height is adjustable and it may be tilted.

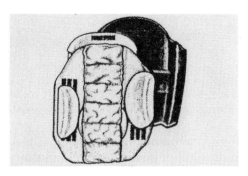

Figure 5.2 Jay back support.

Ulti-mate

The Ulti-mate cushion is a recent innovation from Canada, which is cheaper than either the ROHO or Jay cushions yet provides excellent pressure distribution. Early tests indicate a distribution of pressure comparable with that of the Jay cushion (Pyc, 1990).

The Ulti-mate is a composite cushion with a polyurethane foam base, 'pre-stressed high-resilient foam ischial relief insert', a middle layer of slow moulding visco-elastic foam and a fire-retardant, high-resilient, polyurethane foam top layer. The Ulti-mate is anatomically designed, conforming to the user and producing even pressure distribution. Leg channels promote correct leg positioning and enhance stability. A waterproof, fire-resistant neoprene rubber protects the foams. The outer cover is designed to draw moisture from the surface, reducing the effects of heat and humidity.

Weighing less than 1.4 kg, the Ulti-mate is portable and easy to manoeuvre. Early reports comment favourably on the enhanced stability provided by this cushion and its low maintenance.

Sumed bath cushion

The Sumed bath cushion provides excellent pressure relief while sitting in the bath or on shower chairs or bath hoists. Heavier than water, the cushion sits in the bottom of the bath or can be secured using suction cups.

Mattresses

ROHO produce a mattress that provides excellent pressure relief for those most at risk or who are healing existing pressure sores.

The Stanmore Vaperm mattress is a composite foam system, which will reduce the incidence of pressure sores, providing accepted nursing practices are followed (Scales *et al.*, 1982). The Vaperm mattress is waterproof yet water-vapour permeable and conforms to strict fire requirements. The design of the mattress improves load distribution, providing greater pressure relief on high-risk areas. The Vaperm mattress may be used on an adjustable hospital-bed frame in place of traditional mattresses. It is easy for the individual to turn or be turned on this mattress.

Many individuals wish to sleep in a conventional double bed with their partner. It is imperative that the enthusiasm of the rehabilitation team does not lead to provision of a bed system that does not allow for this desire to be respected or considered. The Vaperm mattress, for example, is manufactured in double-bed sizes. Use of a synthetic sheepskin on one side of a double bed will allow a practical and convenient method of enhancing pressure distribution for the person who has a spinal cord injury. The sheepskin should be the full length of the bed.

The synthetic sheepskin will help to reduce friction and shearing forces, eliminate wrinkles (a problem with sheets), dissipate heat and absorb moisture. It should be laundered regularly but not at high heat or with a harsh detergent, as this causes hardening. If matting or hardening does occur, the sheepskin must be replaced.

If the spinal cord injured person needs to spend prolonged periods in bed, has a fever, infection or is malnourished, an alternating air pressure mattress, air flotation mattress, water mattress or gel pad should be considered. Individual responses vary to these mattresses – some find the plastic covers exacerbate sweating even when covered with a flannelette sheet, hence increasing the risk of skin breakdown. People with quadriplegia have complained that water mattresses make them feel cold. Unless the room is very warm, poikilothermic individuals may indeed experience a lowered body temperature on these devices. Care should be taken to ensure that a special mattress enhances both patient comfort and enhanced pressure distribution, although not intruding on his personal life!

Long-term engagement in personal care activities

During the rehabilitation process, considerable time is devoted to retraining in personal care activities, particularly for people with quadriplegia. Few studies have examined whether these activities continue to be performed once the client has returned home. Functional skills which are acquired in a hospital or rehabilitation centre are practiced in an accommodating environment. Following discharge, the person with a recent spinal cord injury will return to a living environment which either enables or restricts occupational performance.

In a study designed to assess the extent that personal care skills learned during rehabilitation are used at 1–4 years after discharge, Rogers and Figone (1980) found that people with C6 or C7 quadriplegia improved their transfer skills and some subjects improved their skills in independent toileting and bathing. In contrast, the group as a whole regressed in grooming, dressing, toileting and bathing skills. The authors suggest that, as community living has daily requirements that are different from those while hospitalized, it is likely that some of the changes represent a reordering of time and energy based on personal priorities.

In a study of engagement in daily occupations among people with spinal cord injuries, Yerxa and Baum (1986) found that people with spinal cord injuries (73% of whom had quadriplegia) spent less time in self-maintenance than did non-disabled subjects. Further study (Yerxa and Locker, 1990) indicated that people with spinal cord injuries (predominantly with quadriplegia) spent significantly less time on self-care activities than did a non-disabled group, probably because other people provided assistance. This contradicts the common assumption that people with disabilities will automatically spend more time in self-care and less in other occupations.

Weingarden and Martin (1989) found that none of their sample of people with C6 quadriplegia dressed themselves routinely at home, despite being able to do so. The reason given for no longer dressing independently was that it took too much time and/or energy. This calls into question the current use of functional assessment tools which rate dressing in under one hour as 'functional' and raises some further issues. As 'successful outcome' following rehabilitation programmes is often measured by the improvement in physical independence attained by clients, it must be questioned to whose benefit these goals are being sought.

Secondly, it is clear that a 'functional' skill must be accomplished within the individual's concept of an appropriate time and/or energy framework to be actually considered functional. Thirdly, there are implications for mutual goal setting. Complete independence in dressing may not be the ultimate goal for people with C6 quadriplegia, if the time and effort entailed interferes with more important goals such as education or other productive occupations. Successful outcome and independence in self-care activities are not necessarily synonymous.

In the light of these studies it is suggested that the rehabilitation process should not only be prepared to teach the skills to enable independence in personal care activities but also be able to prepare people with severe and chronic disabilities to be effective managers of their time and resources. Therapists have placed great emphasis upon the achievement of independence in personal care activities, yet it would appear that people with spinal cord injuries may choose to expend their time and energy in more rewarding pursuits (Yerxa and Locker, 1990). Considerable time and effort during the rehabilitation of people with quadriplegia has been directed towards self-care skills. Indeed, this single component of occupational performance has received a disproportionate amount of attention, frequently to the exclusion of activities related to productivity and leisure. The need to correlate the therapist's objectives with the needs and goals of the client, viewed in the context of his unique sociocultural environment, are especially evident in the light of these studies.

To date, those individuals who have struggled defiantly to perform every self-care task alone have scored highly on functional assessment measures but may have achieved lives of little value or satisfaction. In the future, measures of outcome and of functional abilities should consider appropriate use of assistance and time; and the client's satisfaction with performance.

However, the importance of personal care skills cannot be overlooked. For some people with quadriplegia who wish to live in complete physical independence, personal care skills will be a primary goal during rehabilitation and every effort must be made to try to match the client's abilities with equipment and techniques to achieve this goal.

Other clients may have a different living environment in physical, social, cultural and economic terms. They may prefer to live in a state of interdependence, sharing tasks with others and using their time and energies for goals related to other occupations. Hence therapists must not impose their own interpretations of the client's problems but must seek to understand the life situation of the client, his goals and objectives and tailor intervention towards attaining those goals.

Unfortunately, therapy programmes are more frequently directed towards the physical state of the client than towards his life, and towards self-care activities to the exclusion of other occupations. The wife of a company director made the following comments concerning her husband's therapy programme.

At the Spinal Centre they don't pay enough attention to your mental state. The therapist has you sitting naked on a bed, struggling for half an hour to put your sock on. I was afraid he'd think, 'If this is what life is going to be like – I don't want it'. They thought at the Spinal Centre that the important thing was to be able to transfer. He still can't – but it doesn't matter. He's happy and I'm happy. There are more important things.
(in Hammell, 1991)

It is clear that, in this instance, physical independence in self-care skills was not a priority for either the client or his wife and attention could more usefully have been directed towards attainment of goals which were personally meaningful in the context of their lives and lifestyle. The fact that the client never did learn to transfer independently represents considerable time and effort wasted during rehabilitation and a consequent lost opportunity for pursuing objectives congruent with the client's own goals. Accountability to both client and funding agency is also in question.

Therapists have tended to view personal care assistance as providing the client with help for tasks he cannot do alone. Many clients prefer to view these services in terms of the additional activities it enables them to do. Independence does not exclude making appropriate use of assistance when required or desired.

Outcome measurement of self-care

Evaluation of rehabilitation outcome has spawned many tools for the measurement of activities related to personal care, mobility and instrumental activities of daily living. However, several serious drawbacks have been noted with regard to these outcome measures. These have been outlined by the Canadian Association of Occupational Therapists (1991) and include the following points.

1. Most tools measure functional ability in self-care as opposed to performance.
2. No tools measure performance in self-care activities such as meal preparation and laundry in terms of the client's environment or role requirements.

Future research will necessitate the development of outcome measurement tools which measure performance as opposed to ability; and measure performance in relation to environment, motivation and role requirements.

FUNCTIONAL MOBILITY

Functional mobility is a self-care skill which relates to movement of the body. In the context of spinal cord injury this will be examined in terms of balance, transfers, wheelchair skills and gait training.

Functional mobility training focuses upon improving and maximizing balance, strength, co-ordination and compensatory movements in preparation for other activities and to allow the maintenance of optimal sitting posture. Individual abilities depend upon many variables. A general guide to functional mobility training and expectations is outlined below.

- C1–C4: functional mobility is discussed in Chapter 6.
- C4: head and neck balance, using head control to maintain sitting posture. Learning to avert the head for protection in case of falls. Tilt table used for standing.
- C5: long and short sitting balance (with support). Assisted rolling. May be able to assist with transfers, using a board. Sitting posture with arms palm down on lap to counteract unopposed supination. Passive range of motion at elbow is especially important. Strong elbow flexors and absent extensors present high risk of contractures and loss of function. May be able to propel an ultralight wheelchair with projection hand rims on a level surface. Functional mobility however, will require a powered wheelchair.
- C6: muscle strengthening. Long and short sitting balance; rolling. Transfers, using a transfer board, in same plane, i.e. chair to bed, chair to chair. Changing planes, lying to sitting, sitting to lying. Moving forwards and backwards on mat. Independent in ultralight wheelchair. Able to propel up gentle slopes.
- C7: as above, plus independent transfers may be possible for most individuals, chair to toilet, chair to chair, bed to chair.
- C8: independent transfers chair to bath. Wheelchair independent, although kerbs may present a problem.

- T1–T5: back-wheel balancing, ('popping wheelies'), in wheelchair. Pulling wheelchair into vehicle. Potential use of the Reciprocating Gait Orthosis (RGO). Chair to floor, floor to chair transfers.
- T6–T8: knee–ankle–foot orthoses (KAFOs) for walking short distances on level surfaces.
- T9–L3: KAFOs, gait pattern will vary according to individual abilities (becoming more of a functional option).
- L4–L5: ankle–foot orthoses (AFOs), for functional gait.

Transfers

Transfer training is a problem-solving activity for the therapist and client. No single transfer will suit the physical abilities of every client or their unique needs. Research and experimentation of the many methods available will enable an appropriate and safe choice of transfer to be made.

Many individuals choose to use a transfer board. Several designs are available, the straight board being commonly used. However, as it is more usual to perform a transfer which involves moving through an angle rather than in parallel, a curved board was designed to enable the client to remain in contact with more of the board throughout more of the transfer. Figure 5.3 shows the Oxbow transfer board. The tail of the S is positioned under the client and the opposite tail is pointed towards the direction of movement, i.e. to the right in the figure. The board's design allows for easier positioning under the hip, it clears the large wheel of the wheelchair and provides support for a lateral transfer.

A general guide to transfer expectations was outlined above. In addition, the person with high-lesion quadriplegia must demonstrate the ability to direct safe transfers. This includes use of a mechanical lift such as the Arjo Dextra as well as a manual transfer.

A one-man pivot transfer can be performed with attention to the comfort and safety of the client, the safety and good body mechanics of the attendant. Importantly, it is not possible to drop the client if this manoeuvre is performed correctly. Further, his arms are tucked in and not vulnerable to trauma. To transfer from chair to bed, or chair to chair, moving to the **client's** right, the procedure is as follows.

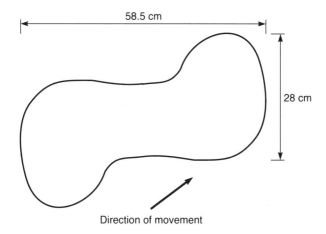

Figure 5.3 Oxbow transfer board.

1. Position the wheelchair beside the bed.
2. Remove the right armrest of the wheelchair and both legrests.
3. The client's buttocks are shifted forwards in the chair (if necessary) so that his feet rest on the floor (or on a low wooden block).
4. The client's arms are flexed so that, as he bends forwards, they lie across his lap, elbows on thighs.
5. He is leaned forwards, his head and shoulders bent to the right of the attendant, i.e. to the client's left.
6. The attendant places her feet in front and a little to the sides of the client's feet. She bends her knees and grasps one hand under each side of the client's chest wall (not axillae), buttocks or transfer belt (whichever position provides the greatest mechanical advantage relative to their body builds).
7. By rocking the client forwards while simultaneously extending her own knees, the client is rocked forwards, rotated to the left and lowered in one smooth movement. The attendant has not lifted the client, twisted or extended her back but has used good body mechanics and quadriceps musculature to complete the manoeuvre.

This transfer is especially useful for a tall client or one for whom spasticity makes a standing transfer dangerous for himself or his care attendant. A transfer disc may also be used for this transfer.

Lateral transfers (with a transfer board for people with quadriplegia and without a board for people with paraplegia) are the most usual choices. The client and therapist together will devise the most appropriate method for getting from chair to/from chair, bed, bath, toilet, car and floor. The most important factors to consider concern protecting the skin from friction and trauma (for example in lifting over, or around the large wheel of the chair) and the unique home and work environments that the client will most commonly encounter. It is sobering to consider, for example, that some indigenous people in countries such as Canada and South Africa have been taught bath transfers when no such facilities exist in their home communities. Transfers, as all treatment interventions, must be appropriate to the life of the individual and his environment.

Wheelchair skills

Achievement of wheelchair skills will be dependent upon good posture. This is as relevant for the client who will operate a powered chair as for the person who propels a manual chair.

Pressure is distributed over a larger area if the footrests are adjusted to the height that allows the thighs to be completely supported. This also allows drainage into a leg bag, if one is worn. Most clients find that maintenance of the hips, knees and ankles at 90° provides the greatest comfort, stability, pressure relief and the least spasticity. However, the optimal position for each client will be determined in collaboration with his therapists. Each client will need to determine the preferred balance between stability and mobility. For example, a wheelchair with a high back provides more stability and trunk support but allows for reduced mobility, as the user cannot reach as far back on the wheels. However, the backrest should be of sufficient height to avoid kyphotic posture and significant long-term disability.

All wheelchair users will need to master the basic skills of wheelchair propulsion, applying and releasing the brakes, making forward and backward turns, negotiating doorways and manoeuvring into awkward places such as lifts. Some safe method must be devised for picking up items from the floor. Additionally, the individual must be able to operate the release mechanism for the legrests and also be able to remove the armrests.

More advanced skills will include the safe operation of the wheelchair over rough terrain, up and down kerbs, up and down ramps and righting the chair and the user in the event of a spill. This latter will be a particularly important skill to master if the person is engaging in basketball or other similar sporting activities. The 'wheelie' has been described as the cornerstone of advanced wheelchair skills (Nixon, 1985). The ability to balance the wheelchair on the back wheel is integral to the ability to negotiate kerbs and rough ground. Some intrepid wheelchair users are confident in negotiating stairs by 'popping a wheelie' and using the stair handrail. Considerable practice is required to assume and maintain a 'wheelie', during which the therapist should ensure safety, as there is an inherent danger of falling backwards.

Choice of wheelchair

There appears to be consensus among clinicians that people with cervical lesions (of C5/6 and below) will achieve the greatest potential for mobility if using an ultralight manual wheelchair. However, in view of the future decades of active wheelchair use which face all people with recent spinal cord injuries it is difficult to make a convincing argument for anything other than an ultralight wheelchair for all people with spinal cord injuries. The considerable upper extremity musculoskeletal problems experienced by people with long-term spinal cord injuries are documented below ('chronic overuse syndromes'). Clinical experience and anecdotal evidence point to time lost from employment, costly physiotherapy treatments and reduced function among those who seek to maintain an active lifestyle from a wheelchair that weighs approximately 20 kg, is difficult to balance, to manoeuvre and to self-propel.

During a recent investigation in England into the social situation of people following spinal cord injuries (Hammell, 1991) the author enquired about the type of wheelchair used by each individual. Although the sample size was small ($n = 15$) the results provide an interesting snapshot of the situation. Of the men with spinal cord injuries (mean age at injury = 37), 93% had purchased their own ultralight wheelchair (predominantly the Quickie) although one man stated that he still used his government-issue wheelchair 'for a really good work out once a day'. The sole subject who used his government-issue wheelchair exclusively, indicated that he leaves his house only three or four times a year.

Major (1990) outlines some of the factors that affect the choice of a wheelchair. These include:

- weight
- straight line control
- stability
- posture control
- energy cost
- durability
- cost
- cosmesis
- comfort
- braking efficiency
- back-wheel balancing facility.

The new, ultra-lightweight wheelchair designs allow the wheelchair to be customized to suit the needs of the individual client. Further, the chair may be modified to suit the needs of various situations. Changing the geometry of the wheelchair by moving the castors, altering the camber and position of the rear wheels, and the angle of the seat in relation to the ground will all affect the overall performance of the chair. It is therefore important that those therapists who are involved with their spinal cord injured clients in wheelchair selection are aware of the design components and their impact upon performance, comfort, stability and balance. It must also be recognised that very low chairbacks contribute to significant spinal deformity and disability. Sling seats are not appropriate and do not provide an adequate base for a wheelchair cushion to function properly.

The ultra-light, high-performance wheelchairs have proved rugged enough for the abuse sustained during sporting activities as well as the rigors of every day living (Figure 5.4).

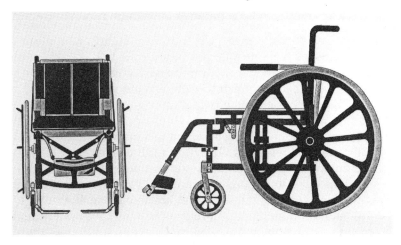

Figure 5.4 Ultra-light wheelchair (Quickie; see also Figures 6.11a and b).

However, it should be cautioned that not all 'ultra-light' chairs are created equally and a racy design does not necessarily equate with enhanced performance and decreased energy costs.

Barnard (1991) reported finding substantially lower energy costs in propelling an ultra-light wheelchair (the Quickie) in comparison to those chairs routinely issued by the National Health Service (NHS) in the UK. The energy cost to healthy, able-bodied subjects of propelling a Quickie (without individual customizing or modification) was 31% lower than that of the NHS chair, which was set to optimal standards.

This raises some important issues. The usual age at spinal cord injury is about 19 years. The life expectancy of people with spinal cord injuries – particulary those with paraplegia, is thought to be close to that of non-disabled people. Hence it may be expected that someone with a recent spinal cord injury will use his wheelchair as a primary means of mobility for five or six decades.

In an era when ultra-light wheelchairs are available for a cost which is not inordinately greater than for a heavier, clumsier chair, the rationale for providing the latter appears flawed.

An ultra-light wheelchair may be customized to ensure comfort, decreases the energy costs involved in propulsion, has enhanced manoeuvrability, stability, straight line control and balance. Most importantly, it provides for greater **functional** mobility, conserving energy for engagement in more meaningful activities than moving the body from A to B, and providing enhanced access to community and recreational resources compared to a chair of greater weight and less manoeuvrability.

Mobility is a basic human right, currently denied to an estimated 20 million people around the world. In developing countries, attention is focusing upon making wheelchairs from locally available materials. The need for a comfortable, affordable, durable, high-performance yet lightweight chair is especially important in regions where there are few roads and no ramps or pavements. Chairs must be effective in both rough urban and rural conditions. Developed nations have been accustomed to sending their discarded chairs to developing countries yet these chairs have proved to be totally inappropriate due to their undue weight, 'standard' size, inherent lack of mobility and the scarcity and cost of spare parts. In response, Hof *et al.* (1993) have developed the Whirlwind wheelchair which can be manufactured in developing countries to meet local needs and which can also be repaired locally.

In the UK, Fyfe and Wood (1990) report: 'The low tetraplegic [quadriplegic] requires a chair of such construction as to reduce to the absolute minimum the force necessary to initiate and maintain forward motion, and finely balanced to facilitate negotiation of irregular surfaces.' This must surely be the requirement of all people with disabilities who rely upon a wheelchair for their functional mobility. Therapists must work with their clients to ensure that the optimal wheelchair is provided for every individual, advocating for changes in policies where these are required.

Pushing mitts

Trauma to the hands while propelling a wheelchair can be greatly reduced by the use of pushing mitts. These may be commercially manufactured from heavy-duty suede leather with the addition of Dycem palms for extra traction. Alternatively, mitts can be made to measure or adapted from industrial gloves such as those used in the logging industry. Some people find the type of fingerless gloves used by cyclists to be satisfactory. These have reinforced palms, Velcro closures and have the advantage of being comparatively cheap and easily obtainable. However, this design may be more difficult to don and doff for people with limited hand function.

Gait training and ambulation

Few aspects of the rehabilitation programme are as controversial as that of upright ambulation following spinal cord injury.

Many people with spinal cord injuries have the physical potential to achieve upright mobility, using orthoses (calipers) and crutches, sticks (canes) or walking frames (walkers). Hence many physiotherapy programmes have included intensive, expensive training to meet this goal. Indeed many private clinics have been developed (especially in the USA) to cash in on the desire of people who wish to achieve upright mobility.

However, research and experience have shown that most people will opt for wheelchair mobility following discharge to the community, as this provides a more practical, faster means of mobility, with less energy expenditure. Further, many individuals recognize that upright mobility using orthoses and crutches does not equate to their originally stated goal of 'walking'. Many professionals question whether considerable time, energy and money is usefully spent on acquiring a skill that is unlikely to be used in the long term. Others believe that, as some people do not give up ambulation using extensive equipment, all people with spinal cord injuries should be given the chance to try this form of mobility. Wheelchair mobility then becomes a matter of personal choice, representing independent and convenient mobility, rather than symbolizing disability (Somers, 1992). Somers suggests that some individuals may attain psychological benefit from gait training even if they ultimately choose to use a wheelchair. Until given the opportunity to try ambulation and to experience how difficult it is, some people may be left with the feeling that they could have succeeded if only they had been allowed to try.

Controversy is at least as keen among people with spinal cord injuries. For example, Oliver (1993), a professor of disability studies (who also has a spinal cord injury), describes walking as being more than a physical activity but one that has cultural symbolism. He cites the example of charities who spend a great

deal of money in pursuit of cures for 'non-walking'. 'The problem is, of course, that throughout the history of human kind,
the number of cures which have been found to these "chronic
and crippling diseases" could be counted on the fingers of one
hand and still leave some over to eat your dinner with'. Oliver
sees the rehabilitation process as the exercise of power by one
group over another and that 'the exercise of power involves the
identification and pursuit of goals chosen by the powerful and
these goals are shaped by the ideology of normality'.

This theory sees the rehabilitation industry as being focused
upon assisting the individual to become 'as normal as possible' –
largely by trying desperately to walk.

> In terms set by the rehabilitation enterprise . . . non walking
> can be tolerated when individuals are prepared to undergo
> rehabilitation to nearly walk or to come to terms with their
> non-walking. Not walking, or rejecting nearly-walking as a
> personal choice . . . exposes the ideology of normality and it
> challenges the whole rehabilitation enterprise.
>
> (Oliver, 1993)

However, the quest for 'nearly walking' is not, as Oliver
would seem to suggest, limited to rehabilitation professionals
and researchers. Many people who have sustained spinal cord
injuries vehemently reject the medical pronouncement that they
will never walk again and are prepared to find their own therapists, to spend substantial sums of their own and others' money
and gruelling six-hour daily schedules of exercises in an attempt
to achieve upright mobility. Although this is clearly an individual choice, it is unfortunate that much of the publicity and
fund-raising material that emanates from these projects conveys
the impression that everyone with a spinal cord injury could
walk if they only tried hard enough, and further, that 'normal'
walking is a realistic and achievable goal. Although it may be
worthwhile to some people to spend all their time and energy in
physical exercise to mobilize slowly on sticks, splints and
walkers, this is not everyone's primary goal.

There is no clear answer to a debate that has some people with
spinal cord injuries arguing that 'walking' is an agenda established by professionals to restore 'near normality', whereas
others, similarly injured, argue as vehemently that not enabling
upright ambulation is part of an unjustified medical conspiracy.

Somers (1992) proposes that any spinal cord injured person who wishes to attempt ambulation should be given the opportunity to do so – if possible postponing the purchase by the individual of expensive orthoses until the potential and desire for functional ambulation have been demonstrated. There can be few more clear examples of the need to correlate the therapist's interventions with the goals and aspirations of the individual client.

Many centres advocate regular standing as a means of preventing contractures, reducing spasticity, aiding renal function and stimulating circulation (Bromley, 1991). Debate has also centred upon whether standing minimises the development of osteoporosis and subsequent risk of long-bone fractures among people with spinal cord injuries but this remains undetermined. Standing may be achieved using a tilt table for people with higher lesions, a standing frame or parallel bars for people with lower lesions.

There is general agreement upon the need for active hip flexors (i.e. a lesion below L1/L2) before walking with orthoses can be considered to be 'functional'. However, despite evidence that even those individuals who have active hip flexion will generally use a wheelchair for mobility to gain greater speed for less energy expenditure, many patients will go to considerable lengths to find a facility where someone will agree to brace them (Nixon, 1985).

Gait expectations at different levels of complete injury may be broadly outlined as follows.

- T1–T5: walking in parallel bars using a swing to gait. Potential for using a rollator and KAFOs but this will be solely for exercise and self-esteem and not for functional mobility.
- T6–T8: potential for walking short distances on level surface using rollator and KAFOs.
- T9–T12: potential for walking on level surfaces, using KAFOs and walking frame or forearm crutches, using swing-to or swing-through gait.
- T12–L3: potential for independent ambulation using KAFOs and forearm crutches, using swing-to, or swing-through gait on level surfaces, up-ramps and stairs.
- L4–L5: wheelchair not required. Ability to walk indepen-

dently using AFOs and forearm crutches or walking sticks on all surfaces and elevations.   (Nixon, 1985)

Incomplete lesions will result in varying degrees of additional functional potential.

The reciprocating gait orthosis (RGO) and hip guidance orthosis (HGO) are custom-made braces designed to enable people with spinal cord injuries to reach functional standing and efficient ambulation. However, reports indicate that the physiological cost index (PCI) for RGO walking is substantially greater than that of wheelchair propulsion while achieving speeds of about a quarter that of wheelchair use. The RGO is prone to continual breakdown and the subsequent time involved with repairs will substantially interfere with quality of life. The HGO is reported to be more reliable but is also more bulky.

Ogilvie *et al.* (1993) examined the physiological benefits for people with paraplegia of upright weightbearing and walking over a two-year period (using a RGO). They report that their results were disappointing. The expected improvements in physiological function did not occur. Despite the rehabilitation lore that holds that vertical weightbearing posture bestows improvements in respiratory mechanics, urological drainage, bone density and lower limb blood flow, there is little scientific data to support this view. Ogilvie concludes that the physiological benefits to people with paraplegia of using walking orthoses are not as great as has generally been claimed in the medical literature. Despite this, people who wish to use such an orthosis should not be denied the opportunity but it must be clearly explained that this is 'not the panacea for all their ills' (Ogilvie, 1993).

In conclusion, it must be emphasised that people with low, or incomplete spinal cord injuries who wish to try gait orthoses should be given the opportunity to do so. Those with higher, complete lesions may also wish to experience gait training. Before such a trial, all people with complete spinal cord injuries should receive thorough training in wheelchair skills, as this is most likely to be the choice for functional mobility on a long-term basis.

Clearly most wheelchair users would much prefer to be able to walk normally. However, the type of walking currently available using these orthoses is not normal, and is expensive in terms of time, money and effort.   (Whittle *et al.*, 1991)

Functional electrical stimulation

Functional electrical stimulation (FES; functional neuromuscular stimulation, FNS) has been extensively researched for two decades in an attempt to stimulate the neuromuscular system and achieve functional ambulation. FES has been the subject of considerable media attention, which has unfortunately conveyed the impression that it enables functional, 'normal' walking. However, in spite of international efforts and enormous financial expenditure, success is limited and only a few, very fit young people, with spastic low-lesion paraplegias (i.e. above T11) are able to stand up and walk using FES (Isakov, 1992). Isakov reports that: 'Although some paraplegics gained the capacity to walk, they were able to do so only for short distances and mainly within the laboratory environment'.

Although considerable progress has been made, it is doubtful whether the term 'functional' can yet be appropriately applied to this technology. The orthoses are bulky and take 30–45 minutes to don correctly and attach to the wiring system (Zejdlik, 1992). The energy expenditure is significant, fatigue is a severely limiting factor, ambulation is slow and unsafe on uneven ground. The costs involved are substantial. Research subjects to date have been a small number of carefully selected patients. There is a major commitment of time and energy by those people who use FES.

Although proponents of FES cite improved health benefits as potential outcomes, there is little scientific data to support these claims (Zejdlik, 1992). Studies have, however, suggested positive functional gains in some individuals with incomplete spinal cord injuries, including increased voluntary muscle strength, increased stride length and decreased physiological cost of gait (Granat *et al.*, 1992, Granat *et al.*, 1993). The potential for health problems also exists with soft tissue damage, postural deformity and increased spasticity.

It is of the utmost importance that people with spinal cord injuries are provided with realistic explanations regarding the present use of FES and its present potential. Barr (1993) indicates that the greatest subjective benefit from an FES standing programme was psychological. Subjects reported increased self-esteem and a realization of the extent of their disabilities and the practicalities of the wheelchair, following the FES programme. However, the cause and effect relationship is unclear. It is difficult to discern whether the FES itself produced these reported benefits or if it was the increased attention and time from therapists and researchers that led to a subjective sense of wellbeing. At an estimated cost of over US$33 000 (£22 000) for a one-year FES programme (Phillips, 1989), it must be questioned whether this is the most effective or appropriate means of enhancing psychological wellbeing.

It is not known how much potential FES realistically holds in enhancing functional mobility for people with spinal cord injuries. Yarkony *et al.* (1990) caution: 'It is essential that investigators in this field do not provide patients, laymen, and the mass media with expectations that exceed present knowledge or experience with FNS'.

Further issues arise from the application of this technology for walking. Does FES promote the false hope of 'normal walking' among people with recent injuries and does this encourage the injudicious spending of huge amounts of money? Does society's considerable stigmatization of people with disabilities lead to an attempt to appear more 'normal'? Is FES the primary research goal of people with spinal cord injuries? If successful, will it be available to a few, well-insured spinal cord injured individuals in a handful of developed nations or will it have practical application for people with various forms of spinal cord damage from all ethnic and socioeconomic groups? By focusing upon high-technology 'solutions' to handicap, the rehabilitation research community risks total alienation from a growing disability rights movement which seeks equal opportunities for all its members (not only young people with low-lesion, traumatic paraplegias) and the removal of social, economic and architectural barriers to full societal participation.

In the USA, where considerable profits are to be made from apparent innovations in the treatment of people with spinal cord injuries, some disabled people are speaking out about their experiences and their concerns about 'walking' programmes. Criticisms centre upon the unrealistic expectations of patients who surrender tens of thousands of dollars to profit-based clinics, which capitalize on the common ambitions of newly injured people to 'walk away' from the rehabilitation centre. Some say the operators of these facilities are 'high-tech snake-oil salesmen, selling denial and false hope, often for an enormous price, to vulnerable people . . . who refuse to accept that they'll be disabled for the rest of their lives'. Further, 'They're telling people the only way you can be acceptable as a member of this society is to be striving with all your might to walk' (O'Keefe, 1992).

A new FES system, expected to cost about US$15 000 (£10 000) to enable slow walking for short distances on flat surfaces, 'hopes for a 40% market share of the estimated 10,000 new spinal cord injuries each year' (Spinal Network Extra, 1992). It is evident that significant prestige and substantial profits are riding on these devices.

There have been great advances in the use of electrical stimulation for such functions as diaphragm pacing and bladder control. The future may hold great potential for functional hand control for people with quadriplegia and for functional standing and walking – for significant distances at functional speeds and on various surfaces.

It must be clearly understood by all people who undertake FES programmes at the present time (1994) that this work, after 20 years, remains 'investigational' and is still considered to be 'research'. Physiological benefits may indeed be derived from FES, orthotic systems and intensive muscle training but functional walking remains sadly elusive. Reports from people with spinal cord injuries in the USA indicate that such explanations may not always have been forthcoming. Although noting that everyone who has sustained a spinal cord injury wants to try to walk, Subbarao (1991) notes: 'Functional Electrical Stimulation and other new orthotic designs have not notably increased the number of persons able to walk after a spinal injury'.

If the fantasy is walking, then walking programmes prolong and strengthen it, extending the painful denial process that follows every spinal cord injury. That's why I call these programs the Denial Merchants. Cashing in on people's terror at leaving a rehab. hospital while promising to work miracles is not only despicable, but damaging to the person's eventual return to a full life . . . Call it 'targeting marketing', call it 'ripe for picking', call it what you want. I call it the unconscionable

exploitation of people too stunned to know which way to
turn.   (Kennedy, 1992)

History will decide whether the misgivings of these
Americans with spinal cord injuries are proved to be correct or
whether FES, new orthotic designs and intensive muscle re-
education programmes will prove to have significant benefits for
large numbers of people with disabilities.

Chronic overuse syndromes

The upper extremities of people with long-term spinal cord
injuries are subject to considerable stress due to their use not
only for prehension but for mobility.

During wheelchair propulsion the shoulder is forced through
an arc against resistance. During transfers, bodyweight is trans-
ferred across the soft tissues around the shoulder, resulting in
high pressure and abnormal distribution of stress (Bayley *et al.*,
1987).

Research studies have revealed the high incidence of shoulder
pain among people with chronic spinal cord injuries, with
approximately 33–35% of people with paraplegia and quadriplegia experiencing either persistent pain, or pain during transfers
(e.g. Silfverskiold and Waters, 1991).

Several studies have reported the high incidence of carpal
tunnel syndrome among people with paraplegia, the incidence
increasing with the duration of spinal cord injury.

People with paraplegia are considered to be at high risk for
developing carpal tunnel syndrome due to repetitive trauma
while propelling the wheelchair and to the use of press-ups to
relieve ischial pressure. This latter manoeuvre requires the
elbows and wrists to be locked in full extension while transferring the weight of the body through the arms. The use of
crutches also requires the weight of the body to be borne by fully
extended wrists.

The findings of these studies indicate the pain that results
from frequent use and increased stress on the upper extremities.
The consequences of this pain and subsequent impairment are
of greater functional consequence to someone with a spinal cord
injury than would be the case for an able-bodied person who
does not rely upon the upper extremity for mobility.

Chronic pain, reduced mobility and loss of function have potentially serious consequences to the quality of life of the individual. Hand function is dependent upon full, painless shoulder range of motion. Consideration should be given to providing alternative means of mobility for those with chronic shoulder problems, such as powered wheelchairs and electric hoists, where appropriate. Transfer boards reduce the stress on shoulder joints and may also help to reduce pain during transfers.

Further research should identify strategies for prevention and management of shoulder pain syndromes and carpal tunnel syndrome amongst people who use their upper extremities for long-term mobility.

The results of the studies outlined above provide those involved in the provision of wheelchairs with a clear mandate to engage in timely prophylaxis of upper extremity pain and dysfunction. People with spinal cord injuries may expect to live for many decades with their impairments and it is imperative that they are provided with every mechanical advantage to prevent a seriously handicapping condition.

Irrespective of level of lesion, people with spinal cord injuries should clearly have the opportunity to use wheelchairs that require the least possible effort to propel. Any loss of remaining upper extremity function because of persistent pain can cause a marked decrease in functional mobility and personal care. Hence future costs for attendant care services must be included in the cost-benefit equation. Requisition of an ultra-lightweight wheelchair may be viewed as a constructive step in the prevention of upper extremity overuse syndromes.

COMMUNITY MANAGEMENT

Self-care requires more than attention to personal care and functional mobility. Adult self-care activities will also include occupations such as shopping, handling money, accessing transportation, paying bills and using a telephone (Law *et al.*, 1991). Community management for people with spinal cord injuries may also entail accessing community resources such as Independent Living Centres (see Chapter 8), spinal injury associations and personal care attendant agencies. Becoming comfortable in community management is as much a part of rehabilitation as learning to transfer. Independence in personal care and mobility is of little value unless the individual can access transportation and achieve independence in his business affairs and purchase choices.

Communication

Advances in technology have enabled all people with spinal cord lesions, at any level, to operate a telephone independently. Adapted equipment is available from telephone companies and from aids and equipment suppliers (see also Chapter 6).

People with quadriplegia at C5 may be able to write using a long opponens or Futuro splint to support the wrist and a writing attachment. A right angle holder will allow use of a typing stick to access a keyboard.

People with lesions at C6 may use a short opponens splint and pen holder, a writing splint and typing stick. Those with lesions at C7 or below will not require special equipment for writing but may choose to lace a pen through their fingers (C7) to enhance their grasp. These skills may be practiced early in the rehabilitation process by completing hospital menu sheets while lying prone on the Stryker frame.

Community visits

Following a spinal cord injury, the individual re-enters the community with specific impairments that impact upon his previous experiences of community interaction. The physical accessibility of the environment and the social, cultural and economic obstacles which may or may not be present will determine how disabling and handicapping will be future community interactions.

Community living requires the ability to solve problems and direct others verbally when assistance is required. Early and regular returns to the community during rehabilitation will enable each individual to gain experience and skills required upon discharge. Initially accompanied by a therapist and/or someone who has already successfully re-integrated into the community, the client with a recent injury will have the opportunity to learn how to negotiate physical barriers in the environment, what provisions must be in place before a building or facility can be considered to be wheelchair accessible and how to change those which are discriminatory.

People with cervical lesions may need practice in handling money and may wish to carry a writing splint with them in case they wish to write a cheque or sign a credit card receipt.

Experimentation may identify the most appropriate method for carrying valuables and purchases securely. If a back pack is used, practice may be needed to retrieve and stow items. A pouch attached to the side of the chair may be useful for carrying writing aids and other small items. Many people use a pouch attached between the top of the legrests, behind the legs, for carrying money and credit cards safely.

All community visits will entail planning, solving problems and evaluation. Preparation for successful return to community living will clearly require more than a home visit. Excursions may be made to banks, shops, restaurants, work places, sporting facilities, theatres, pubs, night clubs – a broad sample of the places that were routinely visited before injury.

The spinal cord injured individual will decide where he wishes to visit based upon his past interests and future goals. He is responsible for planning and preparing for the visit, for timing catheterisations, arranging transportation, using the therapists as resources and analysing the success of the trip upon return to the rehabilitation unit. The rehabilitation process is about making decisions, solving problems and active learning. It is also about teaching the therapist about what it means to be disabled in the community. Community visits are the chance to realize these objectives.

Transportation

Driving

The ability to drive provides great opportunities for access to vocational, social and recreational activities. Spinal injury centres that have recognised the tremendous impact of driving upon the opportunities for social integration and employment of people with spinal cord injuries are providing the opportunity for driver training for those who are unable to drive and the chance to become competent with hand controls for those who already have a licence. Official testing will be arranged before discharge so that the newly injured person is able to re-enter the community with one of the most important skills required for full access to community participation.

Although individual abilities will vary, people with lesions at C6 and below are usually able to operate a vehicle safely. Hand controls are used for braking and acceleration. A wide variety of hand controls are made, so research may be necessary to determine the most suitable for each individual. Steering wheel adaptations are available and some people may find power steering to be a beneficial feature. Vans may be fitted with electric lifts, all controlled by switches which are accessed from a panel on the side of the vehicle. These enable people with quadriplegia to access their vehicle without having to transfer into a driver's seat and try to pull their chairs in behind them. Some people with quadriplegia may choose to transfer from the wheelchair into the driver's seat when in the van. Others may have a system that secures the wheelchair and allows them to drive without transferring. Powered wheelchairs are available which fold into the space where the driver's seat in a car would normally be positioned, enabling the wheelchair user to drive without transferring.

Air travel

Air travel is now possible for all people with spinal cord injuries, including those who use powered wheelchairs and ventilators. In general, international airlines have become more accommodating to passengers who have special needs, with services including special meals and wheelchair-to-aircraft seat transfers (i.e. with no need to use a special chair to access the aircraft). Although it is still rare to find wheelchair-accessible toilets, these are now available on some aircraft. Alternative arrangements must be made for the majority of aeroplanes which do not have accessible facilities. Since 1984, Air Canada has implemented a 50% fare reduction for personal attendants travelling with a disabled person, within North America.

Airlines will need to be informed in advance that someone who uses a wheelchair will be travelling. Special arrangements may be required for handling batteries and ventilators. A medical certificate may be required.

Two publications provide excellent information concerning

travelling with a wheelchair – including valuable advice regarding airline travel.

- Noble, C. (1985) *Handi-Travel*. Canadian Rehabilitation Council for the Disabled, Toronto, Ont.
- Anon. (1990) *The World Wheelchair Traveller*. Automobile Association and Spinal Injuries Association, London.

Public transportation

The Americans with Disabilities Act (1990) has provided legislation which states that no one may be denied access to public facilities on the basis of their disability. From 1992, the Act prohibited the purchase and lease of new buses, rapid rail vehicles or light rail vehicles which are not readily accessible to people with disabilities. Further, each public entity must develop a plan for a paratransit system.

It is to be hoped that less enlightened administrations will enact similar legislation to allow people with disabilities equal access to their societies and communities. Chapter 8 examines the negative correlation between life satisfaction, engagement in productive occupation and leisure pursuits and the lack of accessible transportation.

In North America, car rental agencies will readily install hand controls for disabled drivers. Portable hand controls have also been developed. In Vancouver, Canada, the public transit systems (buses, taxis, ferries and monorails) are accessible to people who use wheelchairs. Vans equipped with wheelchair lifts may be rented at all major Canadian airports.

In other places, tax-paying citizens who have disabilities subsidize transportation services to which they themselves are denied access. Until this situation is changed, people with spinal cord injuries will need to research the resources available in their own communities and countries so that they can achieve maximum mobility in their environments.

Accessing community resources

Before leaving the rehabilitation facility, the person with a spinal cord injury will need to be familiar with the resources available to him in his community. These may include financial benefits or subsidies, wheelchair-accessible recreational facilities, wheel-chair sports associations, accessible housing, transportation and medical services. Many spinal centres maintain an updated information kit containing current knowledge regarding com-munity resources. It may be several months before the newly injured person is ready to access these resources and it is there-fore useful to have the necessary information in booklet form so that it is available as and when it is required.

In addition, the client must be aware of how he can access information concerning changing programmes and technology, so that, once he is discharged, he can keep up to date with new equipment, publications, treatment options and benefits. Knowledge is not static and part of the learning process during rehabilitation is focused not just upon transfer of information but of teaching how to learn.

Sadly, many people with spinal cord injuries do not know how to access the information which could be relevant to their situation and hence remain oblivious to new technologies relating to such aspects as wheelchair design, options for parenthood or legislation concerning benefits.

Community management is not a static skill and the ability to access relevant and current information is an important part of the knowledge to be gained during the rehabilitation process.

Social skills

It is unfortunate that the topic of social skills needs to be addressed in a book concerning spinal cord injury. As the great majority of people who sustain these injuries are in their late teens or in adulthood, the skills that enable appropriate func-tioning in a social context have already been mastered. In view of the fact that spinal cord injury does not produce speech impairments, deafness or cognitive impairments which might alter previous patterns of interaction, a problem with social skills might not appear to be an issue.

However, it is an unfortunate reality that social, interpersonal and cultural barriers present a very formidable obstacle to people with physical disabilities.

The constitution of Disabled Peoples' International (DPI, 1985) defines **handicap** not in terms of the disabled individual but rather as the 'loss or limitation of opportunities to take part in the normal life of the community on an equal basis with others due to physical and social barriers'. Hence, it is the barriers that are erected by society which are viewed as preventing full participation in society, equalization of opportunities and full societal integration. Although it is clearly the role of all rehabilitation professionals to address directly the legal, political, economic, social, cultural and physical barriers that exclude people with disabilities from achieving the same rights accorded to other members of society (see Chapter 10), it is also our mandate to enable the newly injured client to discover the tools to facilitate interactions with the social environment as he will find it at the present time.

Two new situations present themselves to the newly injured person. One relates to the reactions of others to their disability; the other pertains to the need to ask others for help.

Healthcare and rehabilitation staff have a great affection for submissive and compliant behaviour from their patients. Work load and accountability are both decreased and the pervading ambiance of passive co-operation is very pleasing. However, these are not the behaviours that will best serve the client in his community and social interactions, and are not the behaviours to be reinforced during the rehabilitation process. Indeed, passivity is to be discouraged from the earliest stages of professional intervention.

Assertiveness will require the individual to express and assert his needs with both confidence and directness. Although typically regarded as a personality problem in rehabilitation facilities, assertiveness is the behaviour most appropriate to establishing and maintaining relationships and achieving objectives and goals in the community.

Assertiveness is a behaviour that is derived from self-respect and self-esteem. As the early months following injury predominantly consist of interactions with healthcare and rehabilitation personnel, these professionals have a considerable role to play in encouraging the client to view himself in positive terms. Staff who convey attitudes of pity and sympathy or who assume an aloof and superior distance from their devalued clients will negate their efforts to maintain a positive sense of self.

Much communication and human interaction depends upon eye contact. The desirability of establishing or maintaining eye contact may be especially pertinent for someone who is seated in a chair. Using others with spinal cord injuries as role models, new means of physical expression and non-verbal communication may be learned.

People with disabilities may be confronted by others whose opening gambit is 'What happened to you?' The response 'Why do you ask?' seems to be the most appropriate, as it provides the opportunity for further dialogue with someone whose relative may recently have been injured. The decision whether to respond to the purely nosy person will clearly be a personal one!

Frequent visits in the community will enable the individual with a spinal cord injury to gain confidence in asking strangers for help if and when the need arises. Establishing eye contact and being quite specific about the request will enable the other person to understand exactly what is required. Most people like to help others but need clear directions on how to go about doing this constructively.

There will also be occasions when no help is required or desired and an offer must be declined. This is especially encountered by people with paraplegia who may be frustrated by the attempts of others to push their wheelchairs, to lift the chair into a vehicle or to assist in other tasks they would prefer to perform independently. A clear and direct decline, with thanks for the offer will save both parties from embarrassment.

Although many people find their previous social skills, personality and confidence are more than adequate to their needs following injury, others will benefit from practice and role modelling. Some centres use role playing in sessions designed to teach social skills and assertiveness. Although these courses are also available at community colleges for members of the general public, role play techniques are not comfortable for everyone and should be left to individual choice.

Many research studies have found that people with disabilities do not enter social and community environments as frequently as do other people. Although barriers to full participation undoubtedly exist in society, enhancing social skills may provide one avenue towards achieving interaction and integration into society and to enhancing comfortable interpersonal interaction. Community management is an essential aspect of self-care skills for all adults and social skills comprise a component in the successful performance of such activities.

In a recent study of people living in the community, Hammell

(1991) reported that several men with spinal cord injuries stated that they had needed to learn how to initiate and maintain comfortable social contact with other people. Further research might identify ways in which the rehabilitation team can assist these people in gaining the skills necessary to overcome societal barriers and to interact socially in the community. Trieschmann (1988) further proposes: 'It seems likely that persons with quadriplegia need to develop a greater skill at coping with interpersonal relationships than persons with paraplegia because the former group's very survival often depends on their ability to get along with those around them.'

DISCHARGE PLANNING

Discharge planning is discussed in a small minority of works concerning spinal cord injury, yet it is difficult to conceive many topics more instrumental to assuring positive outcome and ensuring appropriate follow-up.

Discharge planning is not the final step in the treatment and rehabilitation programme. Rather, this is an integral part of the entire process. Throughout the period of hospitalization the client will have been encouraged to establish personally meaningful long-term goals and these have formed part of the discharge planning process. Learning and problem-solving activities have been part of the discharge process, as have the frequent community excursions, the mastery of self-care skills and the planning for engagement in productive and leisure occupations. Discharge planning will also incorporate such aspects as driver training, evaluation of the home environment and obtaining necessary aids, equipment and physical modifications.

Discharge planning is a collaborative effort, with the client and his close friends and family actively involved in making decisions with members of the rehabilitation team. Success in this effort will be dependent upon clear lines of communication, stemming from the early, active involvement of the client's close friends and relatives throughout the rehabilitation process.

The discharge plan should be consistent with the individual's goals, his functional abilities and impairments, likely prognosis and the available community resources (CAOT, 1991).

The termination of active therapeutic intervention and

resumption of full community participation can either be a traumatic and threatening event or a smooth transition. Rehabilitation staff can facilitate this transition in several ways, not limited to the following.

1. Thorough assessment with the client of his future home and work/study environments both to identify potential barriers and to have modifications, aids or equipment in place before discharge.
2. Early and frequent community visits, enabling the client to identify the social and physical barriers in his environment and devise appropriate management strategies. These visits are an opportunity for experiential learning and enable the individual to become familiar with the possibilities for social interaction and community participation.
3. Early links with peer groups from his local area. These individuals may provide invaluable information concerning local facilities and resources in addition to providing support and continuity between institution and community.
4. Early links with community services such as community occupational therapists and community health nurses, providing these professionals with the opportunity to learn more about spinal cord injury management and to facilitate their communication with the client.
5. Planning care services for people who wish to use care attendants. The rehabilitation facility and staff may act as resources in locating and training attendants, according to the needs and wishes of the client. Guidance may be requested regarding job descriptions, hiring and managing attendants (see Chapter 9).
6. Studies indicate that inactivity, poor social support systems and the lack of opportunity to participate in social and community interactions have a negative impact upon the health of people with spinal cord injuries and may affect survival itself. Awareness of these factors throughout the rehabilitation/discharge planning process will ensure that every effort is made to enhance social support systems and encourage early and frequent engagement in leisure and productive occupations.
7. Clients who are being discharged should be provided with written manuals, commensurate with their level of reading

skill, and dealing with aspects of management related to spinal cord injury. Clear, factual information will reinforce the learning acquired during hospitalization and may help to prevent or identify potential complications. In conjunction with this, a guide to resources should be available so that the client may keep well informed about support groups, benefits, equipment and other community and commercial resources.

In documenting a discharge summary, the therapist will include such aspects as the functional status of the client, his goal attainment, his unmet goals and plans for meeting these goals, the plans for ongoing or follow-up services and any further recommendations (CAOT, 1991). Such a report should serve both to protect the privacy of the client and to provide pertinent information for those involved in follow-up services.

Integral to the concept of discharge planning is the provision of excellent follow-up services; indeed, it is proposed that a spinal unit should ultimately be judged by the standard of its follow-up system (see Chapter 9).

RE-ADMISSION TO HOSPITAL

A recurring complaint among persons with disabilities is that, if they use a primary care physician, they must constantly educate their physician about the idiosyncracies of their impairment and how it needs to be taken into account when prescribing treatment. (DeJong *et al.*, 1989)

Study of hospital use in the USA indicated that people with spinal cord injuries had the highest rates of re-admission to hospital of any diagnostic group. In a 12-month period the frequency of repeated admissions among total hospitalizations for people with spinal cord injuries was 97% (Zook *et al.*, 1980). Hence, it is indicated that initial, acute hospitalization will not be as costly as the illnesses and problems that necessitate so many subsequent admissions.

In a study of people with spinal cord injuries who had been discharged from initial rehabilitation for one year, Davidoff *et al.* (1990) found that 39% had been re-admitted to hospital during that year. They indicate that re-admission for secondary complications of acute spinal cord injury are both common and very expensive. A previous cross-sectional survey of people living independently with spinal cord injuries showed 57% to have been hospitalized during the previous year (Meyers *et al.*, 1985).

Re-admission is a major obstacle to independent living and to quality of life. It is a barrier to employment, to education, community re-integration, psychological equilibrium, personal relationships and family interaction. Although people who have been discharged from rehabilitation programmes are not generally ill, they do have a narrow margin of health and many acute health problems such as urinary tract infections, respiratory infections and pressure sores do not surface until after discharge from a medical programme. Two of the leading causes of re-admission – urinary tract infections and pressure sores – are largely preventable.

Little emphasis has been placed on meeting the healthcare needs of people with disabilities after they have been discharged from rehabilitation facilities. Studies have suggested that people with spinal cord injuries may be hospitalized following inability to access primary medical care. The shortage of affordable and accessible transportation may prevent access to a clinician. Many community practitioners' offices are not accessible to wheelchairs and data also suggest 'the inadequacy of current health and social services, and the public policy that supports those services, to meet the needs of those with high-level SCI [spinal cord injury]' (Meyers *et al.*, 1985).

In a study of America's working-age people with disabilities, DeJong and associates (1989) reported that over 45% of people with spinal cord injuries had difficulty in the previous 12 months in finding a physician who was knowledgeable about the particular healthcare needs related to their disability. Further, 50% of those with spinal cord injuries reported that had they gained timely access to a healthcare provider who was knowledgeable about spinal cord injury and its idiosyncracies, that one or more hospital re-admissions could have been averted in the previous 12 months.

Meyers *et al.* (1985; 1987; 1988) report on an alternate model of care delivery established to provide accessible primary care to people with major physical disabilities in a manner consistent with the philosophies of the Independent Living Movement (see Chapter 8). This community-based programme involves nurse practitioners (who evaluate medical problems and visit clients in the office or their own homes) and primary physicians who provide emergency consultation at home or in the office, 24 hours a day, seven days a week, and who also provide managed hospital care and specialty consultation. Meyers' studies indicate that some clients will experience a reduction in emergency visits and in-patient care and that managed and accessible home care may reduce the overall need for care. However, these positive results could not be generalised to the whole group. Factors such as poor social interaction and depression were positively correlated with repeat hospitalizations, indicating that attention to psychosocial and mental health services might contribute to a reduced demand on in-patient medical facilities.

Meyers' group indicated that one of the factors most strongly correlated with high numbers of hospital admissions was that of people who left their homes less than once a day. The impact of an inaccessible environment upon ill health and upon the production of handicap, and the reduced opportunity for social interaction and community participation, may be a critical factor in the causation of this variable. Meyers (1989) indicates that, although not all predictors of medical care use are amenable to intervention (for example, age or years since injury), the means for increasing social interaction and meeting instrumental activity of daily living needs (grocery shopping, transportation) are obvious. Improved transportation services, removal of architectural and programmatic barriers and expansion of personal care services requires only political will.

REFERENCES

Ainsley, J., Voorhees, C. and Drake, E. (1985) Reconstructive hand surgery for quadriplegic persons. *American Journal of Occupational Therapy*, **39**(11), 715–21.

Barnard, I.S. (1991) *An Investigation into the Energy Expenditure in Self Propelling Wheelchairs*, MSc thesis (Rehabilitation Studies), University of Southampton, Southampton.

Barr, F.M.D. (1993) Functional Electrical Stimulation: patient perceptions. Proceedings of the Society for Research in Rehabilitation Scientific Meeting (abstract). *Clinical Rehabilitation*, **7**, 79.

Bayley, J.C., Cochran, T.P. and Sledge, C.B. (1987) The weight bearing shoulder. The impingement syndrome in paraplegics. *Journal of Bone and Joint Surgery*, **69**, 676–8.

Bromley, I. (1991) *Tetraplegia and Paraplegia – a Guide for Physiotherapists*, 4th edn, Churchill Livingstone, Edinburgh.

CAOT (1991) *Occupational Therapy Guidelines for Client Centred Practice*, Canadian Association of Occupational Therapists and Health Services Directorate, Health Services Promotion Branch, Health and Welfare Canada, Toronto, Ont., pp. 83, 157.

Corbet, B. (1980) *Options*, Hirschfeld, Denver, CO, p. 15.

Davidoff, G., Schultz, J.S., Webb, T. *et al.* (1990) Rehospitalization after rehabilitation of acute spinal cord injury: incidence and risk factors. *Archives of Physical Medicine and Rehabilitation*, **71**, 121–4.

DeJong, G., Batavia, A.I. and Griss, R. (1989) America's neglected health care minority: working age persons with disabilities. *The Milbank Quarterly*, **67** (Suppl. 2, Part 2), 311–51.

DPI (1985) *Disabled Peoples' International Constitution*, 1, DPI Development Office, Winnepeg, Man.

Fisher, J.M. and Hunter, J. (1992) Adapted make-up kit for persons with C5 and C6 quadriplegia. *Canadian Journal of Occupational Therapy*, **59**(5), 268–75.

Ford, J. and Duckworth, B. (1987) *Physical Management for the Quadriplegic Patient*, 2nd edn, F.A. Davis, Philadelphia, PA.

Fyfe, N.C.M. and Wood, J. (1990) The choice of self-propelling wheelchairs for spinal patients. *Clinical Rehabilitation*, **4**, 51–6.

Garber S.L. (1985) Wheelchair cushions for spinal cord injured individuals. *American Journal of Occupational Therapy*, **39**(11), 722–5.

Garber, S.L. and Dyerly, L.R. (1991) Wheelchair cushions for persons with spinal cord injury: an update. *American Journal of Occupational Therapy*, **45**(6), 550–4.

Gilsdorf, P., Patterson, R. and Fisher, S. (1991) Thirty-minute continuous sitting force measurements with different support surfaces in the spinal cord injured and able bodied. *Journal of Rehabilitation, Research and Development*, **28**(4), 33–8.

Granat, M., Keating, J.F., Smith, A.C.B. *et al.* (1992) The use of Functional Electrical Stimulation to assist gait in patients with incomplete spinal cord injury. *Disability and Rehabilitation*, **14**(2), 93–7.

Granat, M.H., Ferguson, A.C.B., Andrews, B.J. and Delargy, M. (1993) The role of functional electrical stimulation in the rehabilitation of patients with incomplete spinal cord injury – observed benefits during gait studies. *Paraplegia*, **31**(4), 207–15.

Grundy, D. and Swain, A. (1993) *ABC of Spinal Cord Injury*, 2nd edn, British Medical Journal, London, p. 54.

Hammell, K.R.W. (1991) *An Investigation into the Availability and Adequacy of Social Relationships Following Head Injury and Spinal Cord Injury: a Study of Injured Men and their Partners*, MSc thesis (Rehabilitation Studies), University of Southampton, Southampton.

Hill, J.P. (1986) *Spinal Cord Injury – a Guide to Functional Outcomes in Occupational Therapy*, Aspen, Rockville, MD.

Hof, H., Hotchkiss, R. and Pfaelzer, P. (1993) Building wheelchairs, creating opportunities. Collaborating to build wheelchairs in developing countries. *Technology and Disability*, **2**(2), 1–14.

Isakov, E., Douglas, R. and Berns, P. (1992) Ambulation using the Reciprocating Gait Orthosis and Functional Electrical Stimulation. *Paraplegia* **30**(4), 239–45.

Johnstone, B.R., Jordan, C.J. and Buntine, J.A. (1988) A review of surgical rehabilitation of the upper limb in quadriplegia. *Paraplegia*, **26**, 317–39.

Kennedy, N.B. (1992) The denial merchants cash in. *Spinal Network Extra*, Winter, p.47.

Krajnik, S.R. and Bridle, M.J. (1992) Hand splinting in quadriplegia: current practice. *American Journal of Occupational Therapy*, **46**(2), 149–56.

Lamb, D.W. (1992) The current state of the management of the upper limb in tetraplegia. *Paraplegia*, **30**, 65–7.

Law, M., Baptiste, S., Carswell-Opzoomer A. *et al.* (1991) *Canadian Occupational Performance Measure*, Canadian Association of Occupational Therapists, Toronto, Ont.

Lee, A. (1988) Survey of Rancho flexor hinge splint users. *British Journal of Occupational Therapy*, **51**(6), 197–8.

Major, R.E. (1990) Some aspects of wheel geometry related to manually propelled wheelchairs. *Physiotherapy*, **76**(10), 663–5.

Maslow, A.H. (1970) *Motivation and Personality*, Harper and Row, New York, NY, pp. 15–23.

Meyers, A.R., Branch, L.G., Cupples, L.A. *et al.* (1989) Predictors of medical care utilisation by independently living adults with spinal cord injuries. *Archives of Physical Medicine and Rehabilitation*, **70**, 471–6.

Meyers, A.R., Cupples, A., Lederman, R.I. *et al.* (1987) A prospective evaluation of the effect of managed care utilization among severely disabled independently living adults. *Medical Care*, **25**(11), 1057–68.

Meyers, A.R., Cupples, A., Lederman, R.I. *et al.* (1988) The epidemiology of medical care utilization by severely disabled independently-living adults. *Journal of Clinical Epidemiology*, **41**(2), 163–72.

Meyers, A.R., Feltin, M., Master, R.J. *et al.* (1985) Rehospitalization and spinal cord injury: cross-sectional survey of adults living independently. *Archives of Physical Medicine and Rehabilitation*, **66**, 704–8.

Nixon, V. (1985) *Spinal Cord Injury – a Guide to Functional Outcomes in Physical Therapy Management*, Aspen, Rockville, MD.

Nosek, M.A. (1993) Personal assistance: its effect on the long term health of a rehabilitation hospital population. *Archives of Physical Medicine and Rehabilitation*, **74**, 127–32.

Nosek, M.A., Parker, R.M. and Larsen, S. (1987) Psychosocial independence and functional abilities: their relationship in adults with severe
musculoskeletal impairments. *Archives of Physical Medicine and
Rehabilitation*, **68**, 840–5.

Ogilvie, C., Bowker, P. and Rowley, D.I. (1993) The physiological
benefits of paraplegic orthotically aided walking. *Paraplegia*, **31**(2),
111–5.

O'Keefe, M. (1992) Walking programs – rehab or razzle-dazzle? *Spinal
Network Extra*, Winter, p.34–40.

Oliver, M. (1993) What's so wonderful about walking? *Spinal Injuries
Association Newsletter*, 68, 3–5.

Phillips, C.A. (1989) Functional Electrical Stimulation and lower extremity bracing for ambulation exercise of the spinal cord injured
individual: a medically prescribed system. *Physical Therapy*, **60**, 842–9.

Pyc, G. (1990) Seating pressure. *Caliper*, **XLV**(4), 27–9.

Rogers, J.C. and Figone, J.L. (1980) Traumatic quadriplegia: follow up
study of self-care skills. *Archives of Physical Medicine and Rehabilitation*,
61, 316–21.

Roth, E.J., Lawler, M.H. and Yarkony, G.M. (1990) Traumatic central
cord syndrome: clinical features and functional outcomes. *Archives of
Physical Medicine and Rehabilitation*, **71**, 18–23.

Scales, J.T., Lowthian, P.T., Poole, A,G. and Ludman, W.R. (1982)
'Vaperm' patient support system: a new general purpose hospital
mattress. *The Lancet*, P 1150–52.

Shepherd, C.C. and Ruzicka, S.H. (1991) Tenodesis brace use by persons with spinal cord injuries. *American Journal of Occupational
Therapy*, **45**(1), 81–3.

Silfverskiold, J. and Waters, R.L. (1991) Shoulder pain and functional
disability in spinal cord injury patients. *Clinical Orthopaedics*, **272**,
141–5.

Somers, M.F. (1992) *Spinal Cord Injury Functional Rehabilitation*,
Appleton and Lange, East Norwalk, CT.

Spinal Network Extra, (1992) Walking to the market place. *Spinal
Network Extra*, Winter, p.42.

Subbarao, J.V. (1991) Walking after spinal cord injury: goal or wish?
Western Journal of Medicine, **154**(5), 612–4.

Tough, A.J. and Chandler, C.S. (1992) A comparison of three high
pressure relief wheelchair cushions (abstract) *Clinical Rehabilitation*, **6**
(Suppl.), 68.

Trieschmann, R.B. (1988) *Spinal Cord Injuries. Psychological, Social and
Vocational Rehabilitation*, 2nd edn, Demos, New York, NY, p. 267.

Trombly, C.A. (1983) *Occupational Therapy for Physical Dysfunction*, 2nd
edn, Williams and Wilkins, Baltimore, MD, pp. 395–7.

Vanden Berghe, A., Van Laere, M., Hellings, S. and Vercauteren, M.

(1991) Reconstruction of the upper extremity in tetraplegia: functional assessment, surgical procedures and rehabilitation. *Paraplegia,* **29,** 103–12.

Weingarden, S.I. and Martin, C. (1989) Independent dressing after spinal cord injury: a functional time evaluation. *Archives of Physical Medicine and Rehabilitation,* **70,** 518–9.

Welch, R.D., Lobley, S.J., O'Sullivan, S.B. and Freed, M.M. (1986) Functional independence in quadriplegia: critical levels. *Archives of Physical Medicine and Rehabilitation,* **67,** 235–40.

Whittle, M.W., Cochrane, G.M., Chase, A.P. *et al.* (1991) A comparative trial of two walking systems for paralysed people. *Paraplegia,* **29,** 97–102.

Yarkony, G.M., Jaeger, R.J., Roth, E. *et al.* (1990) Functional Neuromuscular Stimulation for standing after spinal cord injury, *Archives of Physical Medicine and Rehabilitation,* **71,** 201–6.

Yerxa, E.J. and Baum, S. (1986) Engagement in daily occupations and life satisfaction among people with spinal cord injuries. *Occupational Therapy Journal of Research,* **6**(5), 271–83.

Yerxa, E.J. and Locker, S.B. (1990) Quality of time use by adults with spinal cord injuries. *American Journal of Occupational Therapy,* **44**(4), 318–26.

Zejdlik, C.P. (1992) *Management of Spinal Cord Injury,* 2nd edn, Jones and Bartlett, Boston, MD, pp. 262, 501–3.

Zook, C.J., Savickis, S.F. and Moore, F.D. (1980) Repeated hospitalization for the same disease: a multiplier of National Health costs. *Milbank Memorial Fund Quarterly,* **58**(3), 454–71.

Further information regarding development of wheelchairs for developing countries

Wheeled Mobility Center, Division of Engineering, San Francisco State University, 1600 Holloway Avenue, San Francisco, CA 94132, USA.

6

Management of high lesions

> If a society has the technology to keep this patient
> alive, then it must consider the human being and
> adapt its technology to respect the dignity of the life it
> has saved.
>
> (*Burnham and Werner, 1979*)

INTRODUCTION

Brian Clark's brilliant and insightful play, *Whose life is it anyway?*
(1978) surrounds a former sculptor, currently a C4 quadriplegic,
who questions whether a life of complete physical dependency
and inactivity can have any value, quality or pleasure. He elects
to die rather than have an active brain and no opportunities for
that brain to direct anything.

In 1992, in Canada, a landmark judicial decision granted a
ventilator-dependent quadriplegic woman the right to refuse
medical treatment and to be disconnected from her respirator,
thereby ending her life. The petitioner, known in the media
as Nancy B, had irreversible neurological damage and was
paralysed from the neck down following Guillain-Barré disease.
She had been in hospital for two and a half years. Her death, at
age 25 and the decisions which she took in exerting her rights to
determine her own treatment and to achieve her goals, sparked
debate and controversy across the country.

Advocates of the 'Right to Life' movement deplored the action
taken by Nancy B. and by the court, yet contributed nothing to
the debate concerning how healthcare professionals and others
can ensure that the lives which they preserve and prolong have
quality, value and worth for each individual.

Polatajko (1992) proposes that 'life' and 'living' are not necessarily the same thing and that healthcare providers must not only

prolong the quantity of life but also prolong the quality of life and hence the will to live.

In the 4th century BC, Aristotle wrote that 'the quality of a life is determined by its activities'. Polatajko further explores this concept by suggesting that life without the ability to 'do' is not worth living.

The previous illustrations should not be interpreted as pessimistic with regard to the rehabilitation of the person with a high-lesion quadriplegia. On the contrary, the author is enthusiastic about the possibilities for activity, for environmental interaction and for quality living which may now be accomplished by this client group. It is crucial however, that healthcare professionals recognize the extreme importance to a body, which is largely deprived of sensory and motor stimulation, of achieving meaningful activity. A simplistic vision of rehabilitation as the teaching of physical skills (such as transfers and self-care activities) has enabled rehabilitation staff to abdicate their considerable responsibilities to people with high-lesion quadriplegia. For the majority of adults, independence in self-care forms a very minor facet of life. Of greater value and meaning are social activities, purposeful activity and creative leisure pursuits. These are the very areas that may also be explored to enable those clients with high-lesion quadriplegia to attain a life of quality and value. It may not be the client who lacks 'rehabilitation potential' but the vision of the rehabilitation professional which is limited!

Functional assessments have the potential to connote a person's worth (Kielhofner, 1993), hence people with high-lesion quadriplegia are often considered to be 'not worth' a rehabilitation programme. Krishnan and Watt (1993) propose an alternate mandate:

> There is a considerable onus upon the professions, having intervened to save life by means of assisted ventilation, to do everything possible to maximize the quality of life, and this includes the objective of discharge from hospital to home as well as harnessing the latest technological advances in the name of greater independence.

It should be a point of shame to healthcare professionals that specialized rehabilitation services have frequently been denied to people with high cervical cord lesions, on the basis that these clients lack the potential for independence in self-care skills. Many spinal injury units do not admit people with high lesions, preferring instead to admit paraplegics who will require shorter stays, hence achieving greater 'throughput' and who will be able to make use of gymnasium and sports facilities. Some spinal units do not accept people who use ventilators due to a lack of staff training. It is suggested that, as families and friends can be trained to care for these individuals, spinal unit staff should also be trainable. 'Only when all injured patients have an equal opportunity for rehabilitation will the trauma of cervical spinal cord injuries be diminished' (Roye *et al.*, 1988).

Additionally, staff who have not had previous experience with someone with a high cervical lesion who has achieved a meaningful and purposeful life, may feel that the newly injured client with high cord damage would have been better off if he had died. This attitude of sadness and pessimism will be transmitted to the client who may hence view his situation as meaningless and hopeless. The staff attitude may in reality become a self-fulfilling prophecy. It is therefore essential that individuals with high cervical lesions have access to rehabilitation services of excellence which will emphasize options in productivity and leisure and will work with the client in achieving a life that has quality. A ground-breaking programme in Vancouver, Canada employs the skills of therapists and the expertise of people with high-lesion spinal cord injuries who live in the community, in a project to facilitate the transition of people with high-lesion quadriplegias from institutional dependence to self-managed community living.

Although it is undoubtedly costly to provide comprehensive rehabilitation and equipment for people with high-lesion quadriplegia, we must consider whether it is humane not to offer such services. If the decision has been made to save a life, the commitment must be in place to ensure that life has dignity and purpose. Not to do so is an immoral misuse of our technological achievements and of the financial resources already expended in preserving and prolonging that life – an exercise of technology and not of humanity.

This chapter will outline some of the resources which are currently available to people with high-lesion quadriplegia and their therapists in achieving a quality lifestyle. The intention is not to describe specific manufacturers' equipment, as improvements are being made continually but rather to provide more general descriptions of the available equipment options.

HIGH-LESION QUADRIPLEGIA AND REHABILITATION

It is only within the past decade that crisis intervention and sophisticated medical diagnosis and treatment have enabled the survival of significant numbers of people with high-lesion quadriplegia.

The description **high-lesion quadriplegia** is used for a person who has sustained a severe neurological deficit caused by a lesion or damage to the cervical spinal cord at C1, C2, C3 or C4.

It is estimated that each year in the USA, 166 people sustain an injury at C1–C3 and that 540 people sustain an injury at C4. This equates to an annual incidence of 3.15 per million per year (Menter, 1989). It is unlikely that British figures will be as high, due in part to the lack of commitment to a public education programme of cardiopulmonary resuscitation. It should be noted, however, that disease causes many more cases of high-lesion quadriplegia than does spinal cord trauma (Kirby, 1989).

A literature review reveals few references to the rehabilitation of people with high-lesion quadriplegia. Journal articles have focused upon the medical aspects of the crisis and subsequent care but have rarely addressed the issues of achieving a meaningful and active lifestyle. However, studies of patient outcomes from specialized centres have revealed positive results. A study in the USA (1985, in Menter, 1989) demonstrated that people with high-lesion quadriplegia were leading fulfilling lives, interacting socially, living at home and participating in a range of activities both at home and in the community. Notably, they reported high self-esteem, good quality of life and were glad to be alive. Menter notes that the positive reports of the patients themselves contradicts the common expectations of healthcare professionals: that the lives of high quadriplegics are so awful that no one would wish to endure such suffering. Further study in Southport, England has revealed a similar, positive outcome, with every ventilator-dependent quadriplegic surveyed reporting to be glad to be alive (Glass, 1993). Bach (1991) suggests that healthcare professionals usually overestimate the negative impact of ventilator use on people with severe disabilities and underestimate the satisfaction with quality of life reported by the clients themselves.

It is usual for textbooks concerning the rehabilitation of people with spinal cord injuries to examine the situation of those with lesions below C5. It is essential, however, that professionals also attend to the rehabilitation of those with higher lesions. As medicine advances, such individuals will surely survive in ever increasing numbers. High-lesion quadriplegia is the result not only of trauma, but of vascular insult, tumours and disease. Accordingly, the location of treatment may not be a specialized spinal unit but a general hospital. When the potential for control, activity and a life of quality exist it is incumbent upon rehabilitation professionals in every location to address the needs of these clients and to rise to meet the very considerable challenge that these individuals represent.

DEFINITION

As a general guide, injury or damage to the spinal cord at C1 or C2 will prevent independent functioning of the diaphragm and these individuals will need to be artificially ventilated at all times. Injury at C3 may leave weak functioning of the diaphragm so that the individual may manage without mechanical ventilation for prolonged periods. At C4, the patient is likely to be able to breathe using his diaphragm at all times. All complete cervical lesions will paralyse the other muscles of respiration.

EARLY INTERVENTION

Rehabilitation should not be considered to be a process reserved for the late stages of treatment but rather as an integral part of the entire treatment process. Intervention should begin at the earliest possible moment, while the patient is still on the intensive care unit. Early focus should be upon enabling control of the environment and hence upon facilitating interaction with the environment.

Orthotics

Protocols for splinting tend to vary, especially between North America and the UK. The author proposes the following model for splinting but recognizes that procedures may vary.

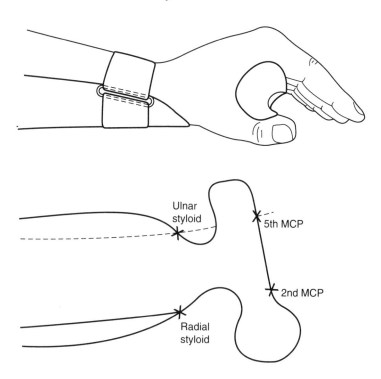

Figure 6.1 Long opponens splint. Indications: weak wrist extensors (C4/C5 lesions). Splint: extends two-thirds up the forearm (i.e. within approximately 6 cm of the elbow); pronate (palm down) for forearm moulding; thumb – metacarpophalangeal (MCP) opposition, thenar eminence free, thumb in abduction, directly under second MCP joint; wrist – 0–30° of extension; adequate web space; maintain palmar arch; ensure MCP flexion is not impeded. Straps: may be crossed at wrist to reinforce extension (Rehabilitation Institute of Chicago, 1985; Malik 1979).

Following a full assessment, a long opponens splint (Figure 6.1) is made for all patients with serious cervical cord damage. Splinting should be begun immediately upon admission, certainly within 48 hours following acute admission. The orthoses should be worn 24 hours a day and should be removed both for passive range-of-motion exercises and also, importantly, to check for pressure areas every two hours when the patient is turned. Even if the severity of the injury would seem to indicate that there will be no significant neurological return

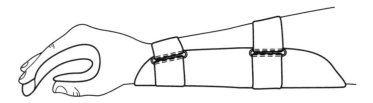

Figure 6.2 Resting splint. Fabrication: wrist – 15–30° of extension; 30–45° of MCP flexion; slight interphalangeal flexion; thumb – abduction; first MCP directly under second; leave thenar eminence clear; splint extends two-thirds up the forearm, i.e. within approximately 6 cm of elbow (Rehabilitation Institute of Chicago, 1985; Malik 1979).

to the wrist extensors or hand, the patient is given the benefit of the doubt until spinal shock has subsided.

When it is clear that no muscle function will be likely to the wrist extensors, resting pan (paddle) splints (Figure 6.2) will be made to prevent flexion contractures and joint deformities (the 'claw hand') and to maintain the normal curvature and appearance of the hand. Early orthotic fabrication provides the occupational therapist with an opportunity for contact with the patient and the beginning of an active dialogue.

Overcoming sensory deprivation

The occupational therapist will also work with the client in achieving functional communication and may use an eye-gaze board for the respirator-dependent person. The person who is treated with tongs on a Stryker frame experiences a time of severe sensory deprivation and psychological trauma, especially if he requires respiratory support which prevents him from speaking.

(The Stryker frame, which may be used to maintain alignment of the healing spine, consists of narrow anterior and posterior sections, between which the patient is confined, like a sandwich. A circular turning mechanism pivots the patient about a longitudinal axis, to allow an alternation between the supine and prone positions. Skeletal traction can be maintained while on the Stryker frame by the use of calipers inserted into the skull and the application of a traction force of several kilograms).

Visual deprivation for the patient who must alternate between a view of the ceiling and a view of the floor, with no opportunity to turn his head in any direction, may be partially overcome by the careful positioning of mirrors on stands and on the floor. Prism glasses may be used during supine lying.

Environmental control

A basic environmental control system, interfaced by eyebrow switch, tongue switches, leaf switches or pneumatic switches, will be required to allow the patient to call for help. The intensive care unit should be equipped with electronic systems to allow patients to summon assistance and these may be adapted to the needs of the high quadriplegic. If the patient is likely to be on the intensive care unit for longer than a few days the environmental control system may be used to operate an electric page turner, positioned on the floor (for prone lying), or to control a radio and television.

The occupational therapist is able to provide careful training in the use of such equipment and realistic information about what options will be available later on. A high cervical cord lesion precipitates an unexpected and abrupt change from vigorous activity and independence to a state of infantile physical dependency. This dependency is accentuated by mechanical equipment required to stabilize the spine and by any intrusive devices that provide mechanical ventilation. It is therefore essential to provide this individual with the means to control some aspects of his environment to reduce the sense of powerlessness and helplessness that may otherwise be present. Simple technological devices now exist to assist these clients and constitute a small proportion of the cost of other services provided on the intensive care unit. By provision and training in the use of basic environmental control systems, the occupational therapist has early contact with the patient in helping him to regain control over, and interaction with, his environment.

Mobility

Once the patient is permitted to progress to sitting, it is the author's belief that he should have the opportunity to be in a reclining powered wheelchair. If chairs are not available for loan, this may not be possible, as the optimal method of control or type of wheelchair will not yet have been established.

However, independent mobility provides for some degree of control over the environment and this should be initiated as early as possible.

Wheelchair sitting is started gradually, with the chair reclined and the patient sitting on a suitable cushion to provide for pressure relief in the ischial and sacral regions. If a mechanical lift has been used in transferring the patient, the lift sheet must be of the type that can be removed once the patient is in his chair, so that there is no interference with the functioning of the pressure relief cushion. If the patient requires ventilation, the bedside respirator can be used or a portable unit can be mounted under the chair.

Blood pressure should be monitored because postural hypotension is common in high cervical lesions (see Chapter 4). Due to low vasomotor tone, blood may tend to pool in the abdomen or legs, resulting in decreased blood pressure. High-quality pressure stockings and an elastic abdominal support may be worn initially to minimize this effect. The abdominal support provides additional assistance for breathing for a quadriplegic person who is seated. The reclining angle of the wheelchair may be gradually decreased if the blood pressure remains within normal parameters. The aim is to achieve 80–90° to provide for good weight distribution and upper body function.

It is of great importance – and a courtesy to the patient, to inform him, before elevation into sitting, that he is likely to feel dizzy and nauseous but that this will gradually diminish. Patients have recounted tales of experiencing nausea and blackouts, without any indication from the staff that this would not be a permanent feature of their future life. These individuals state that they felt so awful during the process of learning to sit up that they felt they would be better off to remain permanently lying down. Such needless anxieties can be relieved if it is clearly explained to the patient that he will eventually be able to sit up for very many hours at a time without experiencing any discomfort.

If the patient is unable to support his head when in a sitting position, a foam support and headrest can be used for this purpose. The arms should be supported by adjustable height armrests, a tray or arm troughs to maintain the integrity of the glenohumeral joint and prevent subluxation, stretching of muscles and pain.

Range of motion

Early in the treatment process, the therapists will assist the patient with passive and active range of motion (see Chapter 4). By strengthening the facial and neck musculature by isotonics and isometrics, the therapist prepares him for the use of control switching mechanisms, driving mechanisms for a powered wheelchair and encourages him to increase his endurance, before performing mouthstick activities.

Respiratory care

The skills of the physiotherapist or respiratory therapist will be required in the management of respiratory problems associated with high-lesion quadriplegia.

Pulmonary complications are a major factor in the morbidity and mortality of people with spinal cord injuries both in the acute period and throughout life. In view of the fact that not all people with spinal cord injuries are treated at a special unit and that many will attend their local hospitals for future care, related or not related to their spinal injury, physiotherapists in any hospital can expect to be involved in the emergency, acute or long-term respiratory care of this client group.

Clough *et al.* (1986) list the problems that lead to respiratory compromise:

- decreased inspiratory capacity
- decreased forced vital capacity
- reduced expiratory reserve volume
- inspiratory and expiratory muscle paralysis
- diminished chest wall mobility
- reduced lung compliance
- loss of an effective explosive cough
- increased energy cost in breathing
- paradoxical chest wall movement
- abnormal ventilation – perfusion relationships and loss of the sigh reflex.

Thorough and comprehensive assessment is essential before treatment is initiated.

Guidelines for respiratory rehabilitation of people with high spinal cord injuries have been described in the literature

(Clough *et al.*, 1986; Brownlee and Williams, 1987; Zejdlik, 1992). This includes:

- diaphragmatic strengthening exercises, ventilatory muscle training;
- use of an abdominal support or binder when sitting to correct the position of the diaphragm, increase tidal volume and decrease shortness of breath;
- chest mobilization to maintain compliance of the chest wall, by such methods as deep breathing (including incentive spirometry) and glossopharyngeal breathing.

To improve bronchial hygiene:

- assisted coughing by manual abdominal thrust;
- suctioning (portable suction equipment must be carried with the client at all times);
- postural drainage and position changes, especially positioning in prone if this is possible.

Carter (1989) provides a thorough outline of the choices available for ventilatory support.

If a tracheostomy is used, some form of communication must be devised. A speaking tracheostomy tube is a single, cuffed tube designed with an external airflow line. Non-verbal communication such as lip reading, communication boards, typing or computer-generated systems are laborious and do not facilitate easy communication and expression of feelings and ideas. Communication is an essential component of good treatment. Leder (1990a; 1990b) outlines specific rehabilitation techniques to provide optimal care for the ventilator-dependent person who has a tracheostomy and is cognitively intact.

If a patient uses artificial means of breathing support he must always have an Ambu-bag with him in case his portable respirator breaks down. All accompanying family members, friends or staff must know how to use this device.

Sensory and motor stimulation

The person who has sustained traumatic quadriplegia may be perceived by others as being physically frail and fragile. For this reason, physiotherapy sessions have sometimes focused more upon range-of-motion exercises, strengthening of remaining musculature, use of the tilt table and teaching transfers than upon a more vigorous activity programme. Gilinsky and McIntyre (1989) describe programmes that increase sensory and motor stimulation for this client group. These programmes provide a sense of being handled and of movement which do much to reduce the perception of fragility. This produces an important sense of bodily integration and proves to the client that his body can be touched and manipulated without discomfort to himself, or displeasure to others.

OCCUPATIONAL THERAPY

Occupational therapy, 'the art and science which utilizes the analysis and application of activities specifically related to occupational performance in the areas of self-care, productivity and leisure' (CAOT, 1991) is also a crucial service for the high quadriplegic. Through use of an assessment measure, such as the Canadian Occupational Performance Measure (COPM) (Law *et al.*, 1991), the client and therapist together determine goals, define a strategy and assess outcome. An individualized measure such as the COPM can be used in the instance of a physically dependent client to enable evaluation of his degree of control over his environment.

Self-care components of occupational performance may consist of some of the following activities.

- Personal care: directing others in satisfactory performance of toileting, washing, dressing, dental care and taking medications.
- Functional mobility: directing others in pressure relief measures, transfers in and out of the wheelchair and in and out of transportation vehicles.
- Community management: using public transportation, for example, aeroplanes, trains, special-needs transportation, taxis, arranging for services such as wheelchair repairs, shopping and dealing with money.

This is not an exhaustive list but it does indicate some of the many areas in which people with high-lesion quadriplegia may achieve independence by directing their own care.

Productivity components of occupational performance may include activities such as planning for return to employment, studying and household management activities, such as buying groceries, planning meals and directing others in home cleaning, laundry and minor repair jobs. With increased time available for leisure activities, productivity may now incorporate occupations such as painting, developing computer literacy or dealing with correspondence for a voluntary organization. **Leisure** activities may include quiet recreation such as listening to music, playing games, writing letters, reading and watching television. Active recreation and socialization are also important to consider and therapists must ensure that the client is not only able to control his own telephone and television but also able to gain access to films, restaurants, pubs, clubs, parks, religious facilities, transportation, museums, libraries, sporting venues and other social events (Law *et al.*, 1991). Hence, the site of therapeutic intervention cannot be solely the confines of an institution but must incorporate the parameters of the community and environment to which the client plans to return.

Functional activities training

The sensitivity and skills of the occupational therapist may be required in assisting the patient to recover his psychological equilibrium. The psychosocial adjustment needed following the onset of a high-lesion quadriplegia is major and although this by no means dictates that all such individuals will be depressed (see Chapter 7), mood state may effect the initial timing of a functional activities training programme.

Prolonged sensory deprivation, concomitant head injury, grieving for others who may have died in the accident that caused the quadriplegia, medications, total immobilization and severe pain may all contribute to a state in which it is difficult to assimilate new information.

Collaborative assessment by the occupational therapist and client will have determined the vocational and avocational interests of the client and this will influence the functional activity which is to be tried. Chapter 1 examined in depth the issue of establishing goals and objectives, in a collaborative partnership. Although solving problems and taking risks are inherent rights of the individual, it is suggested that the earliest activities for this particular group of clients consist of something achievable. It is important that the client be given the opportunity to succeed at the task to achieve some early sense of accomplishment in gaining a new skill.

Equipment and functional training

For any piece of equipment to be useful, it must be cost-effective, reliable and easy to use. Studies have shown that items which do not meet this criteria are discarded and no longer used following discharge. The patient's motivation to use the equipment can be aided by the positive attitude of the therapist. If the therapist has a good working knowledge of the equipment and can solve problems with the patient, this will also help to instill confidence in both the equipment to be tried and the therapist.

Mouthsticks

The item that can provide the person with high-lesion quadriplegia with the greatest access to functional activities is the mouthstick. There are many choices for design, depending upon such factors as oral dental status, range of motion and stability of the head and neck. Low vital respiratory capacity will have a detrimental effect upon endurance.

Many professionals have directed attention towards the design of mouthstick orthoses for people with severe disabilities, including dentists, occupational therapists and biomedical engineers and several useful articles can be found in the professional literature of these groups. It is important that occupational therapists involved in the provision of mouthsticks increase their knowledge of oral safety and the standards for mouthstick design which have been established by dentists.

A mouthpiece that must be held between the teeth allows for a good range of movement but produces fatigue after short periods of use. This may be the most suitable choice, however, for drawing and painting because the stick can be manipulated easily to reach a wider area. However, a mouthstick that contacts only the anterior teeth can cause oral problems, including changes in the periodontal tissue, stretching of ligaments and damage to teeth. A large stick may produce temporomandibular joint dysfunction (Smith, 1989).

If plastic is to be used to cover the end of the stick which is to be held in the mouth, it is essential that this be non-toxic. The

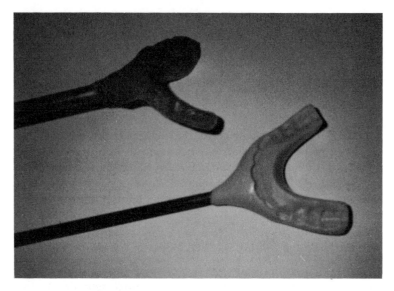

Figure 6.3   Mouthstick pieces. Constructed by a dentist, these provide for distribution of forces across several teeth but, to allow for easy access and removal, they do not cover all the lower teeth.

same is true for any adhesive used to attach the mouthpiece to the stick. A dentist will be able to advise regarding suitable, non-toxic substances.

A dental plate that fits over the bottom teeth will allow the patient to speak, breathe easily and swallow during use. It does not need to be clamped onto by the teeth and has the advantage of mobility by using jaw movements (Figure 6.3). Such mobility is not possible if a top dental plate is constructed. In the presence of a top dental plate or damage to the top teeth, a lower plate for the mouthstick is particularly recommended. This type of mouthpiece is less fatiguing for lengthy use than one which must be grasped by the teeth but it also requires more head mobility than a stick that can more easily be manoeuvred around in the mouth.

The shaft of the mouthstick needs to be strong enough for depressing switches, or pushing a game piece or book around on the lap tray, yet light enough to prevent fatigue and muscle strain. Acrylic, plastic, bamboo or fibreglass shafts have been used but these cannot be bent to suit individual requirements.

Some people prefer an angled shaft to provide enhanced visibility at the tip. Aluminium tubes have been used with good success, combining strength and lightweight with the ability to be bent. An aluminium arrow shaft (size 1816) is especially appropriate for this purpose. These are cheap to buy, or may be donated by local archery groups when they are no longer accurate enough for archery. The type of eraser that fits the end of a pencil will fit the aluminium shaft snugly, to provide friction against a page for turning.

Modular mouthsticks are available commercially, which allow the user to access different attachments, for example, pen, paint brush and turning end. Telescoping mouthsticks are also available from commercial manufacturers. These allow the user to adjust the stick to various lengths independently.

Alternatively, it is possible to construct a lightweight, telescoping mouthstick at minimal cost (Figure 6.4). This requires an aluminium arrow (size 1816) which has a lower dental plate attached by a dentist. Another, thinner aluminium tube, such as an arrow shaft (6031) is needed, which will slide into the first. Using one white, plastic, interchangeable holding tip from a commercially available mouthstick package, the smaller tube is inserted into the wider tube and locked in place using an Allen wrench (Allen key) in the holding tip. The Allen wrench is glued firmly into the threaded Allen bolt on the holding tip, using Superglue, so that the longest end of the wrench is free. The user may then push this wrench end against a fixed object to loosen the Allen wrench and the inner tube may be adjusted independently to a longer or shorter length. This allows the user tremendous freedom in determining the length of the stick which is appropriate for any given task, for example, a short stick for signing a name or for painting, medium length for turning book pages and long for turning newspaper pages.

A docking station is also necessary, where the mouthstick can be rested. No independent use of the mouthstick can be accomplished if the user cannot even access his stick! There are many possibilities, including an adjustable, angled plastic cylinder, a small broom clamp or a commercial model, which allows for several mouthstick ends to be stored in an adjustable, angled unit (Figure 6.5). The docking station may be elevated on a gooseneck, attached to a work surface or mounted on the powered wheelchair, if this is the most convenient option.

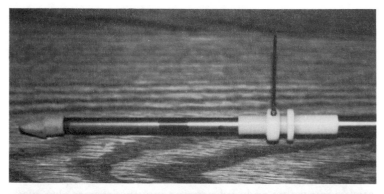

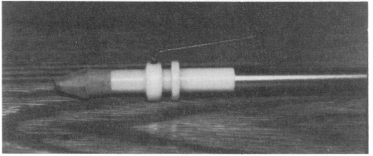

Figure 6.4 Adjustable length mouthstick constructed from two aluminium arrow shafts. (a) Extended; (b) retracted.

For specific activities, it may be worth considering commercial products such as a vacuum wand or pincher mouthstick. The vacuum wand enables the user to suck on the mouthpiece to create a vacuum at the other end. This may be suitable for fine work such as sorting stamps but requires considerable breath control. The pincher mouthstick ('bird beak') requires the user to press firmly with the tongue on a trigger which opens up a pincher on the opposite end. This is tiring for the user but is excellent for playing cards, in conjunction with a card holder (Figure 6.6). The pincher mouthstick is also useful for inserting individual sheets of paper into a typewriter or printer.

Mouthstick activities: productivity and leisure

The person with high-lesion quadriplegia who has built up sufficient musculature around the neck to stabilize the head can

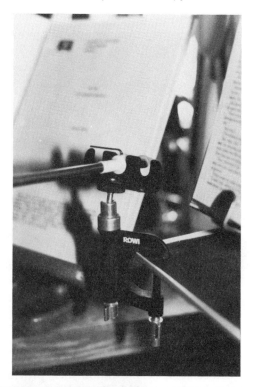

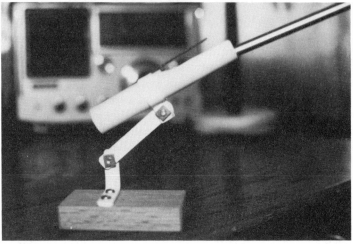

Figure 6.5 Docking station for several mouthsticks. (a) Commercial model; (b) custom-made docking station for single mouthstick.

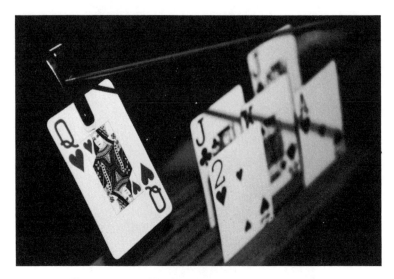

Figure 6.6   Bird beak mouthstick and card holder.

start using a mouthstick for simple activities. Turning the pages of a book elevated on a tilted book stand may be an initial objective, the eraser end of the mouthstick provides friction against the page. The page will be turned by moving the stick diagonally across the page towards the centre, while applying pressure.

Eventually, the client may wish to be able to sign his own name legibly and uniformly, for the validation of legal documents, letters or cheques but this requires great skill. Training can start with painting horizontal and vertical lines, geometric shapes and large pre-writing patterns before progressing to increasingly smaller alphabets and writing. A pen can be either held in the mouth or inserted into the end of the mouthstick shaft or holder. Each individual may wish to experiment to determine the writing instrument of choice. The user may prefer a felt-tip pen, ball-point pen or pen with a rolling ball end.

For painting or drawing, an adjustable easel will allow the client greater access to his work. Electrically driven easels are available which, although expensive, allow the user to alter the angle and position and provide greater access to a larger canvas. The person who gains good control of the mouthstick may wish

to continue to paint or draw recreationally, or perhaps to progress to painting on carved wooden pieces or ceramics. It has
been suggested that acrylic or water colour rather than oil paints
be used by people with high-lesion quadriplegia. There have
been reports of headaches and nausea in association with oil
paint use, because of the close proximity of the face to the work
plane.

Typing, word processing and computing

An electric typewriter, which has easily depressible keys, a self-
correction feature and a self-return key can be accessed using
the mouthstick. If appropriate, this can be tilted towards the
user to allow all the keys to be reached. Paper which is on a roll
can be used in the typewriter, to allow for more independence.

A more convenient tool for writing, note taking and filing is
the word processor. A computer has the considerable advan-
tages over a conventional typewriter of enabling the user to
review easily all that has already been written, store and retrieve
information entered previously, edit text with little effort and
check and correct spelling errors. Computer keys depress more
easily than those of a typewriter, hence reducing neck strain for
mouthstick users. Other methods of input to the computer are
also possible and will be discussed later in this chapter.

A keyguard may be needed by some people, to prevent the
mouthstick from skidding off the key when it is depressed.
Many different styles of these are available, to fit either type-
writers or computer keyboards.

The mouthstick may also be used to access various types of
environmental control units which have pressure pads or buttons for input. Similarly, the mouthstick is used by some individuals to adjust thermostats, control televisions, video cassette
recorders, stereo systems – either by remote control or direct
touch, dictaphones (for note taking or recording information
received over the telephone), or telephone answering machines.

With practice and perseverance, many clients with high-
lesion quadriplegia become adept at using their mouthsticks.
Some become highly skilled at drawing or painting, whereas
others learn to use theirs for such functional activities as inserting and removing floppy discs from a computer.

Communication is not limited to typing or mouthstick use.

Some people with high lesions make cassette tapes to send to their friends instead of writing letters. This is especially useful during prolonged bed rest.

Leisure activities

Exploration of satisfying leisure activities is to be viewed as an important aspect of human occupational performance and hence an important aspect of the rehabilitation process. People with high-lesion quadriplegia may have more time to enjoy satisfying leisure activities than they did previously and there are many options and opportunities for experimentation.

A simple adaptation to the mouthstick will allow it to be used for manoeuvring chessmen, draughts or mah jong tiles and these are all activities that allow for competition and socializing with friends. Playing pieces for backgammon, solitaire and dominoes can be adapted to make them easier to move using the mouthstick.

Small magnetic travel games may be used if the playing surface needs to be tipped to allow the person with high-lesion quadriplegia to reach it with his mouthstick. Electronic or computer games are available and, although removing the social element, may allow for more regular and challenging games.

Using a bird beak or pincher mouthstick, or a suck/blow vacuum wand, the client can learn to manipulate playing cards and insert or remove them from a holder.

Reading

Small newspapers may be independently accessed using a large bookstand or Posturite book ledger. These will hold the paper at a suitable height so that the pages may be turned using a mouthstick. For large-sized newspapers, large, wooden fan-shaped frames are available. The stand is hooked onto a table which is of suitable height for turning pages and reading. Even the largest size papers can be supported on these devices. It has been found that making a hole with a hole punch through the entire paper at a distance of about 3 cm from the top corner, and inserting a large, round, loose-leaf ring will enable the paper to be hung from the top of the newspaper stand. By this method the paper is held quite securely and the person with high-lesion

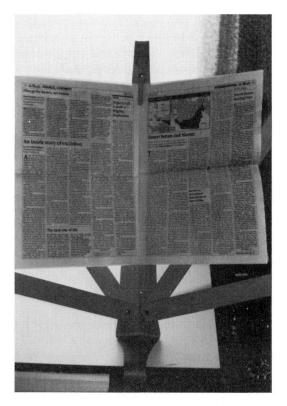

Figure 6.7 Newspaper holder.

quadriplegia who has good head mobility is able to turn the pages using a mouthstick (Figure 6.7).

There are several companies that make electric page turners for use by people with severe disabilities. These have a variety of control interfaces. Unfortunately, this still appears to be unsatisfactory technology and the ideal machine has yet to be developed. As these are expensive items of equipment, it is important to ascertain that no other method of page turning is available and that the model to be purchased has been thoroughly tested for suitability by the potential user, under the same circumstances as the intended use. The page turner should allow for various thicknesses of magazines and books (both hardback and paperback) and should ideally turn pages backwards as well as forwards, especially if it is to be used for studying. Trial should also be made to ensure that a single page will be reliably turned by the machine at all parts of the book and not just at the centre. The electric page turner may be a viable option for the person with a severe disability, especially if long periods of time are spent in bed.

Bookstands

A good bookstand is a necessity for most people with high-lesion quadriplegia and there are many excellent ones to choose from. Some are designed for the mass market, such as for supporting cookery books or work manuals and these tend to be the cheapest. Some stands are designed specifically for people with quadriplegia and are springloaded to hold the book securely in place. These are suited to both hardbacks and paper-backs. The pages may be easily turned using the mouthstick.

Cassette tape books

A large number and variety of books are now available on cassette tape and these may be especially enjoyed by people who spend much time in bed. Many cassette recorders and stereo systems have easy touch buttons that may be operated using a mouthstick. Alternatively, an environmental control unit may be used to control the functions of the cassette player.

Photography

Devices are available to allow someone with high-lesion quadri-plegia to operate an electronic camera. This may be mounted on a tripod that stands on the lap tray, or alternatively, a mobile arm can be mounted on to the side of the wheelchair.

Spotting scope

If the person with high-lesion quadriplegia is interested in bird-watching, horse racing or some other activity that normally requires binoculars, he may wish to consider mounting a spotting telescope on a camera tripod. Many models of both telescope or tripod are available and some tripods will allow the user to move the instrument from side to side and tilt it up and down. Minor modification may enable independent adjustment of focus, provided this is located on the proximal end of the scope.

Hunting, shooting and fishing

In the USA, hunting rifles have been modified to enable a person with high-lesion quadriplegia to use a mouthpiece to control movement of a rifle from side to side and up and down. The gun fires when the user sips on a vacuum tube. These adaptations have been used to enable target shooting in addition to trophy hunting.

Fishing equipment has also been adapted successfully to enable people with high-lesion quadriplegia to operate a rod with a combination of chin and pneumatic controls.

Remote control vehicles

A simple joystick control, manipulated by the mouth or chin can be used to operate remote control vehicles such as yachts or cars. In places where races for yachts are held, for example, the person with quadriplegia is able to compete at an outdoor activity alongside his able-bodied peers.

Music

Playing the mouth organ (harmonica) may be an option for some people and this may additionally constitute a form of incentive spirometry! Music stores sell the self-supporting harness for the mouth organ, as these are also used by guitarists whose hands are not available to hold the instrument. Computer-generated music is becoming an increasingly viable option.

Blow darts

Several leisure activities have already been outlined with regard to mouthstick use. Many leisure occupations tend to be cognitively oriented, for example, reading and playing draughts and chess. Other typical forms of entertainment for people with high-lesion quadriplegia tend to be visual – spectator sports, films and the theatre – but there are few outlets for competitive physical activities.

Batavia (1987) has discussed the merits of using a short blow gun for target shooting darts. This requires some respiratory exertion and may not, therefore, be suitable for those with severely compromised respiratory systems. However, for those who have active diaphragms, the physical exertion may help to increase respiratory strength.

If there is a fear of injury from the darts, Velcro darts can be used in their place. This is an inexpensive form of recreation and may allow for some expression of the competitive drive which has been typical of this client group.

SELF-CARE: PERSONAL CARE

Drinking

Drinking is one self-care activity that may still be performed at the client's pace and convenience.

The wheelchair bracket and distal arm of a mobile arm support may be attached to the wheelchair at shoulder height and a round wooden box with a centre pivot constructed to fit on to this. The box holds a cup or can securely and eliminates the risk of spills. A small piece can be cut out of one side to accommodate the handle of a cup (Figure 6.8).

Using a disposable, bendable, plastic straw suitable for both hot and cold liquids, the client with no function in his arms will be able to gain easy access to his drink and consume this at his own speed. The drink will not spill even if the chair is being driven, as long as the terrain is fairly smooth.

Many people who have sustained a spinal cord injury require a high level of liquids during the day to maintain their health. To provide for more independence in gaining access to a drink, a long gooseneck can be used (Figure 6.9). With a clamp on one end to secure it to a table, the gooseneck can be directed towards the client, where he can reach it easily. A thin vinyl tube runs up the centre of the gooseneck and is placed in a jug of water. The user sucks on the other end of the tubing to draw the water into his mouth. A strong amount of suction is required initially to draw the water up the tube but, once it is flowing, it is little

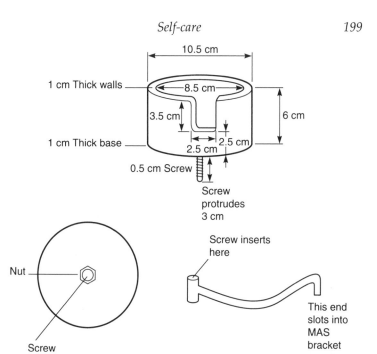

(a)

(b)

Figure 6.8 Drink box (designed by the author). (a) Construction; (b) in use.

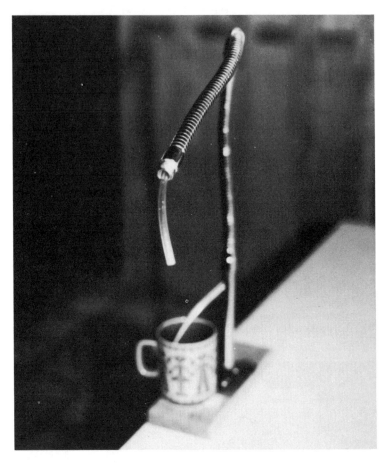

Figure 6.9 Gooseneck and straw.

effort to continue drinking. The vinyl tubing is removable for cleaning and replacement. The apparatus provides for independent access to a drink, both from the wheelchair and in bed.

Self-feeding

Another personal care activity which may be considered is self-feeding with the use of **mobile arm supports** (MAS; formerly termed 'ball bearing feeders' or 'balanced forearm orthoses').

The MAS needs to be installed by a skilled and experienced clinician and is suitable only for the highly motivated user, as much adjustment and training is required in the early stages.

Physical requirements are as follows. The client must have stability and endurance in sitting, be able to co-ordinate the contraction and relaxation of innervated muscles at will and have little or no upper extremity spasticity. He needs to have fundamental control of shoulder movement patterns and a small degree of elbow flexor sparing.

However, given the above prerequisites, which may be met by some individuals with C4 quadriplegia, the MAS can provide for independence in a key area of daily living. It is not necessary to outline here the fitting and training for the MAS, as this has been well covered by Wilson *et al.* (1974), Thenn (1975) and Trombly (1983).

The MAS is used in conjunction with a scoop dish or plate guard, a Dycem friction mat to stabilize the plate and possibly a raised platform to bring the plate up to a suitable level.

Swivel cutlery is also used. Initially, a spoon is used during training but a spork or fork may be preferred once the basic technique has been mastered.

In the early stage of training the user may have problems in retrieving food from all parts of the plate. With practice and increased muscle strength and co-ordination, however, it is possible to choose food types from every part of the plate and thus derive greater satisfaction and pleasure from the dining experience.

In this, as in all other care activities, it is essential that the client be able to instruct others in donning the MAS. The use of mirrors during the training and adjustment process enables the client to participate actively when modifications are being made, to solve problems and to develop an awareness of the location of the various components and their relationships to each other.

The mobile arm support is designed for use by people with a variety of medical diagnoses which affect the upper body. Problems may arise when the device is used for people with high-lesion quadriplegia, as the arm trough is only 254 mm or less in length and this will be insufficient to support the hand and wrist. A T-bar addition is available from manufacturers but this alone will not support a completely denervated wrist. To overcome this problem, an adapted design uses a custom-

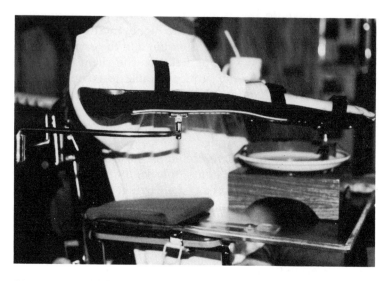

Figure 6.10   Mobile arm support. Commercial hardware and custom-made arm trough to support flaccid wrist and hand (see Whalley, 1981).

moulded plastic arm trough for a client with long arms, weak elbow flexors and absent wrist extensors (Whalley, 1981). This plastic trough extends from finger tips to elbow and replaces the manufacturer's short forearm trough (Figure 6.10). This appliance has been used satisfactorily for a decade but can be replaced by a thermoplastic trough formed by an orthotist, to a cast of the client's arm. Such an orthosis makes mobile arm supports available to a client group who would otherwise be unable to feed themselves. However, it must be emphasised that considerable experience is required to fit, adjust and adapt mobile arm supports and technical support from a prosthetic/ orthotic department may be required.

The mobile arm support bracket is designed for use on wheelchair tubing of 22 mm diameter. The bracket may need to be adjusted or longer bolts used, if the tubing is fatter than 22 mm. Alterations to the seatback upholstery may also be necessary to allow the bracket to be fixed to the chair at a suitable height.

It is unlikely that people with high-lesion quadriplegia will be able to use this equipment for other functional activities, as they tend to experience fatigue after using the MAS for feeding.

FUNCTIONAL MOBILITY: WHEELCHAIRS

The choice of a suitable wheelchair is one of the most crucial elements in providing independence to someone with high-lesion quadriplegia.

A manual wheelchair is required as a back-up chair and for ease of transportation. This will need a semi-reclining or full-reclining back because of the lack of postural musculature available to maintain a stable, upright posture. Sling seats are unsuitable and incompatible with good pressure relief and posture. A removable headrest will be needed, especially if the user is tall. Adjustable height armrests are usually necessary to protect the vulnerable shoulder joint. Full-length armrests may be used in conjunction with moulded arm troughs, which support the arm, maintain the hand and wrist in good position and help in maintaining good posture and balance.

Legrests should also be of the elevating type and may combine H-straps, heel and/or toe straps to control spasms and preserve good posture. (If the user buys his trousers with leg lengths of about 8 cm more than he did when he was standing, these will sit nicely down over the feet and cover these additions to the footrests).

The manufacturers of ultra-lightweight and sports chairs have developed lightweight wheelchairs which will either tilt or fully recline (Figure 6.11). These chairs are considerably easier to manoeuvre than traditional models. Their light weight makes transportation and lifting of the chair much less hazardous for an attendant. The recliner folds for enhanced portability.

A lap board (tray) will usually be required for both the manual and powered wheelchair, especially if arm troughs are not used, if the client plans to use a mobile arm support for self-feeding or wishes to perform activities with a mouthstick at close range. A clear Plexiglass tray, securely fastened to the wheelchair (using rubber O-rings and a D-ring) is preferable because this allows a view of the feet when driving. This also helps the client to overcome sensory deprivation and presents less of a barrier between the client and other people.

An Obus or Jay back support cushion may be required to maintain excellent alignment of the spine and support the trunk, especially in tall individuals. Slingback upholstery is not

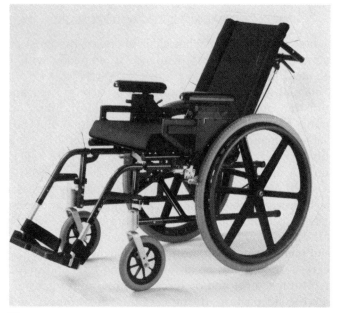

(a)

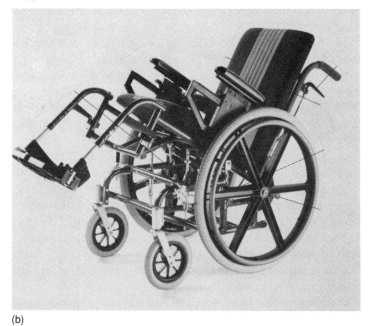

(b)

Figure 6.11 (a) Quickie recliner wheelchair; (b) Quickie tilt wheelchair.

suitable. More sophisticated custom-made means of support may be required by some people.

A chest strap is required, especially if travelling in a vehicle.

Cushions

An excellent cushion is required for pressure relief. The choice of cushion may depend upon factors such as allergies (e.g to foam), flaccidity, spasticity, amount of perspiration and seated stability.

For the majority of people with high-lesion quadriplegia who are unable to perform their own weight shift, a soft cushion is required to enable them to sit for long periods of time. The high-profile ROHO is often chosen, as this does not absorb moisture, is washable, does not promote perspiration in most people and allows for extended periods of sitting. Most high-level quadriplegics will require either a high-profile or Enhancer cushion. Its inherent lack of lateral stability – a problem for paraplegics, is unlikely to be a problem for this client group. Use of the Enhancer cushion increases lateral support because of the variety of height of the air cells. However, there is certainly no one optimal cushion that can be universally prescribed for all clients with spinal cord injuries and the Jay cushion, in particular, has high user acceptability (see Chapter 5).

Powered wheelchairs

Powered wheelchairs are the current focus for development of many manufacturers and there are several new designs and innovations on the market, some tried and tested, some still subject to critical flaws and problems. Some of the most promising new developments in powered chairs are by the manufacturers of lightweight wheelchairs. These smart, new powered chairs combine all the new innovations with increased speed, enhanced control, yet no loss of manoeuvrability.

In Britain, some powered chairs have been designated 'indoor' or 'outdoor' and have been supplied to be used according to those descriptions. With the advent of more modern, compact wheelchair designs over the past two decades, such designations are largely redundant and someone who requires a powered wheelchair can use this both inside and outside. For someone who is dependent upon a powered chair for mobility, it is clearly impractical to change chairs upon entering or leaving a building – and the costs involved would be prohibitive. Manoeuvrability of many powered wheelchairs is excellent and this has provided the opportunity for enhanced community access and independence.

Some companies in North America and Scandinavia have experimented with a power-based chair which has a modular base, separate seating systems and four small wheels. The low centre of gravity makes it difficult for an attendant to assist in turning the chair should difficulties arise and it is generally unsuitable for mounting ventilatory equipment – this has to be placed behind the chair, thus increasing its length and the space required to turn the chair. The seating surface is more unstable than the conventional chair design due to the single centre-post mount and can therefore increase postural instability. Some concerns have been expressed by disabled people's transit systems because of the problems involved in securing these chairs in the event of an accident.

New models of powered chairs now have direct drive systems on a more conventional frame design and provide power without the use of belts. Microcomputer controls allow acceleration speed and joystick sensitivity to be pre-programmed. In addition, these new chairs allow different sizes of ventilator trays to be fitted and have environmental control interfaces.

It is essential that trial be made to ensure that the powered wheelchair of choice is suitable for the mode of transportation available.

Powered wheelchair frames may be provided with a semi-reclining backrest. This is necessary for the majority of people with high-lesion quadriplegia who experience respiratory insufficiency or tend to fall or slouch forwards if they sit at a 90° angle. Some individuals will only have the backrest reclined a few degrees but this will be sufficient to provide stability in sitting.

A powered reclining mechanism is an option on many chairs and allows the user independently to adjust his position. This may be advantageous to those with cardiopulmonary difficulties but it may also trigger spasms, thus causing the user to misplace his control mechanism. Shearing will occur as the chair is moved from a right angle to a full recline and this may cause wrinkling of clothes and subsequent pressure problems. Newer chairs have anti-shear features for powered recline but some degree of shear will still be inevitable and may be a problem. Powered reclining chairs must have legrests that will elevate at the same time to provide some protection from the shearing process.

Options on the modern powered chairs (of both frame types) include an automatic tilt feature, whereby the user can independently tip the chair back on its frame to relieve pressure. This may be of especial benefit to someone with reduced respiratory function or who is respirator-dependent, as the change of position can facilitate breathing. The shear factors, which may preclude auto-reclining features, will not be as evident with tilting.

The physiological benefits of user-operated tilt and recline mechanisms include increased sitting tolerance, pressure alteration, enhanced breathing and the subsequent reduced requirement for attendant care. More important is the increase in independence achieved when someone can adjust their own position and achieve greater comfort without help.

Some chairs also offer an automatic braking mechanism. However, it is important to test out a chair under normal conditions of use, as on some models every additional feature (including braking) that requires additional drawing of power from the batteries will result in a corresponding reduction in the hours that the chair can be used. Examples have been given in which the chair can no longer be driven all day on a charge because of the increased drag on the battery potential. Clearly, this does not provide for enhanced independence but the exact reverse and may be a significant detriment to the active user.

It should also be noted that, if a portable respirator is required, it must have its own separate battery system. It must not be run from the wheelchair batteries.

Control options

The control device for many powered wheelchairs may also be used to activate an environmental control system.

The person with high-lesion quadriplegia has several control options and should be given the opportunity to test each one to make an informed decision before a wheelchair is ordered.

In the USA, pneumatic control is frequently used. This

interface activates a microswitch system. Control of the chair requires no active head movement and the chair can still be operated from a reclined position.

Proportional controls provide the best manoeuvrability of the chair and can be activated by a chin control. (The chin control can be proportional or non-proportional). The chin control is common in the UK but has the combined disadvantages of poor head/neck posture when driving and an unsightly and obtrusive barrier close to the face which may inhibit social interaction.

The Canadian head rim control provides proportional control with the use of a small active range of motion of the head. The device is unobtrusive and does not need to be moved for eating, drinking or conversing.

The presence of severe flexor or extensor spasms and the risk of fainting and falling either forwards or backwards may influence the selection of either the chin or head rim controls. It may not be possible for the user to operate these controls if he is in a fully reclined position.

The on/off and forward/reverse switches can be activated using shoulder shrug or by tilting the head to operate cheek leaf-switches.

Microswitches have been incorporated into headrests to provide a head-controlled switching system. This allows for selection of desired speed and of environmental control interface but is not as immediately responsive as the proportional control. Thus, turning spaces may be larger and there is no opportunity for spontaneous movement, as is the case with proportional control systems.

It is possible, in addition, to have an attendant-controlled switching mechanism.

After examining the various options, the selection of a chair depends upon client choice, motor function, spasticity, respiratory status, susceptibility to sores, functional activity and perception. Cost may, unfortunately, also be a limiting factor in the selection of this piece of equipment, proving, again, that handicap is not solely a product of an impairment but of the barriers which prevent achievement of full potential.

The choice of a control mechanism also depends upon where the chair is to be used, the level of function and awareness of safety. Finally, the acceptability of the control to the user is the most important factor.

The powered wheelchair allows the person with high-lesion quadriplegia to achieve independence in functional mobility and restores some measure of control over the environment. Sadly, the cost of these chairs has prohibited their use by many individuals who do not enjoy the benefits of being members of supportive societies which place a high value upon human rights and healthcare. Lathem *et al.* (1985) estimated that 51% of people with C1–C4 quadriplegia did not receive any form of powered wheelchair when they were discharged from their spinal centres in the USA – this despite being members of the richest society in the world but one which, in 1993, still provides no health insurance for an estimated 37 million of its citizens.

ENVIRONMENTAL CONTROL SYSTEMS: SELF-CARE, PRODUCTIVITY AND LEISURE

The development of the environmental control system (ECS) has done more than anything else to allow the severely disabled person to regain privacy, control over the environment and interaction with the environment. Studies suggest that ECS users are more active, independent and spend more time engaged in educational activities than non-users. The provision of these essential pieces of equipment may help to reduce the costs of staffing and personal care attendants and leads to enhanced relationships between the client and his care providers, increased physical and psychological independence and employment opportunities for some individuals.

The ECS consists of four elements:

- input switch
- control unit
- feedback (auditory or visual)
- appliances.

The system may also be accessed from a wheelchair control, by single or dual switches, by a computer or by voice.

The positioning and type of switch vary according to the individual's needs, abilities and preferences, range of motion and accuracy. There is a large selection of switches that may be tested to assess individual suitability. These include: rocker, dual button chin, lever, pneumatic, pillow, cylindrical, tongue, eyebrow and voice. Some of these switches may be activated by the smallest degree of controlled movement. The switch can be mounted on a gooseneck or angle arm to provide for easy access.

Appliances/functions

Virtually any electrical appliance may be activated using an environmental control system. The most common uses are:

- operating the functions of an electric hospital bed. By raising or lowering the head of the bed, the person with quadriplegia may initiate spasms which will help to relieve pressure and thus provide for enhanced independence;
- using an emergency call system, especially important for people who are respirator-dependent, and while the client is still on the intensive care unit;
- operating a fan;
- turning a radio on and off, adjusting the volume and tuning;
- turning a television on and off, adjusting volume, changing channels. A satellite dish may also be controlled – turned, tuned and adjusted for horizontal/vertical polarity;
- using an intercom;
- telephone dialling, placing and receiving of calls, re-dialling and number storage;
- dictaphone playing, recording and rewinding.
- drawing curtains;
- using the ECS to operate a computer (including printer) or vice versa;
- opening doors;
- turning pages with an electrical device;
- operating light switches and dimmers;
- playing a stereo, including all functions of a modern system – CD player, dual cassette player – rewind, fast forward, play, record and auto-reverse, radio (all functions) and record player;
- operating heating controls;
- adjusting air conditioning;
- using a video cassette recorder (VCR), including all functions – record, play, rewind, fast forward etc.

There is a tremendous range of choices and prices among ECSs and it is essential that these be thoroughly investigated and their options be given careful consideration. Choice may depend upon the need for visual or auditory feedback. Some of the original systems have been upgraded but not sufficiently to allow for a wide variety of electrical gadgetry – all the functions of a VCR, for example. It is important to consider carefully any future use the client may have for his ECS and whether the unit can really be expanded to meet these needs. Medical diagnosis alone does not determine candidacy for an ECS. Each individual will need a full functional assessment (range of motion, strength, endurance, sensation, co-ordination, visual/aural perception), a needs assessment and an assessment of the unique environment where the ECS is to be used (Dickey and Shealey, 1987).

It is of the utmost importance that every time the client is turned or undergoes a nursing or care procedure, the switch is returned to a position where it can be reached.

The ECS may be operated from any room, from the wheelchair control itself, or via a control system mounted on the chair. Several units are available which are portable and can therefore be taken to another building. Some basic and economical systems can be purchased from electrical dealerships. These consist of a power control box and individual X10 modules, which are attached to appliances throughout the house and operate on electrical frequencies. Others allow control over electrical appliances in the home by vocal command. More than one input can be located in the home so that the user can control his appliances from his bed, or in any room, from his wheelchair.

A cheaper and more flexible system may be achieved by combining compatible elements from different systems. For example, electrical devices listed above may be controlled via a programmable infrared control (for example the TASH Relax, 95 mm–190 mm) which may be interfaced with an X10 control-type module receiver (Figure 6.12). This system can be operated by any single input switching system. The infrared control can be easily programmed by the user to control any infrared remote device. An individual user could have a push-button remote controller in one room (for use with a mouthstick), a pneumatic control for access from a wheelchair in the bedroom and another pneumatic control positioned for use in bed. Every one of the 17 functions (and more) listed above can be operated, the modules can be controlled via the computer and most importantly,

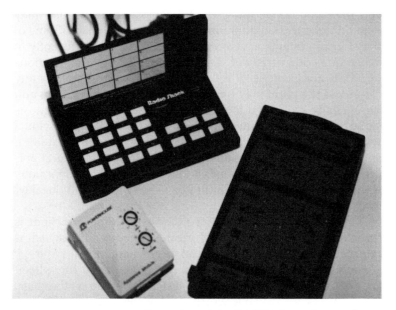

Figure 6.12   X10 controller and module, TASH infra-red controller.

because this is not all obtained from a specialized company, the whole system, in 1994, costs about £500 (US$730 or C$1000). This sort of combination of commercially available technology is clearly far cheaper and more flexible than even the cheapest modular unit available from companies which deal solely with equipment for people with disabilities.

The provision of an ECS is essential in allowing the severely disabled individual to have some independence and safety, while also allowing privacy and positive interaction with the environment.

Training

There should be proper orientation to the ECS equipment to ensure full acceptance and use. Family and care givers should also be oriented as to its functions and potential and involved with the client in solving problems. Each component should be explained, examined and fully tested. Periodic re-evaluation of use is also recommended because switches may be inappropriate or positioning inadequate. The aim of the training for and the provision of the ECS is to provide the client with maximum independence and the care giver with maximum relief.

TELEPHONES

The telephone is a vital link between the patient and his family and friends, in addition to his business, financial and social contacts. It can be accessed via the computer or ECS, using a hands-free or speaker telephone.

Some institutions in Canada have a small room with a pressure-sensitive floor pad. When a wheelchair rolls onto the pad, a speaker telephone automatically turns on and connects the user to the switchboard operator. The operator will place the call for the client, who communicates via the speaker telephone.

Less sophisticated options are also available. Hands-free speaker telephones are economical and can be operated using a mouthstick, as can automatic dialling units and answering machines. The receiver can be mounted on a gooseneck, if this provides more privacy for the user. The new cellular telephone technology has provided portable telephones that are voice-activated and hands-free. These telephones can be pre-programmed to dial a selection of numbers automatically on a one-word command, or to be answered on command.

COMPUTERS: PRODUCTIVITY AND LEISURE

Advances in computer technology have allowed people with severe disabilities to participate equally with able-bodied people, and have presented them with options and opportunities previously unrealized.

Voice control of the computer is a form of input that is being developed by many researchers. Reports of success in achieving a fast, accurate and reliable method of input by voice control tend to vary. Although there are still some problems in achieving consistent performance at the present time, this is undoubtedly a promising area. Choice of a voice-controlled system will depend upon factors such as background noise, voice consistency, software compatibility, voice amplitude and required range of vocabulary. With current equipment, it is possible that the ventilator-user may not achieve a consistent enough voice tone for successful operation. However, input options such as eye-gaze or speech recognition are likely to be the way of the future. Unfortunately, costs are currently prohibitive, although there are several other methods of input from which to choose.

An ultrasonic headset (Headmaster) enables the user to operate any standard programme on some models of computer, in addition to an ECS. Movements of the head control a pointer on the screen and selection is made by blowing into a tube which is attached to the headset and curved towards the user's mouth. For word processing, a keyboard layout is displayed on part of the computer screen. There is the inherent disadvantage that the user cannot don or doff the headset without help and this precludes spontaneous use of the computer.

If the client wishes to use his mouthstick to activate the keyboard, there are various options to enable more than one key to be struck at once. One solution is to attach key on/off switches to the keyboard and another is to install one of the several excellent software programmes which removes the requirement to hold down more than one key at a time.

To reduce the amount of head movement required to key punch using a mouthstick, ergonomic keyboards are commercially available. In these systems, the keys used most frequently are nearest the centre of the small board and those least used are around the edge. The keyboard is curved slightly (concave) to allow all the keys to be operated. The shift and control keys will latch automatically. This type of keyboard may present less neck strain than the usual 'qwerty' board.

An interfacing scanning system may be used and can be accessed using a pneumatic switch, brow switch or several other alternatives already mentioned as methods of activating an ECS.

If the user has good cognitive abilities, a pneumatic device mounted on a gooseneck can directly operate the computer using military Morse code. This coding system has been enlarged to include all punctuation marks and all the function keys of the computer. Clients who use this option are able to touch-type while reading a document (unlike the mouthstick or headset user). They are also able to achieve great speed and accuracy and avoid the problems of neck and eye strain associated with headset or mouthstick use. There are optional speeds for input. The switch cable attaches to the computer via the joystick, parallel or serial port.

Several options allow the user to access the computer from

bed, which is essential if he is prone to sores, infection or has poor sitting tolerance.

Whether the individual wishes to write letters or poetry, play games or write music, run a business or balance his cheque book, the computer presents both options and opportunities. These opportunities must be fully explored or the client may be tempted to dismiss the computer as not relevant to his goals without having first understood its potential.

To facilitate learning of the new technology, the functions of the computer and the full scope of its potential, it is essential that the client be provided with a knowledgeable instructor. This could be his therapist, or perhaps a university student or other interested person who is fully computer literate and can explore with the client the potential and the available programmes.

Computer technology can be daunting to people who have not learned to apply it but to the person with high-lesion quadriplegia it can be the key to a wealth of opportunities and the chance to compete equally with able-bodied people.

WORKSTATIONS

With all the equipment available to the person with high-lesion quadriplegia, it is essential that his workstation be designed to allow him easy access.

Many designs of worktable are available but the client and therapist may collaborate to re-design or modify these to suit individual requirements. If a commercially available table is to be used, this must be high enough and wide enough to allow the wheelchair to fit underneath. If there is a crossbar to support the table legs, this must not be in a position likely to cause pressure on the legs of the client. If the crossbar or strut is very low it may interfere with the legrests of the chair. The table will need to be high if it is used to gain access with a mouthstick.

Large, rotating tables are available to allow for access to, for example, a calculator, dictaphone or bookstand. The rotating part of the table can be moved using a mouthstick. Smaller turntables can be used to give access to two or more items of equipment. A rotating, four-sided bookstand may be of especial use for students. The type of radial arm designed to support a computer monitor may be used for mounting a bookstand. The angle and position of this is adjustable and the platform is large enough to hold two bookstands, back to back. This may be rotated using a mouthstick. Such a device can also enable the user to read in bed. Adjustable height workstations, mounted on castors may enable a client to access all his equipment from bed.

Electronically controlled office components may enhance independence for people with severe disabilities. Such devices allow the user independently to open mail, access files, store and retrieve books and staple papers. These developments may be prohibitively expensive for many people but do allow someone to work more independently with less reliance upon a carer or co-worker.

ROBOTICS

Technological advances have allowed people with high-lesion quadriplegia to communicate and to be mobile. Attention is now focused upon the ability to manipulate, using robotics. There appear to be two main objectives. One is to provide assistance at a stationary workstation, performing repetitive, programmed movements, such as passing a cup of coffee, selecting files, taking pages out of a printer or turning the pages of a book. These lightweight arms will perform repeat pre-programmed tasks.

Another focus of attention is upon designing a unit that is not confined to one area and can be directly controlled by voice recognition. A wheelchair-mounted system may be the most practical but any system that is to be of benefit must be cheap and available to many people. This may prove to be the hardest goal to meet.

This chapter does not constitute an exhaustive study of the options for engagement in occupation by people with high-lesion spinal cord injuries – just some of the possibilities. People are researching such possibilities as music synthesizers and computer-generated art and design. Each individual will be able to do his own investigation into areas not currently envisioned.

COMMUNITY RE-ENTRY AND COMMUNITY MANAGEMENT

Chapter 5 included a more detailed study of how rehabilitation staff can assist the person with a spinal cord injury in learning to access community resources and successfully re-enter the community in an altered physical form. Brief mention will be made here regarding the special circumstances of people with high lesions.

The first barrier may be the expectation of the staff that high-lesion quadriplegia requires institutional living. In many societies community living is regarded as the norm for respirator-dependent quadriplegic people, rather than the exception. Living with family, friends or care givers provides enhanced quality of life, choice and consumer control at less cost (Laurie *et al.*, 1989; Colgan, 1989). It must again be emphasized that the responsibilities of the rehabilitation team do not stop at the door of the institution but must incorporate the parameters of the client's environment – not the professional's.

Following extended hospitalization, the client who has sustained a traumatic, high-lesion quadriplegia prepares to re-enter the community with a dramatic alteration in his physical ability to meet the challenges that the community poses.

During the rehabilitation process, the person with high-lesion quadriplegia must have learned how to give direction to his companions or care givers on how to help him with his care needs. It is the client himself who must become ultimately responsible for his own care. He must particularly be able to identify the earliest signs of autonomic hyperreflexia, as this is a potentially life-threatening emergency, and he must be able to instruct clearly whoever is at hand to help him (see Chapter 4).

Early trial visits out into the community, accompanied by members of staff and other clients help the individual to overcome his initial fears and increase his sense of competence and self-esteem. At the same time, these visits prepare the client for some of the physical and social barriers that must be confronted. Initially facing attitudinal and architectural barriers with others who can assist, helps to prepare the client in becoming more independent. In having his care needs met, he will have to be both assertive and considerate of the needs of others who may accompany him. This is an instance where peer learning (Chapter 2) may be especially appropriate. The newly injured person can learn much about how to handle problems in the community by accompanying someone who has been living in the community for some time since their injury. This can also be a valuable learning experience for the therapist.

The client is expected to take the lead in the planning and implementation of these visits. Mutual collaboration of therapist and client may produce a list of objectives for a visit, or choice of location but it is the client who must assume responsibility for telephoning in advance to check for accessibility, ordering transportation and arranging to have catheterizations or medications timed to suit the outing. These are normal, independent adult behaviours and responsibilities and these decision-making and problem-solving abilities must be enhanced by the rehabilitation process, not eliminated. On completion of the activity in the community, the client should be able to demonstrate:

- planning skills for self-care and safety
- creative problem solving
- mobility skills
- most importantly, reflection, self-evaluation and suggestions for alternative future actions.

Visits may include many of the places that the client will want to go following discharge to the community or where someone who is not respirator-dependent may wish to go alone while resident in a hospital or young disabled unit. These may include shopping for groceries or clothes, the use of accessible public transport, including aeroplanes, visiting nightclubs and restaurants, attending sporting events, the theatre, hairdresser, educational facilities or public houses. This also helps to expand the awareness of leisure and recreational activities which are available in the community – both for the client and his therapist.

The therapists and social workers will have an important role to play in home visiting before discharge and liaising with community support services in facilitating this transition. If the client is preparing to live with his family, back up and respite services should be routinely offered as part of a comprehensive care plan. Families should not have to apologize for requesting respite care.

The person with high-lesion quadriplegia will have other skills to learn. If he is hiring care givers, he will need to be able to advertise, to interview, to train and to arrange for payment. The care givers will need to be able to perform a transfer without a lift or hoist, as there may be times when one is not available, for example, when travelling or on admission to an acute care facility. He will need household management skills – planning meals, buying groceries, directing others in minor repairs or cleaning tasks. From others who are in a similar situation he can learn new forms of communication. Unable to gesture with his hands for expression, he may use facial expression and other forms of body language. Unable to touch another person to enhance meaning he may learn to be more vocal, more demonstrative and more expressive. DiPasquale (1986) outlines a successful group programme for people with high-lesion quadriplegia. This consists of education regarding self-care, health and leisure activities involving a multi-disciplinary approach and including group exercises.

EMPLOYMENT

Glass and colleagues (1991, unpublished) reported on a collaborative venture between a spinal unit and a local college. Seven people with high-lesion quadriplegia undertook training with accessible computer systems in word processing, databases, spreadsheets, desktop publishing, computer-aided design and other electronic media. At the time of the report, four of these people were employed, two were in college or undertaking further studies and one person had decided that computers were not for him.

The client may have gained some marketable vocational skills during his occupational therapy programme which he can enhance following discharge. Giving clear verbal instructions, typing and word processing, using a computer and calculator and using a dictaphone for recording messages and dictating letters have enabled some individuals to return successfully to the workforce. Western societies value independence and productivity but frequently deny people with disabilities the opportunities to achieve these goals. Opportunities will usually be dependent upon the level of education which has been attained. The brilliant English scientist, Professor Stephen Hawking, is a famous example of what can be achieved by a fine mind – and a supportive environment.

This is an age when technological advancements have provided the tools which allow for a level of independence that could not have been imagined only a decade ago. It is now imperative that all involved in the rehabilitation of people with high-lesion quadriplegia – from whatever cause – work to ensure that this technology is available to everyone who requires it, and that a supportive environment is created which allows for full integration into the community of all people with disabilities, in accordance with the United Nation's resolution (34/154, para 1, 17 December 1979), calling for 'full participation and equality' for people with disabilities.

It is especially encumbent on the occupational therapist entrusted with the rehabilitation of these individuals to assist them in maximizing their opportunities, harnessing technological options and ensuring that the person with high-lesion quadriplegia has the opportunity to explore his possibilities for achieving a greater quality and not just quantity of life.

ACKNOWLEDGEMENT

Much of this chapter is based upon Whalley Hammell (1991) and is reproduced with permission.

REFERENCES

Bach, J.R. (1991) Alternative methods of ventilatory support for the patient with ventilatory failure due to spinal cord injury *Journal of the American Paraplegia Society*, **14**(4), 158–74.

Batavia, A.I. (1987) Blowdarts. *Paraplegia News*, October, p. 43.

Brownlee, S. and Williams, S. (1987) Physiotherapy in the respiratory care of patients with high spinal injury *Physiotherapy*, **73**(3), 148–52.

Burnham, L. and Werner, G. (1979) The high level tetraplegic: psychological survival and adjustment. *International Journal of Paraplegia*, **16**, 184–92.

CAOT (1991) *Occupational Therapy Guidelines for Client Centred Intervention*, Canadian Association of Occupational Therapists and Health Services Directorate, Health Services Promotion Branch, Health and Welfare Canada, Toronto, Ont., p. 140.

Carter, R.E. (1989) Available respiratory options, in *Management of High Quadriplegia*, (eds G.G. Whiteneck, C. Adler, R.E. Carter *et al.*) Demos, New York, NY, pp. 149–72.

Clark, B. (1978) *Whose Life is it Anyway?* Amber Lane Press, Charlbury, Oxford.

Clough, P., Lindenhaur, D., Hayes, J. and Zekarny, B. (1986) Guidelines for routine respiratory care of patients with spinal cord injury. *Physical Therapy*, **66**(9), 1395–402.

Colgan, M. (1989) *Breathing Easy: a Guide for Ventilator Dependent Individuals Moving into the Community*, Independent Living Resource Centre, Winnipeg, Man.

Dickey, R. and Shealey, S.H. (1987) Using technology to control the environment. *American Journal of Occupational Therapy*, **41**(11), 717–21.

DiPasquale, P. (1986) Exhaler class – a multidisciplinary program for high quadriplegic patients. *American Journal of Occupational Therapy*, **40**(7), 482–510.

Gilinsky, G. and McIntyre, J. (1989) Occupational and physical therapy, in *Management of High Quadriplegia*, (eds G.G. Whiteneck, C. Adler, R.E. Carter *et al.*), Demos, New York, NY, pp. 198–200.

Glass, C.A. (1993) The impact of home based ventilator dependence on family life. *Paraplegia*, **31**, 93–101.

Kielhofner, G. (1993) Functional assessment: toward a dialectical view of person–environment relations. *American Journal of Occupational Therapy*, **47**(3), 248–51.

Kirby, N. (1989) The individual with high quadriplegia. *Nursing Clinics of North America*, **24**(1), 179–91.

Krishnan, K.R. and Watt, J.W.H. (1993) Ventilator dependence and high tetraplegia (editorial). *Paraplegia*, **31**(3), 141–2.

Lathem, P., Gregorio, T. and Garber, S.L. (1985) High level quadriplegia – an occupational therapy challenge. *American Journal of Occupational Therapy*, **39**(11), 705–14.

Laurie, G., Headley, J.L. and Mudrovic, W.M. (1989) *Rehabilitation into Independent Living*, Gazette International Networking Institute, St Louis, MO.

Law, M., Baptiste, S., Carswell-Opzoomer, A. *et al.* (1991) *Canadian Occupational Performance Measure*, Canadian Association of Occupational Therapists, Toronto, Ont.

Leder, S.B. (1990a) Importance of verbal communication for the ventilator dependent patient (editorial). *Chest*, **98**(4), 792–3.

Leder, S.B. (1990b) Verbal communication for the ventilator-dependent patient: voice intensity with the Portex 'Talk' tracheostomy tube *Laryngoscope*, **100**, 1116–21.

Malik, M. (1979) *Manual on Static Hand Splinting*, Harmarville Rehabilitation Center, Pittsburgh, PA.

Menter, R. (1989) Introduction to high quadriplegia care, in *Management of High Quadriplegia* (eds G.G. Whiteneck, C. Adler, R.E. Carter *et al.*) Demos, New York, NY, p. 2.

Polatajko, H.J. (1992) Naming and framing occupational therapy: a lecture dedicated to the life of Nancy B. *Canadian Journal of Occupational Therapy*, **59**(4), 189–200.

Roye, W.P., Dunn, E.L. and Moody, J.A. (1988) Cervical spinal cord injury – a public catastrophe. *The Journal of Trauma*, **28**(8), 1260–3.

Smith, R. (1989) Mouthstick design for the client with spinal cord injury. *American Journal of Occupational Therapy*, **43**(4), 251–5.

Thenn, J.E. (1975) *Mobile Arm Supports. Installation and Use: a Guide for the Occupational Therapist*, Fred Sammons, Brookfield, IL.

Trombly, C.A. (1983) *Occupational Therapy for Physical Dysfunction*, 2nd edn, Williams and Wilkins, Baltimore, MD, pp. 273–80.

Whalley, K.R. (1981) Feeder arm for a quadriplegic patient. *Canadian Journal of Occupational Therapy*, **48**(5), 223–7.

Whalley Hammell, K.R. (1991) Occupational therapy in the management of high level quadriplegia. *British Journal of Occupational Therapy* **54**(9) 333–40.

Wilson, D.J., McKenzie, M.W. and Barber, L.M. (1974) *Spinal Cord Injury: a Treatment Guide for Occupational Therapists*, Charles B Slack, Thorofare, NJ, pp. 53–73.

Zejdlik, C.P. (1992) Living with high quadriplegia, in *Management of Spinal Cord Injury*, 2nd edn, (ed. C.P. Zejdlik), Jones and Bartlett, Boston, MA, pp. 257–303.

FURTHER READING

Bromley, I. (1991) *Tetraplegia and Paraplegia: a Guide for Physiotherapists*, 4th edn, Churchill Livingstone, Edinburgh. (Excellent section on respiratory care).

Budning, B.C. and Hall, M. (1990) A practical mouth stick for early intervention with quadriparetic patients *Journal of Canadian Dental Association*, **56**(3), 243–4.

Colgan, M. (1989) *Breathing Easy: a Guide for Ventilator Dependent Individuals Moving into the Community*, Independent Living Resource Centre, Winnipeg, Man. (Canadian resource, providing information regarding various independent living options and models of care delivery).

Colgan, M. (1992) *Breathing Support Options: a Consumer Perspective*, Independent Living Resource Centre, Winnipeg, Man. (Canadian consumers' guide to invasive and non-invasive means of ventilatory support).

Garber, S.L., Lathem, P. and Gregorio, T.L. (1988) *Specialised Occupational Therapy for Persons with High Level Quadriplegia*, The Institute for Rehabilitation and Research, Houston, TX.

Laurie, G., Headley, J.L. and Mudrovic, W.M. (1989) *Rehabilitation into Independent Living*, Gazette International Networking Institute, (*Rehabilitation Gazette*, **29**(1) and **29**(2). This small book contains accounts of the lives of individuals who have used ventilators for many years).

Smith, R. (1989) Mouth stick design for the client with spinal cord injury. *American Journal of Occupational Therapy*, **43**(4), 251–5.

(Excellent review of the literature concerning mouth sticks and an outline of the considerations for fabrication).

Whiteneck, G., Adler, C., Carter, R.E. *et al.* (eds) (1989) *The Management of High Quadriplegia. Vol. 1. Comprehensive Neurologic Rehabilitation,* Demos, New York, NY.

Zejdlik, C.P. (1992) *Management of Spinal Cord Injury,* 2nd edn, Jones and Bartlett, Boston, MA.

7

Psychological adaptation

> The sad truth is that man's real life consists of a complex of inexorable opposites – day and night, birth and death, happiness and misery, good and evil. . . . Life is a battleground. It always has been and always will be; and if it were not so, existence would come to an end.
>
> *(Jung, 1964)*

INTRODUCTION

The person with a recent, traumatic spinal cord injury experiences the trauma of one of the most devastating of all non-fatal injuries following which, the goal is not that of medical recovery but of adjustment or adaptation to circumstances that have been drastically changed.

The past decades have seen a burgeoning of interest in the process of adjustment to the trauma of spinal cord injury. A great deal has been written; most of it from the observations of professionals. There have been trends in theories and many contradictions. From a review of the literature to 1980, two main themes may be identified: that emotional adjustment is an important factor in rehabilitation, and that staff attitudes are crucial to the outcome of rehabilitation (Tucker, 1980). This chapter will illustrate that these two themes are not mutually exclusive. Despite the importance of psychosocial issues to the process of rehabilitation and to living with a disability, discussion of the process of adaptation experienced by the spinal cord-injured person is frequently neglected in the major texts concerned with both spinal cord injury, and rehabilitation.

This chapter will review some of the extensive literature concerning adjustment to traumatic spinal cord injury. It will be proposed that these findings have serious implications for the healthcare professional who is involved in the rehabilitation of the person with a spinal cord injury.

PSYCHOLOGICAL THEORIES

Crisis and denial

A traumatic injury to the spinal cord presents a sudden, over-whelming threat to the individual's safety and constitutes a crisis event. At this stage, crisis intervention is directed to survival of the injury – with increasing success. However, the crisis should not be perceived purely in the context of the potential for physical harm to the life of the patient. Parry (1990) describes some responses that may result from the reaction of the person to his crisis. There may be short-term unreality and anaesthesia, sleep disturbance, disrupted appetite and indigestion, muscle tension, aches, pains, skin rashes, infections, anxiety and depression, problems with reasoning, judgement and concentration, avoidance of the problem, mental pre-occupation with the problem, anger, shame and guilt.

The responses to trauma or crisis that Parry describes may be exacerbated by the environment and medical interventions being made to manage the crisis. The patient with quadriplegia, for example, has lost sensory impulses from the shoulders down. He cannot feel or move. If he is being treated with tongs on a Stryker frame he will alternate between a view of the ceiling and one of the floor. Two-hourly turns to prevent the formation of pressure sores will certainly tend to disrupt sleep. Pain may be severe. If he has a tracheostomy, he may temporarily be unable to communicate.

Sensory deprivation may be the result of a total lack of proprioceptive and kinaesthetic feedback from below the level of trauma. Perceptual deprivation may also occur, in which there is a distortion of sensory stimulation caused by restriction of view, monotonous and continual sounds, nasal congestion (due to the physiology of spinal shock), reduced or absent tactile sensation and the disruption of gustatory stimulation, while no food is being given by mouth (Krishnan *et al.*, 1992). Additionally, decrease in the level of motor activity may lead to confusion, disturbed behaviour and distortions of perception. Krishnan contends that a major factor in the occurrence of visual, auditory and body perception disturbances is the absence or low level of family support (see Chapter 4).

Some professionals believe that, immediately after trauma, the patient will deny the problem to cope with it. However, 'denial' implies rejection or refusal and may be a more active process than is actually occurring in the early weeks following injury. Confusion and disorientation may instead be a direct result of the injury and its management. Horn (1989) expands upon the factors that may keep reality at bay, including medications, severe pain, total immobilization and enforced bed rest. She proposes that, as a result, this phase may be passed in a dream-like state in which adaptation cannot begin and new learning is not able to take place.

Several writers have demanded that 'denial' (or rejection of the fact of the injury) not be confused with hope, which may be an important concept for both the patient and his family at this time. Trieschmann (1988) believes that despite much speculation, no data has been found which substantiates the idea of 'denial'. In fact, many patients actively seek information concerning the implications of their injury in the early weeks of treatment.

Stage theorists

Much attention has been focused upon the 'stage theories' concerning adaptation to spinal cord injury. These stages are based upon those proposed by Kubler-Ross (1969) in relation to coping with death and dying: denial, anger, bargaining, depression and acceptance. The stage theory of adjustment has formed part of rehabilitation dogma for two decades. Hohmann (1975) wrote that a 'normal' individual experiences a sequence of attitudes and feelings as he strives to cope with his injury. The stages included in his sequence were denial, withdrawal, hostility and reaction against dependence. His subjective observations have been cited elsewhere in the literature and the implication for an individual who does not proceed through the prescribed phases is that he must, by default, be abnormal.

Versluys (1983) describes distinct phases of adjustment to disability, including **regression**, which is described as a phase in which there is a retreat from standards of adult independence, with more dependence on others and a more infantile level of weakness. This is an interesting theory of a psychological reaction, as it so accurately describes the early physical manifestations of the spinal cord injury itself!

Although the phase theory is accepted in other early works, these studies are based purely upon observation and in general pre-date more objective analyses of the adjustment process. More recent works have provided evidence that experienced professionals have been shown to overestimate the degree of distress experienced by their spinal cord injured clients and further, that these misperceptions actually worsen progressively with the length of clinical experience (Ernst, 1987). There would appear to be dangers in assigning emotions to another person without adequate testing and to regarding people who have sustained a spinal cord injury as being a homogenous group.

Evidence shows that spinal cord injury is not the product of a sensation-seeking trait and furthermore that there is no one premorbid personality trait that could distinguish the spinal cord injured population from the general population. There is a high rate of risk-taking behaviour, abuse of drugs and alcohol and physically active lifestyles among young men and a subset of these individuals will acquire a spinal cord injury (Ditunno *et al.*, 1985; Tunks *et al.*, 1986). However, as many of these behaviours are common in this group, this should not be interpreted as self-selection. It would seem inconceivable that trauma would produce the same response in a heterogeneous group of people. In reality, the only thing spinal cord injured persons have in common is their disability.

Many professionals have a fondness for theories that suggest an orderly and predictable process of adaptation. However, there is a danger in rigidly applying these theories, in attempting to make the person or the treatment fit the theory instead of using theory as an aid in interpreting the reactions which are actually observed. It is surely more usual for adults to experience a range of emotions during the day, rather than remaining in one 'stage' for a defined period of time. The unfortunate outcome of the popularity among rehabilitation staff for an orderly and predictable theoretical model has been that patients have been ascribed emotions they did not feel, or worse, have actually had hospital discharge delayed because they have failed to exhibit depression (Ernst, 1987)! Preconceived ideas regard-

ing the 'typical' response to a traumatic spinal cord injury may
serve to distort the interpretation of what is actually observed.

Challenge to stage theories

Trieschmann's ground-breaking study (1980) concerning adjustment to spinal cord injury was warmly received by persons who
had themselves sustained spinal cord injuries and who had
apparently felt victimized by those professionals who had written about reactions to disability that were based less on fact than
on theory. Trieschmann (1986) proposes that, although the
stage theory of adjustment has been frequently discussed, little
evidence has been offered to substantiate the assertions of the
theory.

Little reliable evidence exists which indicates that negative life
events produce stages of emotional response. The concept of a
stage theory of adjustment must, by definition, include time
since injury as a crucial factor, yet few studies have paid attention to demographic variables such as either time since injury or
age at injury. Shadish *et al.* (1981) documented the results of
using an assessment scale to evaluate psychological problems.
This did not support the belief that there is a uniform emotional
stage reaction to spinal cord injury.

Oliver (1983) sees stage theories as a problem, primarily because they fail to accord with the personal experiences of many
people with disabilities who do not grieve, mourn or pass
through an orderly series of stages of adjustment. He also
believes that there are serious questions to be raised concerning
whether an individual can be viewed in isolation, rather than as
part of a family and social network. Few researchers have examined the issue of interdependence within families and the
impact of the family's reaction to disability upon the person with
a traumatic injury.

Lawson (1978) found that changes in the emotional states
of people with spinal cord injuries did not fit a stage model of
depressive reaction but rather corresponded to day-to-day
events such as receiving visitors or a medical report.

Depression and staff attitudes

Burke and Murray (1975) state that if a newly injured person
does not appear to be depressed then what is actually happen-

ing is a denial of the functional loss and of the social implications of this loss. The inherent implication seems to be that not being depressed is abnormal or deviant. Further, there is the implication that all people with recent spinal cord injuries must either be depressed or in a state of denial. This categorization of all patients into two groupings of psychological disorders does not allow for the wide range of emotions which may be experienced by a diverse group of adults, from various socioeconomic and cultural backgrounds. Burke and Murray likewise postulate on 'dependency', stating that this is a prominent form of adjustment and that there are two general types: overdependence and underdependence. This would seem to imply that there is no balance between these two 'norms' and that either response is a problem. The reality of adult life is perhaps more an example of interdependence. The issue of dependency is a complex one, as the acutely injured person with a spinal cord injury will almost certainly be experiencing a period of physical dependency, particularly if the lesion is a high one.

Krueger (1984) describes depression as being a normal response to traumatic disability. He proposes that, if depression does not occur, even transiently, this indicates that the reality of the loss has not been recognized. Viewing depression as a natural and necessary part of the process of adjustment to traumatic injury was common in early literature on the subject. Goldiamond (1973), who is himself a psychologist and spinal cord injured, wrote that the hospital told his wife to expect him to be profoundly depressed after his injury. The staff were greatly sceptical when she told them that he was not depressed. He also quotes the case of a Marine corporal who underwent surgery for removal of a bullet and learned that he would be paralysed for life (Newsweek. March 5 1973). He was not depressed, but happy to be alive at all, adjusting to the fact so quickly, that he was sent to see a psychiatrist to determine his sanity!

Cushman and Dijkers (1991) studied depressed mood among people with recent spinal cord injuries and found that less depression was noted by individuals with spinal cord injuries than by hospital visitors! Sadness and grief may be normal responses to life events that are painful, life threatening or disabling but should be differentiated from clinical syndromes of depression. Grief is a complex emotional response and, although people who grieve a loss may describe themselves as being 'depressed', they more usually experience a number of emotions, such as sadness, anger, anxiety, despair and guilt, rather than prolonged depressive mood (Judd *et al.*, 1991).

As unrecognised and untreated depressive illness may severely impair rehabilitation, it is important that persistent mood change, persistent loss of interest in families, the self or the environment, and other symptoms of depression such as impaired concentration, memory, thinking and decision making are taken seriously. Studies which have applied stringent diagnostic criteria have indicated a prevalence of major depressive episodes among people with recent spinal cord injuries to range from 10% to 30%. Rehabilitation staff frequently adhere to the mistaken belief that psychological disturbance will be greater with higher lesions and that people with paraplegia or incomplete lesions will suffer less depression and will, in effect, feel 'lucky' in comparison to their quadriplegic peers. This is not supported by research studies, which have found there is no relationship between either level of spinal cord injury or physical dependency and depression (e.g. Fuhrer *et al.*, 1993).

Results of depression inventories must be interpreted cautiously, as some measures have items that may reflect neurological and physical sequelae of the spinal cord injury, (such as faintness, insomnia, numbness, appetite disturbance, weight loss, feeling weak and constipation) rather than the psychological events they are intended to measure. The physical effects of spinal cord injury on the body may also produce abnormally elevated scores on depression scale items, such as: 'having to do things slowly to ensure their correctness', 'feeling low in energy', 'feeling everything is an effort', or responding negatively to the comment 'I find it easy to do the things I used to do'.

Few clinicians would deny the presence of depression in some people with spinal cord injuries. However, this is not the same as ascribing depressive symptoms to every patient and viewing as maladaptive those who do not show evidence of depression.

Cushman and Dijkers (1990) formulated a study to correlate staff and patient perceptions of depression. Each day the patient was asked to rank his feelings of depression. His care providers – nurses, doctors, therapists, compiled the same form indicating their perceptions of his feelings of depression. They found a consistent bias on the part of the staff to overestimate depressed mood, in comparison to the reports of the patients themselves. They believe that staff may hold preconceived ideas concerning the typical response to spinal cord injury and that these ideas then serve to distort what is actually observed. This is consistent with the suggestion that patient behaviour is interpreted according to the prevailing professional ideology. In the instance of rehabilitation personnel, this reflects the theory that depression is a necessary phase of adaptation to spinal cord injury. Perversely, it has also been suggested that optimism among paraplegics is not accepted at face value by the staff.

Although underestimation of the degree of a client's depression is obviously problematic, there is evidence to suggest that the opposite error is more common on rehabilitation units, with a prevailing tendency to overestimate the degree of distress. This can have serious consequences. The client who perceives pity in the attitude of his staff may internalize that same sentiment, resulting in a self-fulfilling prophecy. Other researchers have also found that serious discrepancies exist between the perceptions held by rehabilitation personnel and the psychosocial situations actually reported by their spinal cord injured clients. The clients reported being less depressed, more optimistic but more anxious than their caregivers predicted.

Some facilities adhere so strongly to the clinical lore concerning stages of adjustment that depression is thus established as a criterion for hospital discharge! (Ernst, 1987). Some people with disabilities have stated that the most depressing aspect of their experience of rehabilitation following their injury was of the staff members telling them that they should be depressed! Contrarily, however, research has found that rehabilitation staff reject involvement with a spinal cord injured person who is depressed, preferring instead to work with one who is not depressed.

It was formerly believed that 'adjustment' as a process would not be complete until the person had experienced depression. Trieschmann (1986) states that data suggests the opposite. She proposes that recent research tends to suggest that those people who exhibit the least signs of depression after injury tend to function best during rehabilitation and following discharge. Other researchers corroborate the idea that depression appears to be counterproductive to post-discharge outcome.

This raises a further issue: that staff attitudes are crucial to the outcome of rehabilitation. Bodenhamer *et al.* (1983) agree that among the psychosocial variables which appear to have an important influence upon outcome are the reactions and expectations of the rehabilitation staff. They report that their comparisons of results of patient and staff responses to a psychosocial questionnaire for spinal cord injured persons adds support to the growing body of evidence that there are serious discrepancies between what the staff perceive to be the psychosocial situation of their spinal cord injured patients and what these patients actually report themselves.

Rehabilitation, medical and nursing staff may adopt two opposing attitudes. One is an intolerance of self-pity, self-blame or lack of enthusiasm. These staff may expect gratitude and interest in the rehabilitation process and in other people. Conversely, staff may perceive the individual as the victim of a tragic event, someone whose life has been ruined and who must therefore, by definition, be depressed and in need of psychiatric intervention.

People with recent disabilities who are adapting to their changed circumstances will be extremely attentive to and influenced by the attitudes of others, most especially the attitudes of health professionals (Nordholm and Westbrook, 1986). These researchers indicate that genuine expressions of positive feelings are likely to be discounted and they propose that health professionals should consider whether the conclusions they draw from patient behaviours are justified. Some people with spinal cord injuries have been the recipients of concerns that their attitude is too positive and hence they must not be dealing with the reality of the situation. Such a stance ignores the heterogeneity of response to trauma, individual coping mechanisms and the meaning that the disability holds for the individual. Further, it clearly illustrates the negative viewpoint held by rehabilitation staff who convey their belief that the patient's situation is awful and requires a response of depression and pessimism.

Dijkers and Cushman (1991) reinforce the serious implications for people with spinal cord injuries when staff disregard their optimism and hope, while overestimating negative mood. They describe an intervention strategy which confronts the staff with the assumptions that underpin their erroneous perceptions and provide them with the skills to approach their clients in a more open-minded way. As rehabilitation staff are a powerful determinant of rehabilitation outcomes, it is imperative that they do not contribute to a negative, hopeless environment. Rehabilitation staff attitudes and behaviour exert a powerful effect upon the response of the individual to his injury and this may be more crucial in determining the response to rehabilitation than any other single factor.

Hypothesis of reduced emotional experience

Hohmann (1966) proposed that high spinal cord lesions produce a direct effect upon emotional reactions, suggesting that the nerve lesion produces a dulling of emotional response and expression. Hohmann's correlation of emotional change and extensive autonomic nervous system disruption does not prove causality and other possible psychological or psychosocial explanations of his results are not explored.

Despite the fact that this early study was reliant upon retrospective, subjective data, which is inherently of questionable accuracy, Hohmann's hypothesis is frequently cited as part of the rehabilitation lore regarding people with quadriplegia. Comparisons of emotional experiences before and after injury were separated by an extensive mean period of 11 years. Further, Hohmann was both the interviewer and the formulator of the hypothesis, which raises the issue of possible bias in data interpretation (Bermond *et al.*, 1987).

Bermond proposes that a way to test the hypothesis of emotional excitability and spinal cord lesions is to examine whether an overall reduction in mood state levels occurs. Their study indicated that the only significant difference in 10 mood state levels between people with cervical spinal cord injuries and a 'normal' control group was a higher level of fatigue among the quadriplegic group. They conclude therefore, that their results do not support Hohmann's hypothesis that peripheral feedback is important for the realization of emotional feelings. Hohmann's theory has been refuted in other subsequent studies (Hester, 1971; Nestoros *et al.*, 1982; Lowe and Carroll, 1985; Glass, 1993) yet is still cited as lore in contemporary works. This controversy illustrates clearly the dangers of formulating theories based on the results and hypotheses of only one study.

PERSONALITY THEORIES

Locus of control

Rotter (1966) described those people who believe that they have a high degree of personal control over events as having an internal locus of control. In contrast, those people who believe that they have little control over events and situations, who believe instead in luck or fate are defined as having an external locus of control. Frank and Elliott (1989) found that people with spinal cord injuries who believe that they are primarily responsible for their health show less depression and more adaptive behaviour than those who have more externalized beliefs.

In a study concerning the relationship between locus of control expectancy and adjustment to traumatic spinal cord injury, Mazzulla (1984) supported the view that those individuals who exhibited an internal locus of control were more able to adjust to the onset of spinal injury. This was irrespective of the time since onset or of the level of disability that determined the actual amount of physical control which the patient could exert. It is noted by Trieschmann (1988) that even though a person with quadriplegia may in fact have less control over his immediate circumstances, this does not necessarily change his perception of control over his life, or indeed, his satisfaction with life. Mazzulla (1984) emphasises that the central issue is not the actual reality of control but the belief of control.

Further, Nordholm and Westbrook (1986) indicate that one manifestation of the personality trait of internal control may be that of assuming responsibility for, or blaming oneself for the accident that produced the disability. Several writers have suggested that those individuals who assume responsibility for their accidents make better adjustments following discharge than those who perceived themselves as being 'innocent victims' (Trieschmann, 1988).

The rehabilitation personnel can work with the patient to increase his sense of control over his environment and thus reinforce the belief that control is still a possibility (see Chapter 1). Early interaction with environmental control units for example, introduces the opportunity for control to the patient in the acute setting and will continue as the patient is encouraged to participate actively in setting goals and making realistic choices.

SOCIOLOGICAL THEORIES

Oliver (1981) argues that psychological approaches to individual adaptation to disability have dominated the field to the comparative neglect of the impact upon family life and upon other family members. He suggests that adjustment to sudden, traumatic spinal cord injury is often more difficult for other family members than for the injured person himself. Recent literature has acknowledged that the injury has an impact on the whole family.

Adjustment to spinal cord injury has generally been examined in the literature solely from the viewpoint of the injured person. Little attention has been focused on the family, although several writers stress the importance of strong family support as being a major factor in the process of adjustment.

Oliver *et al.* (1988) believe that the process of social adjustment arises both from the interactions between the individual and his physical and social environment and, more importantly, from the meanings that these interactions have for both the individual and his family.

Outcome can be considered to be a complex, interactional equation of many factors. Compounding factors include age, intellectual capacity, philosophical/religious beliefs, family structure, quality of interpersonal relationships, academic background, previous losses and coping abilities and the symbolic meaning that spinal cord injury has for the individual. Others include medical complications, medications, endurance, strength, co-ordination, pain and degree of impairment. Additionally, environmental variables will include income, transportation, architectural and geographical barriers, educational and vocational resources and family and interpersonal support. The interaction of so many variables will make it impossible to identify a course of adjustment that is predictable, solitary and uniform (Trieschmann, 1988; Butt, 1989). Recent concentration upon the psychological characteristics of the individual has enabled an abdication of the responsibility to examine the more complex environmental issues that have an impact upon adaptation.

In summary, the sociological theorists examine adaptation to disability in the broad context of the social environment of each individual. Successful outcome is felt to relate not only to the physical and psychological attributes of the client but also to his unique physical and social environment.

Social support

Research studies of the relationship between social support and depression following spinal cord injury find that low depression scores are predicted by high levels of those relationships that offer reassurance of worth and social integration support, irrespective of length of time since injury. Relationships which provide reassurance of worth recognize a person's ability, skill and competence (Elliott *et al.*, 1992). This finding presents a challenge to the rehabilitation professional who may temporarily be in a position to provide this facet of support and it indicates again the possible causality of depression when staff make clear that they expect the patient to be depressed. It is further proposed that social support, which places the person in the role of a passive recipient, may serve to erode the sense of self-worth and self-esteem. Studies in the field of epidemiology have indicated the positive impact upon health, self-esteem and life satisfaction that result from a perception of strong social support (see chapter 8). It is a challenge to the rehabilitation team not only to provide positive support but also to facilitate and encourage the maintenance and strengthening of the social bonds which the client has with his partner, family, friends and community.

IMPLICATIONS FOR REHABILITATION PERSONNEL

Goldiamond (1973) queries the psychological theories to which healthcare personnel have tended to adhere. He states that, as the reaction to one's injury is supposed to cause depression, apathy, depression or aggression will be viewed as inevitable developmental stages in adjustment to the injury and hence the healthcare staff can avoid asking how their own actions might have caused the behaviour. There has been a tendency to disregard the effects of the values, assumptions, attitudes, expectations and behaviours of the healthcare staff and their impact upon the patient. Goldiamond believes that, rather than listing 'problems', it is more useful to define those problems in terms of goals and then establish ways of achieving those goals.

He comments that, when a professional refers to the patient as being 'unaware of', 'not realistic about' or 'repressing' his problem, it is often the professional who is being unrealistic. He says that, if the patient does not appear to be 'facing up' to his situation, it may be because he is trying to face in a different direction – one that can help him in achieving his goals.

Literature which concerns itself with the factors that are involved in the family's reaction to spinal cord injury is conspicuous by its absence. Given the acknowledged role which the family plays in the successful outcome of the rehabilitation process this would appear to be an area which could usefully be researched further.

Compliance and control

The primary goal in the rehabilitation of people with cervical spinal cord injuries is to promote independent thought and restore a sense of power through self-directed behaviour: survival skills for the person with quadriplegia (Mahon-Darby *et al.*, 1988). The goals of treatment must be examined to ensure that what is being achieved is indeed independent behaviour. Trieschmann (1988) reflects upon rehabilitation facilities which treat the patient as the passive recipient of units of therapy and queries how the individual can be expected to be an active participant in life outside. The concept of **compliance** encompasses complaisance, yielding and submission. Compliance may not be the most beneficial attribute to a spinal cord injured person upon re-entry to the community. Co-operation with another's goals is not a predictor of independent living. The patient who evaluates his own needs, decides on goals and implements behaviour to meet these goals is frequently considered to be 'demanding' or 'resistant' by staff (Tucker, 1984). Yet these are the very criteria that are described as creating the environment in which people learn best (Chapter 2). This is relevant, as it has already been stated that rehabilitation is a learning process – of learning how to live with a disability in one's own environment.

Frequently, however, rehabilitation staff may communicate conflicting expectations for their clients. Staff members may expect unquestioning compliance, gratitude and passivity from the client. A contradictory message may also be communicated –

that the client must confront his disability, while learning problem-solving and independence skills. Compliance, passivity and co-operation with authority instead tend to foster dependence.

It is proposed that compliance may not always be in the long-term, best interests of the spinal cord injured person, as compliance with externally imposed routines does not teach independence, problem solving and coping with a disability (Trieschmann, 1986). Rather, the reverse may be true. This presents a clear challenge to all rehabilitation personnel.

MODEL FOR REHABILITATION

It has been proposed that adaptation to a traumatic spinal cord injury is not an isolated process but one that involves close family and friends. The objectives of the rehabilitation team should therefore include facilitation of the family's adaptation to their changed circumstances. Moreover, by understanding the variables that are related to the adaptation to traumatic disability, rehabilitation educators and researchers could design both training programmes for rehabilitation professionals and research programmes that would give thorough consideration to the psychological, social and vocational implication of living with a spinal cord injury.

Planning of a rehabilitation service needs to incorporate flexibility to encourage goal choices by clients. In the past, the rehabilitation staff usually decided what the clients' goals should be. There was also a prevailing tendency towards adjusting the disabled person to the social structure of the rehabilitation facility rather than the other way around.

To achieve meaningful life and not just physical survival, more than mobility skills and a high activity of daily living score must be achieved. Other skills must be acquired, such as creative recreation, financial planning, negotiating community barriers (architectural and interpersonal), managing an attendant, creative problem solving, accessing community resources, assertiveness, sexual expression, vocational planning/training, use of community transportation.

The rehabilitation team will need to become more flexible in recognising the heterogeneity of the life values of the individual. The activated client is one who asserts early control over his environment and works with the healthcare professionals in establishing realistic goals. This requires co-operation on the part of the staff, not compliance on the part of the client.

More focus will be upon out-patient services which may assist the spinal cord injured person in finding solutions to problems once these have been identified. In-patient rehabilitation is an environment ideally suited to learning self-care skills. Yet the implications of living in the community with a spinal cord injury can scarcely be anticipated accurately by the newly injured individual or the predominantly able-bodied staff. Comprehensive out-patient and community-based services should ensure that, once problems have been identified, the knowledge and skills of professional and client can be combined to focus upon possible choices for action. The lifelong process of learning to interact with society and the environment is not complete at discharge from an in-patient facility. Rather, this is when true adjustment and adaptation begins.

As early as 1968, Hallin stated his belief that psychological adjustment is the critical factor in determining rehabilitation success. Yet physical and functional goals tend to be the main focus of the rehabilitation process.

Theories are of use in providing a broad framework or guide within which to assess and assist spinal cord injured patients. However, they should not be viewed as being rigid models to which each person must be made to fit. There needs to be a careful balance between over emphasizing the psychological adaptation that the trauma of spinal cord injury necessitates and ignoring it. Woodbury and Redd (1987) emphasize that health-care professionals need to be aware that there is no one 'right' way to adapt to a spinal cord injury. They stress that the job of the rehabilitation professional is to 'facilitate the patient's progress, not dictate it!'

Healthcare professionals involved in the rehabilitation of people with spinal cord injuries have popularized such elements of clinical lore as the stages of grieving, the need to experience clinical depression, the dulling of emotions with high lesions and the view of spinal cord injury as a lone experience, not shared by the family or close others. Unfortunately, it has been suggested that observations are interpreted according to a fondly held theory, rather than viewed in the light of research studies that have clearly refuted these theories and further, that widespread assumptions are particularly resistant to disconfirming evidence.

Research in the field of social psychology has indicated the tendency to seek, recall and interpret information according to strongly held beliefs, in a manner that is impervious to the actual data. Regrettably, attention has been deflected away from identifying the strengths of those people who cope well with spinal cord injury and assisting all patients to maximize their resources based on these findings. Promotion of self-esteem, allowance of normal coping responses and facilitation of the strengthening of social support systems may be a more positive approach than continuing to interpret observations to fit a preconceived assumption concerning adjustment to loss (Silver and Wortman, 1980; Wortman and Silver, 1989).

Society has tended to view traumatic disability as a tragedy, requiring a response of sadness and depression and frequently these attitudes are reflected by healthcare personnel. If an individual with a spinal cord injury breaks out of that mould, he is regarded as being different or special. Sociologists suggest however, that as the majority of people who sustain spinal cord injuries do achieve satisfying and fulfilling lives, that this should be regarded as the norm, not the exception. Intensive rehabilitation services are usually provided shortly after injury, with clients returning for further treatment only if complications arise. From these contacts alone it is difficult for healthcare staff to comprehend clearly what life with a disability entails, particularly as they may never see those who require no further treatment and return to an active lifestyle.

Rehabilitation staff who have little contact with people with spinal cord injuries in the community may be unaware of the high degree of satisfaction with life and the quality of life achieved by these individuals. Studies indicate that even those with lesions above C4 report that they are glad to be alive. Indeed, in the presence of a supportive environment, a study in Sweden found no difference in quality of life between people with quadriplegia, paraplegia or a control population (Siösteen *et al.*, 1990). In the USA, no correlation was found between level of injury and perceived quality of life. Rather, life satisfaction was positively correlated with perceived control, social support, social integration, occupation and mobility (Fuhrer *et al.*, 1992).

It is incumbent upon the healthcare professional to facilitate the process of adaptation and to recognize that it is not the injury itself which is the predictor of response but the characteristics both of the person who has the injury, and their unique personal, social, cultural and economic circumstances. Inclusion of significant psychosocial components in a more complete rehabilitation programme for both patient and family has been shown to lead to more satisfactory community re-integration. Finally, Cushman and Dijkers (1991) suggest that successful adjustment to disability requires the positive characteristics seen in other, successful, well-adjusted individuals. They enumerate these characteristics as being high self-esteem, productivity and the ability to maintain satisfactory relationships. The successful rehabilitation programme will be the one that fosters these positive attributes – not the one that requires mourning, anger and depression for the losses incurred by the injury!

Zola (1982) considers adjustment to be a lifelong process rather than representing an end point at which adaptation to a particular difficulty has been achieved. Instead, problems must be re-evaluated and adaptations made on a continuing basis. Rehabilitation is not solely concerned with learning adeptness at physical skills but rather of learning to interact with the unique physical and sociocultural environment and the demands that these environments place upon an individual who has a disability. In the absence of a supportive physical and social environment it is unlikely that rehabilitation will cease at discharge. Rather, 'problems must be faced, evaluated, re-defined, and re-adapted to again, and again, and again' (Zola, 1982).

ACKNOWLEDGEMENT

Much of this chapter is based upon Whalley Hammell (1992) and is reproduced with permission.

REFERENCES

Bermond, B., Scheurman, J., Nieuwenhuijse, B. *et al.* (1987) Spinal cord lesions: coping and mood states. *Clinical Rehabilitation*, **1**, 111–7.
Bodenhamer, E., Achterberg-Lawlis, J., Kevorkian, G. *et al.* (1983) Staff and patient perceptions of the psychosocial concerns of spinal cord injured persons. *American Journal of Physical Medicine*, **62**(4), 182–93.

Burke, D.C. and Murray, D.D. (1975) *Handbook of Spinal Cord Medicine*, Macmillan, Basingstoke, p. 79.

Butt, L. (1989) Psychological aspects of discharge, in *The Management of High Quadriplegia*, (eds G.G. Whiteneck, Adler, C., Carter, R.E. *et al.*), Demos, New York, NY, pp. 271–9.

Cushman, L. and Dijkers, M. (1990) Depressed mood in spinal cord injured patients: staff perceptions and patient realities. *Archives of Physical Medicine and Rehabilitation*, **71**, 191–6.

Cushman, L.A. and Dijkers, M. (1991) Depressed mood during rehabilitation of persons with spinal injury. *Journal of Rehabilitation*, **57**(2), 35–8.

Dijkers, M. and Cushman, L.A. (1991) Changing staff perceptions of the mood of spinal cord injured patients: a natural experiment *Canadian Journal of Rehabilitation*, **5**(2), 71–80.

Ditunno, P., McCauley, C. and Marquette, C. (1985) Sensation seeking behaviour and the incidence of spinal cord injury. *Archives of Physical Medicine and Rehabilitation*, **66**, 152–5.

Elliott, T., Herrick, S., Witty, T. *et al.* (1992) Social support and depression following spinal cord injury. *Rehabilitation Psychology*, **37**(1), 37–48.

Ernst, F.A. (1987) Contrasting perceptions of distress by research personnel and their spinal cord injured subjects. *American Journal of Physical Medicine*, **66**(1), 12–15.

Frank, R.G. and Eliott, T.R. (1989) Spinal cord injury and health locus of control beliefs. *Paraplegia*, **27**, 250–6.

Fuhrer, M.J., Rintala, D.H., Hart, K.A. *et al.* (1992) Relationship of life satisfaction to impairment, disability and handicap among persons with spinal cord injury living in the community. *Archives of Physical Medicine and Rehabilitation*, **73**, 552–7.

Fuhrer, M.J., Rintala, D.H., Hart, K.A. *et al.* (1993) Depressive symptomatology in persons with spinal cord injury who reside in the community. *Archives of Physical Medicine and Rehabilitation*, **74**, 255–60.

Glass, C.A. (1993) The impact of home based ventilator dependence on family life. *Paraplegia* **31**, 93–101.

Goldiamond, I. (1973) A diary of self modification. *Psychology Today*, **7**, 95–100.

Hallin, R.P. (1968) Follow up of paraplegics and tetraplegics after comprehensive rehabilitation. *International Journal of Paraplegia*, **6**, 128–34.

Hester, G. (1971) Effects of functional transection of the spinal cord on task performance under varied motivational conditions. *Psychophysiology*, **8**, 451–61.

Hohmann, G.W. (1966) Some effects of spinal cord lesions on experienced emotional feelings. *Psychophysiology*, **3**, 143–56.

Hohmann, G.W. (1975) Psychological aspects of treatment and rehabilitation of the spinal cord injured person. *Clinical Orthopaedics and Related Research*, **112**, 81–8.

Horn, S. (1989) *Coping with Bereavement*, Thorsons, Wellingborough, p. 104.

Judd, F.K., Brown, D.J. and Burrows, G.D. (1991) Depression, disease and disability: application to patients with traumatic spinal cord injury. *Paraplegia*, **29**, 91–6.

Jung, C.G. (1964) *Man and his Symbols*, Dell publishing company. New York, NY, p.75.

Krishnan, K.R., Glass, C.A., Turner, S.M. *et al.* (1992) Perceptual deprivation in the acute phase of spinal injury rehabilitation. *Journal of the American Paraplegia Society*, **15**(2), 60–5.

Krueger, D.W. (1984) Issues in emotional rehabilitation, in *Rehabilitation Psychology*, (ed. D.W. Krueger), Aspen, Rockville, MD, p. 9.

Kubler-Ross, E. (1969) *On Death and Dying*, Collier Books, New York, NY.

Lawson, N.C. (1978) Significant events in the rehabilitation process: the spinal cord patient's point of view. *Archives of Physical Medicine and Rehabilitation*, **59**, 573–9.

Lowe, J. and Carroll, D. (1985) The effects of spinal injury on the intensity of emotional experience. *British Journal of Clinical Psychology*, **24**, 135–6.

Mahon-Darby, J., Ketchik-Renshaw, B., Richmond, T.S. and Gates, E.M. (1988) Powerlessness in cervical spinal cord injury patients. *Dimensions of Critical Care Nursing*, **7**(6), 346–55.

Mazzulla, J.R. (1984) Relationship between locus of control expectancy and acceptance of acquired traumatic spinal cord injury. *American Archives of Rehabilitation Therapy*, Winter, 10–13.

Nestoros, J.N., Demers-Desrosiers, L.A. and Dalicandro, L.A. (1982) Levels of anxiety and depression in spinal cord injured patients. *Psychomatics*, **23**, 823–30.

Nordholm, L. and Westbrook, M. (1986) Effects of depression, self-blame and dependency on health professionals evaluation of paraplegic patients. *Australian Occupational Therapy Journal*, **33**(2), 59–70.

Oliver, M. (1981) Disability, adjustment and family life – some theoretical considerations, in *Handicap in a Social World*, (eds A. Brechin, P. Liddiard and J. Swain), Open University Press and Hodder and Stoughton, London, p. 49.

Oliver, M. (1983) *Social Work with Disabled People*, British Association of Social Workers and Macmillan Education, Basingstoke, pp. 17–18, 22.

Oliver, M., Zarb, G., Silver, J. *et al.* (1988) *Walking into Darkness: the Experience of Spinal Cord Injury*, Macmillan, Basingstoke, p. 35.

Parry, G. (1990) *Coping with Crises*, British Psychological Society and

Routledge, London, p. 29.

Rotter, J.B. (1966) Generalised expectancies for internal versus external locus of control of reinforcement. *Psychology Monograph*, **80**, 1–28.

Shadish, W.R., Hickman, D. and Arrick, M.C. (1981) Psychological problems of spinal cord injury patients: emotional distress as a function of time and locus of control. *Journal of Consulting and Clinical Psychology*, **49**(2), 297.

Silver, R. and Wortman, C. (1980) Coping with undesirable life events, in *Human Helplessness: Theory and Applications*, (eds J. Garber and M. Seligman), Academic, New York, NY, Ch. 12, 16.

Siösteen, A., Lundqvist, C., Blomstrand, C. *et al.* (1990) The quality of life of three functional spinal cord injury subgroups in a Swedish community. *Paraplegia*, **28**, 476–88.

Trieschmann, R.B. (1980) *Spinal Cord Injuries: Psychological, Social and Vocational Adjustment*, Pergamon, Oxford, p. xii.

Trieschmann, R.B. (1986) The psychosocial adjustment to spinal cord injury, in *Management of Spinal Cord Injuries*, (eds R.F. Bloch and M. Basbaum), Williams and Wilkins, Baltimore, MD.

Trieschmann, R.B. (1988) *Spinal Cord Injuries – Psychological, Social and Vocational Rehabilitation*, 2nd edn, Demos, New York, NY, p. 28, 37, 52, 93, 245–7, .

Tucker, S.J. (1980) The psychology of spinal cord injury: patient–staff interaction *Rehabilitation Literature*, **41**(5–6), 114–22.

Tucker, S.J. (1984) Patient staff interaction with the spinal cord patient, in *Rehabilitation Psychology*, (ed. D.W. Krueger), Aspen, Rockville, MD, Ch. 28.

Tunks, E., Bahry, N. and Basbaum, M. (1986) The resocialisation process after spinal cord injury, in *Management of Spinal Cord Injuries*, (eds R.F. Bloch and M. Basbaum), Williams and Wilkins, Baltimore, MD, p. 388.

Versluys, H. (1983) Psychosocial adjustment to physical disability, in *Occupational Therapy for Physical Dysfunction*, 2nd edn, (ed C. Trombly), Williams and Wilkins, Baltimore, MD, p. 17.

Whalley Hammell, K.R. (1992) Psychological and sociological theories concerning adjustment to traumatic spinal cord injury: the implications for rehabilitation. *Paraplegia*, **30**(5), 317–26.

Woodbury, B. and Redd, C. (1987) Psychosocial issues and approaches, in *Spinal Cord Injury: Concepts and Management approaches*, (eds L.E. Buchanan and D.A. Nawoczenski), Williams and Wilkins, Baltimore, MD, p. 191.

Wortman, C. and Silver, R.C. (1989) The myths of coping with loss *Journal of Consulting and Clinical Psychology*, **57**(3), 349–57.

Zola, I.K. (1982) *Missing pieces: a Chronicle of Living with a Disability*, Temple University, Philadelphia, PA, p. 84.

FURTHER READING

Trieschmann, R.B. (1988) *Spinal Cord Injuries: Psychological, Social and Vocational Rehabilitation* 2nd edn, Demos, New York, NY.

Wortman, C. and Silver, R.C. (1989) The myths of coping with loss. *Journal of Consulting and Clinical Psychology*, **57**(3), 349–57.

8

Living with a spinal cord injury: productivity, leisure and socialization

Successful adult functioning requires more than ADL [activities of daily living] and mobility skills; it requires the ability to interact socially in quite sophisticated ways, to compete successfully with one's peers in social, recreational, educational, vocational and economic spheres.

(R.B. Trieschmann, 1988, p. 24)

INTRODUCTION

Studies have shown that there is no relationship between level of injury and quality of life or between physical independence and quality of life following spinal cord injury (Siösteen *et al.*, 1990; Fuhrer *et al.*, 1992). Quality of life therefore must be dependent upon aspects other than physical skills; and the degree of satisfaction with life following discharge must be attributed to factors other than impairments. These factors could usefully be identified and efforts made to address and enhance them during rehabilitation.

Traditional rehabilitation services have been concerned with maximizing health and physical independence. Counselling has had secondary status and even less emphasis has been placed upon enhancing social skills, sexual functioning and those fulfilling activities and meaningful occupations that are not related to paid employment. Study has suggested, however, that level of activity, more than any other factor, influences survival following spinal cord injury (Krause and Crewe, 1987). Such findings indicate that rehabilitation services must place greater emphasis upon enhancing the skills that the spinal cord injured person will need to become an active participant in life.

Studies have further illustrated the link between activities, occupations and health. Increased satisfaction with activities has been correlated with a decreased incidence of both pressure sores and urinary tract infections. Conversely, those factors that predispose people with spinal cord injuries to urinary tract infections include inactivity, poor social support systems and the lack of opportunity to participate in social and community interactions (NIDRR, 1992).

It is important for rehabilitation professionals to absorb thoroughly the implications of these and other studies. Engagement in meaningful occupations and fulfilling activities is a prerequisite for perceived quality of life, for prevention of disabling medical problems – and indeed, for survival itself.

Although Aristotle noted, almost two and a half thousand years ago, that the quality of a life is determined by its activities, the rehabilitation industry has focused largely upon re-teaching the skills that most four-year-olds have attained – self-care and mobility.

Study shows that people in American society spend just under half their lifetime in self-care activities, while more than half their lifetime is engaged in productivity and leisure activities (19% and 35% respectively) (Reed and Sanderson, 1992). This balance of occupations is an important concept in assessing quality of time use, quality of life and health. 'Health is determined by an individual's purposeful engagement in occupation and by a balance of self-care, productivity and leisure' (Law, 1991).

PRODUCTIVITY

Productivity encompasses occupations related to paid and unpaid work, household management, caring for children; and creative play and school activities, in the case of children. Unfortunately, productivity has commonly been confused with the concept of paid employment and outcome measures have been designed to record information related only to employment status. A successful outcome following rehabilitation is hence implied to be that of the person who resumes paid employment. By default, those who pursue further training or education, who engage in child care, household management or voluntary activities are considered unsuccessful, or unproductive.

Western society places high value upon paid employment. 'What one does' determines who one is, one's social status and value within society. Writers have decried the financial disincentives to employment for people with acquired disabilities but society has yet to address the physical and sociocultural barriers that prevent access to the work place. In the early 1990s, when worldwide unemployment rates have soared and millions are without paid employment, it is especially important to form a wider vision of what 'productivity' really entails and what it means for each individual.

Rehabilitation outcome measures have frequently used **employment status** as the single indicator of rehabilitation success. However, Kerr and Thompson (1972) note that return to work is more likely to be the result of good adaptation to spinal cord injury rather than the causal factor that achieves good adaptation.

Assessment of productivity must follow a client-centred approach. Yerxa and Locker (1990) examined the quality of time use by adults with spinal cord injuries. They found that the same occupation may be classified into as many as four different categories, supporting the need for a perspective on the meaning or purpose attributed to activities. The occupational therapists agreed more strongly with each other than they did with the spinal cord injured subjects in classifying the latter's daily occupations. Clearly the occupational therapists have different perspectives on their clients' occupations than do the clients themselves.

> It refutes analysis of activities according to their inherent qualities and suggests instead that the occupational therapist needs to understand the patient's goals for engagement in occupations. It also raises a question about whether occupation can be understood from a behaviouristic approach, that is, by only observing what people do. This study emphasizes the significance of the subject's experience as important information in an activity analysis.   (Yerxa and Locker, 1990)

Productivity has been defined as 'those activities or tasks which are done to enable the person to provide support to the self, family and society through the production of goods and services . . . in the broader sense, productivity performance is the performance area which covers the activities and roles which give meaning and purpose in life' (CAOT, 1991).

> While gainful employment has always been a focal issue in human service programs, policy makers have come to recognize that there are many other ways in which a person can contribute to family and community life: in homemaking, child care, participation in formal organisations and others.
>
> (DeJong and Hughes, 1982)

McKinnon (1992) provides a broad vision of productivity which will be assumed in the present work. McKinnon's delineation for occupational performance in productivity includes:

- paid work
- domestic and household work
- care of children
- school or education
- organizational, voluntary and religious activities.

Assessment of future goals related to productivity has been a neglected area in rehabilitation planning. Some centres have adopted the view that the client is not yet prepared to discuss future employment, hence he is not encouraged to explore his options for engagement in productive occupations. Neither does he have the opportunity to use his professionals as resources in achieving such goals. It is difficult to comprehend exactly what goals the rehabilitation programme is focused towards if the needs of the client for engagement in productive activities is not part of the agenda. Equally irresponsible is the viewpoint expressed in other centres that paid employment is essential in maintaining the respect of one's children, hence engagement in any other form of productive occupation is morally reprehensible. This is a sensitive area in which the values of the therapist are of no relevance. A client-centred definition of problems and goals related to engagement in productive occupation is essential in planning intervention strategies throughout the rehabilitation process (Law *et al.*, 1991).

Few research studies have examined a broad perspective of engagement in productive occupations, perhaps reflecting the values of the rehabilitation industry in general – that paid employment is the only valid measure of successful rehabilitation. Hence there are few existent models for effectively incorporating activities that relate to productive occupations into the rehabilitation process. However, there have been a few notable exceptions.

Kemp and Vash (1971) found that productivity (i.e. 'activities of a constructive nature') following spinal cord injury is more influenced by goals than by any other variable. Those individuals who expressed many new goals were significantly more productive than those who did not.

This reinforces a perspective of rehabilitation which fosters goal-directed behaviour among clients and which encourages individuals to establish a positive vision of the future, using long-term goals and attainable objectives (see Chapter 1). Unfortunately, many therapists have only ever been employed in institutions and therefore have not had first-hand experience with people who have spinal cord injuries and who are living in the community. This may generate low expectations for what may be accomplished following discharge. Follow-up clinics are more usually held in the sterile environment of the rehabilitation centre than the client's own environment and, under such artificial circumstances, it is difficult for the rehabilitation staff to gain a thorough understanding of the client's real life, his lifestyle and his accomplishments. Timing such clinics to suit the preferred working hours of professionals rather than their clients prohibits attendance by those who may have achieved the highest levels of productivity. The people who are seen in these clinics may not form a representative cross-section of people with spinal cord injuries, and staff may thus gain a negative impression of outcome and productivity following discharge.

Without fully exploiting this opportunity to learn from those with experience of community living, rehabilitation professionals have tended to underestimate both the potential for significant goal accomplishment and the barriers that may prevent goal attainment and which the rehabilitation professions should be addressing directly. People with disabilities have thus voiced the concern that their goals are discouraged by rehabilitation staff and that they are encouraged to reduce their expectations and to establish goals which aim low. As we have known for over 20 years that those individuals who express many goals become significantly more productive than those who do not (Kemp and Vash, 1971), such discouragement and deterrent must surely be counterproductive to the basic philosophies espoused by the rehabilitation team.

Kemp and Vash further indicate that those people who expressed a high number of goals related purely to physical functioning were found to be the least productive. This is of relevance to the discussion concerning FES and walking programmes (see Chapter 5). Creative thinking was found to have a positive correlation with productivity. Hence the innovative, problem-solving approach to spinal cord injury management and to addressing environmental barriers not only enhances the learning process and the attainment of objectives but actually influences post-discharge productivity.

Conversely, lack of self-direction and passivity were found to be negatively correlated with productivity. 'Less productive subjects displayed a passive demeanour and tended to be submissive to pressures, depending more on others for control and direction' (Kemp and Vash, 1971). This clearly indicates that the expectations for compliance and co-operation with the goals of others are directly counterproductive for a positive rehabilitation outcome.

Contrary to what might be expected, productivity has not been found to be correlated with level of injury, either in the engagement in paid employment or in unpaid productive occupations. Education has been found to be positively correlated with productivity. Physical disability limits the amount of manual labour that can be performed. Someone with a higher level of education is more likely to be involved in community organisations and less likely to be disadvantaged in the marketplace. As involvement in further education is itself a productive activity, it may be beneficial for clients who lack a clear vocational direction to enhance their opportunities by increasing their educational level.

Of great concern is the finding that transportation barriers have the highest negative correlation with productivity (DeJong, 1984). Accessible transportation is an aspect of public policy which is vital in fostering an active and productive lifestyle among disabled citizens. The absence of transportation which is equally accessible to all citizens serves to prohibit a target group from participation in the work force, in further education, in community organizations, volunteer activities and leisure pursuits. DeJong proposes that his findings highlight the importance of extending mobility training well beyond the walls of the rehabilitation centre. This would enable the client to identify potential barriers to full community participation and would also focus the therapist's attention upon the real issues concerning 'functional mobility'. DeJong queries: 'Why is it that factors considered so important by disabled persons themselves have been overlooked by so many rehabilitation researchers and writers?' One factor in this neglect may perhaps have been the habit of treating patients solely in the sterile isolation of the institution.

In 1978, disabled people blocked inaccessible buses for 24 hours in Denver, Colorado. The protest spurred accessible transit across the USA. Twenty-five years later, one of the protestors, (a post-polio quadriplegic) noted that, before the protest, buses had not been accessible and private transportation was not affordable. He had not been able to work because he could not afford to get there. Since buses became accessible, he has been working every day (New Mobility, 1992).

Rehabilitation professionals have tended to treat the personal, functional and psychological sequelae of spinal cord injury, focusing upon the 'problems' of the individual rather than those of the society to which he belongs. There has been a subsequent avoidance of focus upon the environmental barriers that may be an equal determinant of disability outcomes.

Little research attention has centred upon the diversity of productive occupations and the ways in which therapists can help to enhance post-discharge engagement in chosen activities. Some thought has been directed towards aids and equipment to help the disabled homemaker to achieve successful household management. Women with disabilities have written about their experiences of childcare and these works may serve as resources for their peers. Therapists have also designed baby slings and have modified equipment to facilitate childcare for parents who have spinal cord injuries.

Many studies have examined employment, vocational interests and vocational rehabilitation and these will be examined below.

Research concerning spinal cord injury has largely overlooked the broader concepts of productivity. Equal access to education (schools, colleges, universities), equal access to religious facilities, to voluntary organisations, or to other groups (such as political, union, fraternal) have not been of burning interest to the rehabilitation community. Even the physical and social barriers which prohibit access to the work place have received scant attention. The focus has been upon impairment and disability – not upon the factors that conspire to create handicap.

Hence, although well over a hundred research papers have examined psychological adjustment to spinal cord injury, few rehabilitation professionals have directed their attention to addressing those factors that may influence their client's abilities and opportunities to become fully productive members of their families, communities and to society as a whole. These issues must be addressed in the near future if we are to be accountable to either our clients or to the society that funds the rehabilitation programmes.

Employment/paid work

Research concerning the employment status of people with spinal cord injuries has tended to focus more upon the characteristics of employed persons than the environmental assets which may facilitate return to work.

It has been shown that level of injury is not necessarily correlated with employment status. However, it is suggested that it may take longer for people with quadriplegia to return to work, as they are less likely to be able to return to their former jobs. Hence, early studies which reported higher employment rates among people with paraplegia than among those with quadriplegia may have overlooked the importance of their comparatively few years since discharge (Krause, 1992).

Education has been found to be the most important factor influencing re-employment. Further, people who improve their education following injury are more likely to obtain employment than those who remain at the same educational level. People with higher levels of education are likely to incur less change in their occupation and leisure activities following a spinal cord injury. They are less likely to be disadvantaged by an inability to perform manual occupations. It is further suggested that people with higher levels of education may be more likely to be self-directed and responsible for their vocational future than people who have less education.

Krause (1992) found that, among people who did not complete school (i.e. who had less than 12 years of education), 38% had worked at some time since injury but only 3% were actually employed at the time of the study. Among those with over 16 years of education (equivalent to a USA degree), approximately 70% were employed at the time of the study and fully 96% had worked at some time since injury. His findings dramatically highlight the importance of higher education to the employment of persons with spinal cord injury.

Locus of control and learned helplessness constructs (see Chapter 1) may have relevance in the employment status of people who have spinal cord injuries. People who have an external locus of control belief, who have a low expectancy of influence over events and who have developed a sense of learned helplessness may be unable to take positive action to address physical and social barriers to attainment of their vocational goals.

Unemployment among people with spinal cord injuries in Alabama was found to be most common among people who were black, had less education and were more severely injured (DeVivo *et al.*, 1987). It could therefore be proposed that there is a mandate to further expand vocational rehabilitation programmes for people of minority status to address their needs for greater access to services. DeVivo reaches the contrary conclusion, that, as vocational rehabilitation success was measurable using a small number of predictor variables (i.e. being young, white, female, with high functional abilities and employed at the time of injury), 'one could defend instances when vocational rehabilitation counsellors could focus their efforts on persons having greatest vocational potential' (DeVivo and Fine, 1982).

It could be postulated, however, that, although such a strategy will guarantee impressive outcome statistics, this 'elite' group of rehabilitants may be achieving employment success without the interventions of these counsellors. Further, providing the opportunity for vocational rehabilitation only to those who are most likely to succeed (perhaps independently of the counsellors) encapsulates the philosophy that views disability as an individual problem which requires individual solutions – possibly defined by the individual's predictor variables. It fails to consider the impact of minority stigmatization, low societal expectations and the particularly poor situation and low opportunities for black people living in the American South. Rehabilitation professionals provide services within the context of their societies. 'The real test of a civilised society is the degree of decency with which it treats its minorities' (Pinker, 1974, cited in Jongbloed and Crichton, 1990).

In Sweden, the reverse philosophy has been adopted, that has seen national legislation enable access to transportation, home care services, technical aids and opportunities to engage in education and gainful employment. By seeking environmental changes to enable equal access to all citizens, rather than by teaching each individual to cope in an unfriendly environment, 80% of people with spinal cord injuries living in the community were gainfully employed or studying (Siösteen *et al.*, 1990; Lunqvist *et al.*, 1991), clearly a more impressive result than that achieved by individual intervention.

> Rehabilitation professionals still have a largely clinical or individualistic ideology and focus very little on improving the circumstances of disabled people through changes in law or social policies. They should be less willing to accept individual explanations for problems which are, essentially, economic, social or political and become more involved in advocacy with persons with disabilities.　　　(Jongbloed and Crichton, 1990)

Rohe and Athelstan (1982) evaluated the vocational interests of people with recent spinal cord injuries. Compared with national norms, the men with spinal cord injuries scored much lower on academic orientation, with good physical skills but discomfort with verbal expression. They scored highly on occupational preferences related to action-oriented activities in preference to those requiring data manipulation or interactions with people. Although there were insufficient women in the sample to draw any firm conclusions, it is interesting to note that the interests of spinal cord injured women least resemble those of nurses, physiotherapists and occupational therapists. This may be a potential source of conflict if the values and interests of the client and her rehabilitation staff are diametrically opposed. This evidence supports the proposition that rehabilitation staff should not seek to set goals for their clients nor try to direct their lives. Given the diversity of interests, goals and values, such intervention would, at best, be worthless.

Although Rohe and Athelstan's findings indicate that the vocational interests of people with spinal cord injuries might be incompatible with the limitations imposed by the disability (e.g. farmer, forester, merchant marine officer), their subsequent study reveals some changes in vocational interests, several years after injury (Rohe and Athelstan, 1985). At an average of eight years after injury, the spinal cord injured subjects had increased interests in areas of social involvement – teacher, psychologist, social worker, lawyer, speech pathologist, for example, and also increased interest in the arts.

These studies emphasize the importance of maintaining contact with people with spinal cord injuries and assuring them of appropriate vocational rehabilitation services on an ongoing basis. As it may take considerable time to develop vocational interests in occupations congruent with a physical disability, researchers' measurements of employment status may have very different results, depending upon the number of years after injury. Krause (1992) found that employment rates improve dramatically with increasing time since injury. Hence he strongly opposes the misleading practice of calculating a single employment rate for all people after spinal cord injury.

However, Rohe and Athelstan (1985) also found that the interests that were present before injury were not diminished following physical disability. They therefore propose that 'rehabilitation counsellors should assess interests, assume that they are unlikely to change greatly, and help devise strategies for acting on interests that are present but no longer physically possible'. This appears to be a more constructive approach than the dismissal of 'impossible' interests. Although some research subjects developed new interests, established interest patterns remained consistent for most subjects.

Analysis of research findings revealed that people with spinal cord injuries tended towards introversion, preferring the concrete, practical and physical rather than abstract ideas, interpersonal interactions and verbal self-expression. It is therefore proposed that a counselling process which encourages the expression of innermost thoughts, concerns and feelings is likely to be threatening, bewildering – and unsuccessful. Instead, an approach based on behavioural techniques and accurate feedback on progress is likely to be more appropriate (Rohe and Athelstan, 1982).

Jellinek and Harvey (1982) illustrate the importance of vocational and educational services for people with spinal cord injuries by increasing from 19% to 75% the numbers of clients attaining employment or attending further education following provision of vocational services.

However, although it may not be appropriate for all people with spinal cord injuries to undergo extensive vocational planning during in-patient treatment, it is important that interests and goals are identified and treated seriously throughout the rehabilitation process. Early identification of vocational goals will enhance treatment planning, optimize collaborative goal setting and foster innovative approaches to problems and environments. It may be possible to engage actively social and community support systems to explore options and evaluate choices.

It is also important that rehabilitation services are not limited to the period immediately following injury but are extended throughout life so that those people who must change job due to declining physical status, for example, can continue to benefit from vocational rehabilitation services. Future research should focus more upon the barriers that prevent people from working following a spinal cord injury. Krause (1992) reiterates that if rehabilitation services are to be successful in helping people return to the workplace following injury, they must address issues such as attendant care and environmental accessibility. Equal opportunities will require legal protection to eliminate job discrimination and to ensure access to jobs in accordance with the capacity of the individual.

Spinal cord injury affects primarily young people who have good potential for significant contributions to society. Discriminatory hiring practices, architectural barriers to employment, prohibitive financial disincentives and inequitable access to transportation add considerably to the financial burden to society which is created by a spinal cord injury. If the disabled individual wishes to attain financial independence and employment status, it is counterproductive not to enable achievement of these goals.

Outcome measurement

Outcome measurement related to productivity performance has focused primarily upon return to paid work, as outlined above. Some studies have included productivity in non-paid occupations but measures have failed to consider the relevance and appropriateness of roles in productivity or at those people who may be underemployed relative to their abilities and qualifications.

Assessment of productivity performance following spinal cord injury will require development of tools to measure multiple aspects of productivity (not solely employment status) and consider the relevance of roles and motivation of the individual; and the impact of the environment (CAOT, 1991).

LEISURE

Leisure activities have been defined as those components of life that are free from work and self-care activities (CAOT, 1991). If occupations related to productivity are considered to be those that give life its meaning and purpose, then leisure activities may be conceptualized as being those elements that contribute to life's quality.

There is an assumption that a balanced life will consist of constructive performance in the areas of self-care, productivity and leisure and further, that imbalances between self-care, productivity and leisure time are problematic for maintaining health and wellbeing. However, 'balanced' time does not mean equal time, and few studies have examined the absolute and relative amounts of time that adults spend on these three occupations. Hence it is not yet possible to identify time-use patterns indicative of imbalance, or to identify variations in time use related to role expectations, sociocultural environments or the meaning attached to these activities (McKinnon, 1992).

Some occupations may be viewed as productivity for some people. For example, painting may be a productive activity for a commercial artist. The same activity may be considered to be a leisure interest by someone else.

Despite the importance of engagement in leisure activities following spinal cord injury, few studies have examined this element of occupational performance. This presents problems to the rehabilitation team who seek to enhance engagement in leisure activities and ensure that the client gains the skills to maintain a balance between the components of daily occupations.

Exploration of leisure interests is part of a comprehensive rehabilitation programme which aims to assist the person with a spinal cord injury to return to a balanced and fulfilling life in the community. Following a spinal cord injury, the client may view his mobility limitations as barriers prohibiting involvement in his former leisure activities. Few people are aware of the range of sporting activities, for example, which are available to people with disabilities. The rehabilitation professionals have an important role to play in providing early exposure to the options and choices that are available to enhance awareness and encourage participation.

It is proposed that the rehabilitation programme should include the identification and use of community recreational resources, exploration of adaptations to enable participation in previous leisure interests, the learning of new leisure skills and the refinement of functional abilities related to specific leisure activities. Staas emphasises the long-lasting benefits of incorporating leisure activities into the individual's lifestyle and further suggests that those people who are able to use leisure time constructively and meaningfully are less likely to become depressed. 'The discovery and development of "quality" in his or her lifestyle has its beginnings in the discovery that many sources of self-satisfaction and re-integration into society remain open' (Staas *et al.*, 1988).

Assessment of leisure interests will examine preferences, skills, interests, enjoyment and satisfaction. Intervention will be based both upon the individual and the environment.

From the individual perspective, efforts may focus upon task modification, utilization of special aids and equipment, locating community interest and recreation groups or facilities and re-learning skills and techniques to maximize residual physical function.

Examination of the range of leisure interests outlined below makes clear that an individual focus for intervention will be insufficient and in many instances, ineffective. Leisure activities, perhaps more than any other, require access to a wide range of facilities and locations. Hence intervention will be directed towards removal of architectural barriers and to equalizing access to enable involvement in social and leisure activities.

For the purposes of discussion, leisure occupations will be divided into those activities related to:

- quiet recreation
- active recreation
- socialization.

Quiet recreation

The following is not an exhaustive list of activities. Rather, it is a guide which may suggest avenues for exploration. Many activities may be performed alone but some, such as hobbies, crafts, games and collections may include possibilities for group involvement and wider community participation.

- Listening to the radio
- watching television
- listening to records, tapes, compact discs
- reading books, magazines, newspapers
- hobbies and collections
- crafts, such as pottery, knitting, weaving
- other creative arts – painting, collage etc.
- playing cards, board games.

Active recreation

People with spinal cord injuries have taught us much about active recreation. While rehabilitation centres were teaching archery and snooker, people with spinal cord injuries in the community were canoeing, skiing, hunting and exploring other avenues for active participation in fulfilling and challenging activities. The following, then, is far from an exhaustive list of activities. However, it does provide some suggestions and hopefully will encourage people with spinal cord injuries and their therapists to recognize the considerable potential which exists for engagement in active recreation and hence to explore the possibilities and opportunities.

Entertainment venues that may be visited include:

- sporting events
- museums, libraries
- ballet, opera or drama
- films and festivals, concerts and performances
- art galleries.

Participatory activities include:

- fishing, hunting
- camping, hiking
- caring for a pet
- recreational driving
- dining out
- photography
- visiting parks, beaches and resorts
- attending religious services
- attending lectures and courses
- travelling
- participating in music and drama
- birdwatching
- participating in, or coaching sports (Law *et al.*, 1991; McKinnon, 1992).

Sporting activities include:

- archery
- airguns
- pistol shooting
- aerobics
- auto racing
- basketball
- bowling – alley/green
- quad rugby
- racquetball
- scuba diving
- ballooning
- stretching
- volleyball
- table tennis
- road racing/marathons
- rowing
- canoeing, kayaking
- skiing – snow/water

- dog sledding
- river rafting
- pulking (sit-skiing; Nilsen *et al.*, 1985)
- horse riding
- sailing, boating
- martial arts
- swimming
- tennis
- flying
- fencing
- weight lifting
- all-terrain vehicle racing (ATVs)
- snooker/pool
- darts
- motor cycling
- fencing
- track and field: discus, javelin, shot put, pentathlon, slalom
- triathlon – rowing, swimming, wheeling
- wheelchair racing – 100 m, 200 m, 400 m etc. (Maddox, 1987).

People with spinal cord injuries may engage in many of these sporting activities alongside other people with disabilities or with able-bodied peers. People who have sustained spinal cord injuries have the same rights to experience risk and to participate in adventure sports as they did before injury – the same rights as other adults. It is recommended that the appropriate wheelchair sports association is contacted regarding recommended equipment, accessories or modifications required for certain sports (e.g. ATVs).

Participation in sports has the same potential multiplicity of benefits for people with spinal cord injuries as for non-disabled people. Although research studies have yet to prove conclusive causality, it is thought that physical benefits include improved physiological functioning, increased cardiopulmonary fitness, increased respiratory function in addition to enhanced strength, balance, co-ordination and endurance. Psychological benefits are believed to include self-confidence, stimulation, competition, decreased stress, improved self-image, sportsmanship, personal mastery and the opportunity to test the limits of ability. Social benefits include decreased isolation, interaction with others, team participation, opportunities for travel, comradeship, increased activity levels and increased community participation (Madorsky *et al.*, 1992). Madorsky provides a thorough exploration of training methods for prospective wheelchair athletes.

The opportunity to participate in sports is especially important when Rohe and Athelstan's (1982) findings are considered. They indicate that the high level of interest in adventure and sports among men with spinal cord injuries had not diminished eight years after discharge.

Although Stotts (1986) found that paraplegic athletes had less kidney infections and skin breakdowns than non-athletes this does not prove the direction of causality or a positive relationship between involvement in sports and maintenance of health. The presence of medical complications may have served to prohibit inclusion in sports for certain people. Similarly, athletes may have different psychological and social characteristics which make them more responsible for health maintenance.

Specific research related to the unique physiology associated with spinal cord injuries and the demands of wheelchair mobility is necessary to enhance performance and reduce injuries.

It has been shown that people with spinal cord injuries are at increased risk for cardiovascular disease and this is a primary cause of death. Brenes (1986) suggests that people with spinal cord injuries, who have the lowest concentrations of high-density lipoprotein (HDL) reported for any population, need to substantially increase their levels of activity to reduce their substantially elevated risks of heart attack. The importance of engagement in athletic activity cannot be overstated in reducing the otherwise inherent inactivity associated with spinal cord injury.

Although the grass roots movement has changed wheelchair sports from a therapeutic activity to the competitive arena, the involvement of those with skills and expertise in sports medicine remains important. Prevention, diagnosis and treatment of athletic injuries, medical examinations before participation and the design of training programmes are all areas in which medical and paramedical personnel may be involved. There is a dual benefit, as those medical staff who are made aware of the level of participation and scope of wheelchair sports will be better able to provide informed advice to newly injured people.

Sports injuries

The most prevalent injuries sustained by wheelchair athletes have been outlined by Madorsky and Curtis (1984), as follows:

- soft-tissue injuries, most commonly at the shoulders, elbows, wrists and hands and including muscle sprains, strains, bursitis and tendonitis. Many such injuries are recurrent, and prevention consists of routine stretching, warm-up and cool-down and an appropriately graduated training programme;
- blisters of the hands and fingers are commonly caused by friction against the wheel rim or tyre, and abrasions may be caused by contact with the brakes or by trapping the fingers. Brakes may be removed from the chair for sporting activities;
- pressure sores are at high risk due to trauma, friction and increased pressure on the sacrum caused by the design of many sports wheelchairs. Sweat and moisture exacerbate the problem which may be alleviated by attention to cushioning, pressure relief, nutrition, hygiene and absorbent clothing. Outstanding athletes, with or without disabilities, will always run the risk of injury as they stress tissue tolerance to its maximum during training and competitions. Nevertheless, most injuries are not serious, sprains and strains accounting for the majority of complications among people with spinal cord injuries who participate in sports (Nilsen *et al.*, 1985).

Socialization

Socialization may be conceptualized as a component of leisure activities, including interactions with family, friends and wider involvement in the community. The importance to health and wellbeing of strong social support systems will be outlined below. Socialization examines the activities by which social bonds are initiated, strengthened and maintained. Opportunities for social interaction are inherent in most of the activities outlined as **active recreation** and some of those delineated as **quiet recreation**. As social isolation is a common experience following a traumatic spinal cord injury, it is of great importance that the elements of satisfying socialization are considered and enhanced during the rehabilitation programme and through follow-up assessment.

Socialization may include:

- visiting, entertaining
- telephone contact
- letters and mail
- planning and attending social functions
- attending bars, pubs and clubs.

From an individualistic perspective on intervention, the importance of enhancing social skills and developing strategies to facilitate interactions was outlined in Chapter 5. However, it is evident that an individual strategy for intervention is woefully inadequate. For as long as bars, clubs, social facilities and community buildings incorporate discriminatory barriers to equal access, people with spinal cord injuries will experience considerable impediments to engagement in social interactions and activities.

In examining the factors that influence leisure activities following stroke, Morgan and Jongbloed (1990) report that, although some activity changes are attributable to reduced function, the interaction of individuals with their total environment is much more important than the severity of the disability. Future research which examines the involvement in leisure and socialization of people with spinal cord injuries will need to consider the impact of a facilitatory or a discriminatory environment.

Investigation of the impact of a spinal cord injury upon social relationships and leisure behaviour will increase our understanding of the complex relationships between actual occupational performance and the social, physical and cultural environment (Morgan and Jongbloed, 1990).

Activity levels in the community

An early study examined the pursuits, before and after injury, of people with traumatic quadriplegia in terms of frequency of participation and enjoyment of activities. Participation in avocational activities following spinal cord injury was found to decline despite a period since discharge ranging from 1.5 to 4.5 years. Those activities reported at greatest decline in participation included sports and exercise, outdoor activities, travel, acquiring new skills and going out for eating and drinking. No activity (including pursuits such as reading) was reported as having a substantial increase in participation. Lack of transportation was identified as a primary obstacle to activity (Rogers and Figone, 1978).

In a study of people following spinal cord injury, Yerxa and Locker (1990) identified the obstacles to community functioning:

- architectural barriers
- lack of friends or social activities
- lack of accessible transportation
- lack of financial resources.

Hammell (1991) reported that men with spinal cord injuries had lower levels of social integration than a comparison group of men with severe head injuries. All the men with spinal cord injuries commented that lack of access prohibited their full participation in society.

However, the number and diversity of activities in which a spinal cord injured person engages during in-patient rehabilitation has been found to predict the number of activities after discharge (Rintala and Willems, 1987).

Close examination must be made of the in-patient milieu, as study by Kennedy *et al.* (1988) suggests that people with spinal cord injuries have a high level of engagement in solitary activities during in-patient rehabilitation. Their results revealed a social ecology of solitary and inactive behaviour, passivity and lack of diversity of activity. This would appear to be totally at variance with the concept of active rehabilitation that is suggested to be the best predictor of positive post-discharge outcome. If the rehabilitation programme is focused towards ensuring a high level of social interaction and activity following discharge, it is imperative that close scrutiny of the in-patient environment reveals a milieu that fosters patient involvement and activity, not institutionalization.

Outcome measurement

Assessment of the components of life that are characterised as 'leisure' may examine interests, or frequency of involvement.

Standardized measurement is made complex by the personal meaning that may be construed by an activity; for example, use of the telephone may be a function of productivity for one person, a form of recreation for another or a vital component of self-care for another. An understanding of the individual's interpretation of his activities is essential to measure outcome accurately. Yerxa and Locker (1990) found that occupational therapists agreed more with each other than with their spinal cord injured subjects when classifying occupations. This again indicates the need to gain an understanding of the client's life, through active dialogue.

Although subjective measures may record ratings of enjoyment, satisfaction and involvement in chosen leisure activities, further research is required to develop outcome measures that assess performance in leisure activities (CAOT, 1991).

SOCIAL SUPPORT

Human beings of all ages are found to be at their happiest and to be able to deploy their talents to best advantage when they are confident that, standing behind them, there are one or more trusted persons who will come to their aid should difficulties arise. The person trusted provides a secure base from which his companion can operate.   (Bowlby, 1973)

Social support is generally defined in terms of the availability of people whom the individual trusts, on whom he can rely and who make him feel cared for and valued.

Many studies have highlighted the importance of social support in attenuating the effects of events that are stressful, hence reducing the incidence of disease or morbidity. The presence of social support has been related to reduced levels of distress and depression.

A study of the factors that influence return to work following a traumatic spinal cord injury concluded that the identification of a strong social network as defined by the presence of one or more confidants was an important correlate of post-injury employment status (MacKenzie *et al.*, 1987).

Broadhead *et al.* (1983) reviewed the many theories concerning the causal link between social support and health. They conclude: 'The goodness of fit between person and environment

depends upon a match between the demands of the environment and the person's abilities to meet them on the one hand,
and the needs of the individual and the resources from the
environment available to satisfy these needs on the other.'

Mental health is associated with having several good friends,
abundant contacts with people both outside the home and
outside the primary group and above all, not one but a number
of attachment figures (Henderson *et al.*, 1978). The emphasis
in examining social support must focus upon the quality of
relationships rather than just their number or type.

Schulz and Decker (1985; Decker and Schulz, 1985) inter-
viewed 100 people an average of 20 years after their spinal cord
injuries. They concluded that those people who had high levels
of social support, who were satisfied with their social contacts
and who felt they had high levels of control over their lives also
reported high levels of wellbeing. Of particular significance was
the finding that 41% of respondents named only one support
person – usually a female spouse. This finding may be relevant
to the subsequent study of the primary care givers of this same
group of people. There was an inverse relationship between the
perceived burden of care and satisfaction with the quality and
quantity of social contacts. The researchers note that this
reciprocal relationship between the spinal cord injured person
and the carer/spouse requires attention not only to the social
support network available to the person with paraplegia but also
to that of the care giver/spouse (Decker *et al.*, 1989).

In further studies of people with spinal cord injuries, social
support has been found to be positively related to life satisfaction and physical wellbeing, and associated negatively with
depressive symptomatology. People with spinal cord injuries
who perceive a high level of social support have been found
to have significantly fewer health problems and hospital
admissions than those who report low availability and adequacy
of social support (Anson, 1993).

What are the implications for healthcare and rehabilitation
personnel of the numerous research reports linking social support to physical wellbeing, life satisfaction, positive mental
health, self-esteem and hope? Clearly, there must be a concerted
effort to enhance the existing social bonds between the client
and his support system but, unfortunately, the literature is not
replete with models for accomplishing this goal. Rintala (1992)

suggests that interventions might include social skills training, counselling or providing recreational and social events to include people with spinal cord injuries and those people who are viewed as important. Research should investigate whether interventions are effective in producing change in the quality or quantity of social support.

Hammell (1991) suggests that examination should be made of the ways in which partners may be included throughout the rehabilitation process and the relationship of this involvement to subsequent emotional wellbeing. From the earliest stage of treatment, efforts should be made to assist both partners in strengthening social supports – by involvement of close family and friends in therapy sessions, social activities and making decisions. Hammell's study found that social integration scores were lower among men with spinal cord injuries than for men with severe head injuries, even many years after discharge. This impoverished social situation was found to be shared by their wives. Although the modal number of weeks of rehabilitation for men with severe traumatic head injuries was zero, all the men with spinal cord injuries had attended a special unit and receive regular follow-up care. It is to be hoped that greater emphasis upon community management, socialization, social supports and social interaction as part of the comprehensive rehabilitation process will improve these gloomy findings and ensure that people with spinal cord injuries achieve full and satisfying social integration.

Studies that suggest that the severity of a disability is not the primary indicator of quality of life and satisfaction with life following injury must encourage researchers to examine the interaction of the client with his environment. Morgan and Jongbloed (1990) propose that the attitudes and behaviours of family members and friends are a vital part of that environment and exert a strong influence on how the individual views his disability and on how social relationships, roles and activities are maintained or altered.

Exclusion of the patient's primary group during acute care and rehabilitation, and inadequate attention to full social re-integration during the rehabilitation programme will be counter-productive to the achievement of maximal social, mental and physical health, to productivity and to satisfaction with leisure and socialization.

CULTURAL ENVIRONMENT

Although rehabilitation practice formerly addressed the individual in isolation from his environment, more recent attention has been focused towards the interaction between the client and his unique environment. It is acknowledged, for example, that someone who has a supportive social environment, an accessible physical environment, a positive economic environment and a progressive political and legal environment is likely to be able to achieve a higher level of productivity and engagement in a greater variety of activities than someone whose personal environment is more repressive.

The beliefs and cultures which are unique and personal to our clients will form part of the complex equation affecting response to spinal cord injury, to responsibilities for health, to roles and to engagement in occupations following discharge.

Culture is used to allude to the beliefs, values and customs of an interacting group. In an increasingly multicultural society it is likely that the beliefs, values and customs of clients will not correspond with those of their healthcare and rehabilitation personnel. If rehabilitation is to direct intervention towards the life of the client rather than towards the individual in isolation, it is important that practitioners seek greater awareness of the cultures of their clients.

> The client-centred orientation of practice which seeks an active engagement on the part of the client in defining problems and in setting goals, requires ongoing development of the understanding of how culture shapes conceptions of, and responses to, illness and disability.   (Dyck, 1989)

Dyck proposes that meaningful therapeutic intervention must be framed within interests, values, goals, roles and habits which may be quite unfamiliar to the therapist. She suggests, however, that an awareness on the part of the therapist of differences in cultural values and beliefs will help to gain the active engagement of the client in the treatment process through avoiding activities that may have little meaning to the client or may even be offensive. Further, therapists need to reflect upon their own cultural values and beliefs, to identify possible discordance and to avoid cultural stereotyping.

A philosophical shift away from the narrow focus of the

medical model or individual, pathology-oriented care towards the multifaceted nature of people's lives will demand a greater awareness and understanding of the context of client's values, beliefs and customs.

To be effective, measurements used to assess outcome should reflect cultural sensitivity rather than the traditional value system and role expectations of the dominant culture.

WOMEN AND SPINAL CORD INJURY

Among people with spinal cord injuries, women are a minority group. For this reason, they have been under-represented to a significant degree in research studies. Even those studies that have aimed to examine a cross-section of people with spinal cord injuries have frequently had insufficient women represented to be able to provide statistically meaningful results.

Literature concerning spinal cord injury has addressed physiological issues concerning menstruation and pregnancy but has rarely acknowledged the psychological and social issues such as the effects of double handicap experienced by those who are both women and disabled. Perhaps the present work has unintentionally contributed to this inequity, by use of the male pronoun to denote all people with spinal cord injuries.

The minority status indicated by the statistic that only 18% of people with spinal cord injuries in developed countries are women masks the prevalence of women with spinal cord injuries in the community. A simple calculation based on the prevalence statistics outlined in Chapter 3 indicates that approximately 7000 women in the UK and 40 000 women in the USA are living with spinal cord injuries. These are substantial numbers and the perspectives and concerns of women in rehabilitation and in the community clearly merit further attention.

In 1978, Trieschmann noted the paucity of research into the experience of women following spinal cord injury. A decade later she reports a similar disregard for this issue and raises some questions concerning the role of women in society, and especially, the role of disabled women: 'How women cope with disability, whether they cope, what levels of accomplishment they achieve have apparently not been of interest to researchers because the status of these women is not important in our society, and health professionals are a product of this society' (Trieschmann, 1988).

Research studies help to shape the attitudes of professionals, the formation of programmes and the direction of interventions. As researchers, it is evident that we have failed to ask the questions that pertain to women's experience of spinal cord injury. We know little or nothing about their experiences of disability, of their interactions with their environments, of their goals for productivity or leisure, or their perceptions of economic, sociocultural and political barriers to independent and quality living. This provides a poor basis from which to shape programmes of excellence to meet the needs of women. It cannot be assumed that women's experience of spinal cord injury is the same as that of men.

Women have reported the inadequate and prolonged treatment they have experienced in general hospitals. Even in specialized spinal units, however, they report little or no help in coming to terms with the emotional upheaval of sudden paralysis.

> The overwhelming message from women's experience of treatment and rehabilitation following spinal cord injury is that, with some exceptions, there seems to be a policy, and there is certainly a practice, of giving very little attention to the emotional aspects of treatment and rehabilitation.
>
> (Morris, 1989)

The Spinal Injuries Association published virtually the only work containing accounts of women's experience of spinal cord injury (Morris, 1989). This provides invaluable insight to rehabilitation and community workers concerning the perceptions of women of their situation and their treatment. Women speak of assaults to their personal dignity as they were expected to ignore the way the nurses left their clothes twisted untidily and uncomfortably about them; of dissolving into tears and therefore being sent back from physiotherapy 'in disgrace', and of having no opportunities to learn from others who were in similar situations. Most particularly, women report the forced jollity of the units, the requirement for a 'stiff upper lip' and a constant smile. They resented the failure of the staff to help them to plan their futures realistically; and the overwhelming emphasis upon gait training and competitive sports rather than addressing their own needs and priorities.

Trieschmann (1988) discusses society's orientation towards youth and beauty and the disenfranchisement that disabled women may experience if they feel that they have lost their physical attractiveness and some aspects of their femininity. This may be a particular issue during acute care and rehabilitation when female patients are exposed to a predominantly young, predominantly female and overwhelmingly able-bodied staff. Women with spinal cord injuries may feel that these staff members will not understand their situation, emotions and needs. Further, Rohe and Athelstan (1982) indicate that the interests of women with spinal cord injuries least resemble those of social workers, nurses, psychologists, occupational therapists and physiotherapists. They report: 'Lack of congruence in interests may lead hospital staff to conclude that those with SCI [spinal cord injuries] are very different from themselves, thus complicating their interaction. This may even lead to patients being labelled problem personalities more often than their actual behaviour warrants.'

Pinkerton and Griffin (1983) provide one of the few outcome studies of women with spinal cord injuries. Their samples were small, but they identified high levels of activity and positive perceptions of life satisfaction although also a disturbing incidence of suicide. Compared with men with spinal cord injuries, the women maintained their health better and had fewer and shorter hospitalizations. The researchers conclude that the incidence of feelings of depression and frustration illustrates the need for more emphasis to be placed during the rehabilitation period on programmes designed to improve coping and social interaction. This echoes the findings of Morris (1989).

There is an urgent need for thorough research to provide insight into the experiences and needs of women with spinal cord injuries and their perspectives concerning the relevance of current rehabilitation programmes. A considerable body of research has been generated which concerns the experiences and needs of men, and these findings have, to a greater or lesser extent, infiltrated the rehabilitation programmes that are ostensibly designed to meet those needs.

Until a similar body of research has indicated clear directions for rehabilitation, some guidelines are apparent. There is a very great need for a holistic emphasis upon psychosocial aspects of disability and not solely upon physical goals. Although this approach has been emphasized throughout the current work, the needs of women to express their emotions, receive support and counselling and focus upon interpersonal relationships make the argument for this approach especially convincing.

There is a clear need for rehabilitation staff to gain an understanding of their female client's values, goals and interests. Essential in the management of all people with spinal cord injuries, this may be especially important if rehabilitation personnel and their female clients have widely divergent interests and values, as indicated by Rohe and Athelstan (1982).

There needs also to be an expanded interest into issues especially important to women; issues of child care, home making and sexual relationships in addition to those issues of education, employment, leisure interests and socialization which are important to all clients. 'Hospitals and the people who run them can be crucial in helping us to confront these issues. Sadly they usually fail us' (Morris, 1989).

Therapists who work with spinal cord injured women in making future plans, in establishing goals and realizing objectives will need to understand clearly the unique roles in which each woman engages, her cultural expectations, her social support systems, her values and her unique needs for support and information.

Because it is acknowledged that women (if admitted to spinal units at all) will be in a minority, it is incumbent upon the rehabilitation staff to facilitate peer counselling so that a woman with an acute injury may learn ways of coping with role expectations and societal demands from someone who has already gained this experience.

CHILDREN AND SPINAL CORD INJURY

Acquired traumatic spinal cord injury is uncommon in children, with less than 3% of all spinal injuries reported to occur to those under 15 years of age. However, reports indicate that anatomical and developmental factors predispose children to upper cervical injuries and subsequent catastrophic neurological loss. Motor vehicle accidents are the most common cause of spinal cord injury among children, with diving injuries, falls and sporting accidents accounting for most of the other injuries (Flett, 1992). The majority of such injuries are wholly preventable.

Although rehabilitation goals will be similar to those for adults, especial efforts must be made to include the whole family throughout the treatment process and to consider the developmental stage of the child. The physical/functional, mental/intellectual, sociocultural and spiritual components of a holistic rehabilitation programme are as important to the child as to the adult but these are growth areas in childhood, and attention must be directed towards facilitating rather than stunting such growth.

Rehabilitation for the child who has a spinal cord injury will be focused upon returning the child to his former school, enabling him to achieve full re-integration, exploring and maximizing his leisure interests, fostering self-esteem and encouraging him to maximize his academic opportunities towards future employment.

Achievement of self-care, leisure and productive activities will, to a very real extent, be influenced by environmental variables. Political, legal and physical barriers to full educational opportunities and re-integration; social and cultural disincentives to full participation, and economic disadvantage may have severely detrimental effects upon the disabled child. Rehabilitation professionals' interventions will be less than effective if directed only towards the child and not towards his environment.

Children with spinal cord injuries will need to engage in rehabilitation programmes that maximize their functional abilities while fostering normal development, social skills and interaction with others. Young children learn through play, hence use of appropriate toys for the developmental level of the child and his physical/functional abilities will be important. Zejdlik (1992) emphasizes the need to foster developmental progress from the earliest stages of treatment. She indicates that the erroneous assumption that medical and surgical interventions must take prior place, with little regard to the child's natural development, has led to serious, sometimes irreversible psychosocial problems, such as regression, social deprivation and delayed development. She stresses the importance of early collaboration among spinal cord injury and paediatric professionals.

Children who sustain spinal cord injuries are at high risk for developing scoliosis and hip and knee deformities. Regular, long-term monitoring is essential, as deformities have serious consequences for health, positioning and self-esteem.

Young and Cocks (1991) outline a programme of occupational therapy interventions with the ventilator-dependent, spinal cord injured child and the parents. Early recreational involvement with their children helps to compensate for the invasive management techniques in which the parents are engaged. Families of children with spinal cord injuries must be assured of substantial support and regularly scheduled respite care for children with high lesions.

ADOLESCENTS AND SPINAL CORD INJURY

Intervention appropriate to age is especially important in the rehabilitation of the adolescent who has sustained a spinal cord injury. Developmental needs must be considered concurrently with physical and functional needs.

The physical sequelae of spinal cord injury have already been examined. In the case of an adolescent, these massive changes occur at a time when the individual is resolving issues related to personal identity, body image, sexual identity, peer relationships and occupational choice.

Adolescence is a phase typified by questioning authority and seeking independence. A co-operative balance between achieving necessary care activities and performing them within the client's time frame may need to be achieved. Rehabilitation will require collaborative goal planning, allowing for increased independence, enhancement of decision-making skills and opportunities for socialization. Thorough examination of interests and exploration of skills will provide options for treatment activities and for future leisure pursuits. The need to establish objectives which are measurable and achievable is especially important for this client group who have a particular need to be able to chart progress and measure accomplishments.

Prolonged hospitalization may produce social isolation and disengagement from peer groups. Rehabilitation staff can facilitate contacts with peers who have been discharged for a year or two, who can act as positive role models and enable a sharing of experiences.

In addition to exploration of leisure pursuits, identifying recreational activities and facilities, encouraging re-integration into former educational settings and investigating career options, particular attention will be given to socialization. Community excursions, such as to the cinema, shopping centres and restaurants, will enable the adolescent to participate in age-appropriate social activities, facilitating social re-integration and enabling experiential learning as community barriers are identified and overcome.

Mulcahey (1992) proposes a broad perspective on rehabilitation for the adolescent with a spinal cord injury. Future productivity, satisfaction with leisure and social interaction will largely be influenced by the success of the re-integration that occurs following rehabilitation. Successful rehabilitation will not be measured by achievement of independence in personal care activities but by the resumption of meaningful lifestyles and enactment of appropriate roles. Social skills such as initiating conversation, negotiating social interactions, resolving barriers in the environment and networking with other patients to foster support systems and facilitate information exchange, will be an integral part of the rehabilitation process.

Successful rehabilitation to community re-integration will depend upon a sensitive understanding of the perceptions and perspectives of the adolescent and a broad vision of the needs to perform productive, leisure and social activities within a unique and personal sociocultural environment.

THE ELDERLY AND SPINAL CORD INJURY

Although spinal cord injury is predominantly a phenomenon of youth, elderly people are not immune to such trauma. Statistics indicate that approximately 5–7% of all such injuries are sustained by people aged 60 or older. These percentages will increase as the population ages.

Hooker (1986) indicates the typical aetiologies of spinal cord lesions among the elderly. A total of 49% of her subjects were injured in falls and 40% had non-traumatic aetiologies. Studies indicate that cervical injuries predominate in the elderly population. Stover and Fine (1986) report that 67% of those aged between 61–75 years sustain quadriplegias, whereas this figure is 88% among those aged over 75.

Reports suggest that a large proportion of people over the age of 55 have significant medical problems which are unrelated to their spinal cord injuries but which may compromise residual functioning.

A high mortality rate is reported for people aged 60 or older at injury, particularly among people with neurologically complete quadriplegias. There is a comparatively poor prognosis for patients in the oldest age group, with few of these individuals achieving independence in self-care activities (DeVivo *et al.*, 1990).

However, rehabilitation programmes still have both the mandate and potential to enhance self-care skills for the spinal cord injured elderly. Achievement of independence in any self-care activity is of great importance to the individual. Even partial gains towards independence will decrease reliance upon care providers.

The elderly person who has sustained a spinal cord injury shares all the potential complications that may affect his younger counterparts. Many of these problems may be exacerbated by additional factors. Contractures, for example, may be at higher risk due to concomitant intra-articular problems. Elderly people are at greater risk of skin breakdown than younger persons. The effects of prolonged bed rest are especially detrimental to elderly people.

The rehabilitation process may be made more difficult by the complexity of the problems facing the elderly person with a spinal cord injury. The high incidence of cervical lesions, decreased tolerance to fatigue, decreased muscle strength and decreased functional abilities may be compounded by an increased difficulty in learning new habits and behaviours. Hooker (1986) indicates that this group may be especially susceptible to developing learned helplessness behaviours, characterized by depression, powerlessness and disengagement. Social support systems are likely to be reduced in quantity and ageing care givers may be unable to provide substantial material support.

Functional mobility will require wheelchair skills, due to the substantial energy costs required for ambulation. Personal care skills may be maximized and the individual will learn how to direct others to meet his care needs. This is important, irrespective of discharge location. Few nursing home staff, for example, are skilled in the care of someone with quadriplegia, so the responsibility for personal care cannot be removed from the individual.

Rehabilitation attention will also be focused upon opportunities for leisure and socialization. McKinnon (1992) reports that on average, elderly Canadians use 7.5 hours per day for leisure activities. As substantial time is devoted to engagement in leisure occupations among elderly people, exploration of leisure options will be likely to be a predominant aspect of rehabilitation for this age group.

The philosophy of client-centred practice is no less important for the elderly client. Early involvement in making decisions, in establishing goals and objectives and in active participation in defining activities will help to reduce the tendency towards learned helplessness and dependence upon staff.

Further research is needed into the specific needs of the elderly person with a spinal cord injury and how the rehabilitation team can best address these needs.

INDEPENDENT LIVING MOVEMENT

The Independent Living (IL) movement emerged in the USA in the 1960s as a grassroots effort on the part of people with disabilities to acquire new rights, full control over their lives and the opportunity to participate actively in every aspect of society.

As a social movement, the IL philosophy has incorporated an agenda consisting of some basic principles:

- consumer control over service delivery
- the 'right to risk' as an inherent component of true independence
- the demedicalization of basic, self-care maintenance activities in the management of medically stable disabilities
- self-determination, as the right of all people to direct their own lives and choose their own lifestyles
- individual choice of service delivery to empower and enable people to pursue active lives. (Oxelgren *et al.*, 1992).

The IL philosophy has become a powerful force for change throughout much of the world and has forced disability professionals and researchers to realign their thinking and research directions. It has helped to spawn new models of service delivery and has helped to meet previously unmet needs, such as peer counselling and service delivery from disabled people.

DeJong (1979) indicates that the IL movement has primarily focused its energies on a selected population – young adults, primarily from the ethnic majority. People with spinal cord injuries are among those at the core of the movement.

In the beginning of the IL movement, disability professionals were viewed as contributing to the oppression of people with disabilities. Now, many members of the professions are working with IL advocates to ensure consumers have input into the delivery of services appropriate to their needs; encouraging the right to risk and the right to self-determination; and actively working to eliminate the forced institutionalization of people with severe disabilities.

Independent Living Centres (Centres for Integrated Living)

IL centres vary in quality and usefulness in the same way as do rehabilitation units – from the truly excellent to the useless. Initially started in California and now common throughout much of the developed world, IL centres have a self-defined mandate to provide information, support and empowerment to people with all disabilities to achieve full societal participation. Although this consumer-based format has proved very successful in some centres and hence could be unreservedly recommended to people with spinal cord injuries and their families, other centres have proved to be little more than job-creation schemes for the first disabled people through the door and of little benefit to people with a range of disabilities.

> There is growing concern in the community of those with disabilities that some of the promise of independent living centres has not been realized. Some have evolved into just another bureaucracy that provides impersonal services and sometimes misinformation. There is tremendous variability in the quality of the services and quality of the programs.
>
> (Trieschmann, 1988)

IL centres aim to provide a wide range of services such as peer counselling, advocacy, training in independent living skills (attendant management, financial management), educational or vocational opportunities, wheelchair repair, information concerning goods and services or housing referrals.

In the USA, several spinal units work co-operatively with consumer based IL centres to enable people with spinal cord injuries to acquire the skills they need to establish an independent lifestyle following rehabilitation. These community-based support services have proved to be effective in facilitating the change from institutional living to independent living (Frieden and Cole, 1985).

Fuhrer (1990) outlines the beneficial results from close relationships between IL centres and medical rehabilitation centres. However, discrepancies in basic philosophies have caused some conflicts. Fuhrer indicates that the medical rehabilitation philosophy is characterized by viewing the client's problems in terms of physical impairments and functional limitations which restrict occupations. They identify the source of the problems as residing within the individual, emphasizing solutions that require professional intervention and expecting that professionals will direct and control service provision.

Conversely, the IL model is characterized as viewing client's problems in terms of unwarranted dependence upon others, identifying the source of problems as residing largely in the environment, emphasizing solutions based on self-help and believing that consumers of services should control provision of services.

At the University of Michigan, a collaborative programme has been developed to provide the client with the most comprehensive approach to rehabilitation. Integration of the rehabilitation and IL paradigms have led to a programme that includes hospital-based care as well as community care. 'The collaborative rehabilitation/independent living program is designed to improve, enhance and increase independent living skills for the person with a spinal cord injury, thus facilitating discharge to community living' (Rasmussen *et al.*, 1989). Rasmussen's group have produced an excellent resource manual outlining their programme for people with spinal cord injuries. Early results indicate the increased levels of activity and of life satisfaction among programme participants.

It is encouraging to learn that professionals and consumer groups can indeed work together and collaborate in programmes. This will clearly enhance the outcomes for clients with spinal cord injuries.

Therapy practice and the IL paradigm

The IL movement has evolved from the experiences of people with disabilities (particularly those with spinal cord injuries) and of their perceptions of their needs and requirements. It behooves rehabilitation professionals to pay close attention and to learn from these experts how therapy practice can achieve greater congruence with the requirements for community living following discharge.

Frieden and Cole (1985) outline the role of the therapist in facilitating independent living. Throughout rehabilitation there must be a recognition that physical skills alone do not constitute independence. Independence means being able to make independent decisions, not doing things physically alone. The therapists' role is of support in helping the client to learn how to solve problems related to environmental interactions: 'There is sometimes far too much emphasis placed on changing the person as opposed to helping the person adapt to the circumstances and change the environment' (Frieden and Cole, 1985).

People with spinal cord injuries who prefer a practical and concrete approach to life rather than a verbal analysis of feelings may especially benefit from the occupational therapist's approach to activity analysis and the maximizing of roles and occupations. Occupational therapists will further enhance skills of self-direction, such as creative problem solving, crisis management, planning, effective communication, identifying resources, setting priorities, comparing choices, making decisions and assessing risks.

Frieden and Cole emphasize that these skills are most effectively taught through experiential learning during activities in the community. This reiterates again the importance of expanding the therapist's horizons to incorporate the client's environment into the rehabilitation equation.

The IL movement has helped to shift the focus of intervention to allow emphasis both upon the need for the person with a spinal cord injury to gain skills and to adapt his activities in addition to recognizing the considerable role of the environment in the production of handicap. Accordingly, many therapists have become active advocates for broad environmental and public policy changes, to remove barriers to societal participation for people with disabilities.

> We have as much responsibility to be agents of social change and institutional transformation as we have to help persons to change. (Kielhofner, 1993)

REFERENCES

Anson, C.A., Stanwyck, D.J. and Krause, J.S. (1993) Social support and health status in spinal cord injury. *Paraplegia*, **31**(10), 632–8.

Bowlby, J.R. (1973) *Separation: Anxiety and Anger. Attachment and Loss*, vol. 2. Penguin, London, p. 407.

Brenes, G., Dearwater, S., Shapera, R. *et al.* (1986) High density lipoprotein cholesterol concentrations in physically active and sedentary spinal cord injured patients. *Archives of Physical Medicine and Rehabilitation*, **67**, 445–50.

Broadhead, W.E., Kaplan, B.H., James, S.A. *et al.* (1983) The epidemiologic evidence for a relationship between social support and health. *American Journal of Epidemiology*, **117**(5), 521–37.

CAOT (1991) *Occupational Therapy Guidelines for Client Centred Practice*, Canadian Association of Occupational Therapists and Health Services Directorate, Health Promotion Branch, Health and Welfare Canada, Toronto, Ont., pp. 124–6, 139, 141.

Decker, S.D. and Schulz, R. (1985) Correlates of life satisfaction and depression in middle aged and elderly spinal cord injured persons. *American Journal of Occupational Therapy*, **39**(11), 740–5.

Decker, S., Schulz, R. and Wood, D. (1989) Determinants of well being in primary care givers of spinal cord injured persons. *Rehabilitation Nursing*, **14**(1), 6–8.

DeJong, G. (1979) Independent living: from social movement to analytic paradigm. *Archives of Physical Medicine and Rehabilitation*, **60**, 435–46.

DeJong, G., Branch, L.G. and Corcoran, P.J. (1984) Independent living outcomes in spinal cord injury: multivariate analysis. *Archives of Physical Medicine and Rehabilitation*, **65**, 66–73.

DeJong, G. and Hughes, J. (1982) Independent living: methodology for measuring long-term outcomes. *Archives of Physical Medicine and Rehabilitation*, **63**, 68–73.

DeVivo, M.J. and Fine, P.R. (1982) Employment status of spinal cord injured patients 3 years after injury. *Archives of Physical Medicine and Rehabilitation*, **63**, 200–3.

DeVivo, M.J., Kartus, P.L., Rutt, R.D. *et al.* (1990) The influence of age at time of injury on rehabilitation outcome. *Archives of Neurology*, **47**, 687–91.

DeVivo, M.J., Rudd, R.D., Stover, S.L. and Fine, P.R. (1987) Employment status after spinal cord injury. *Archives of Physical Medicine and Rehabilitation*, **68**, 494–8.

Dyck, I. (1989) The immigrant client: issues in developing culturally sensitive practice. *Canadian Journal of Occupational Therapy*, **56**(5), 248–55.

Flett, P.J. (1992) The rehabilitation of children with spinal cord injury. *Australian Journal of Paediatrics and Child Health*, **28**(2), 141–6.

Frieden, L. and Cole, J.A. (1985) Independence: the ultimate goal of rehabilitation for spinal cord-injured persons. *American Journal of Occupational Therapy*, **39**(11), 734–9.

Fuhrer, M.J., Rintala, D.H., Hart, K.A. *et al.* (1992) Relationship of life satisfaction to impairment, disability and handicap among persons with spinal cord injury living in the community. *Archives of Physical Medicine and Rehabilitation*, **73**, 552–7.

Fuhrer, M.J., Rossi, D., Gerken, L. *et al.* (1990) Relationships between independent living centres and medical rehabilitation programs. *Archives of Physical Medicine and Rehabilitation*, **71**, 519–22.

Hammell, K.R.W. (1991) *An Investigation into the Availability and Adequacy of Social Relationships Following Head Injury and Spinal Cord Injury: a Study of Injured Men and their Partners*, MSc thesis (Rehabilitation Studies), University of Southampton, Southampton.

Henderson, S., Duncan-Jones, P., McAuley, H. and Ritchie, K. (1978) The patient's primary group. *British Journal of Psychiatry*, **132**, 74–86.

Hooker, E.Z. (1986) Problems of veterans spinal cord injured after age 55: nursing implications. *Journal of Neuroscience Nursing*, **18**(14), 188–95.

Jellinek, H.M. and Harvey, R.F. (1982) Vocational/educational services in a medical rehabilitation facility: outcomes in spinal cord and brain injured patients. *Archives of Physical Medicine and Rehabilitation*, **63**, 87–8.

Jongbloed, L. and Crichton, A. (1990) A new definition of disability: implications for rehabilitation practice and social policy. *Canadian Journal of Occupational Therapy*, **57**, 32–8.

Kemp, B. and Vash, C. (1971) Productivity after injury in a sample of spinal cord injured persons: a pilot study. *Journal of Chronic Disease*, **24**, 259–75.

Kennedy, P., Fisher, K. and Pearson, E. (1988) Ecological evaluation of a rehabilitative environment for spinal cord injured people: behavioral mapping and feedback. *British Journal of Clinical Psychology*, **27**(3), 239–46.

Kerr, W.G. and Thompson, M.A. (1972) Acceptance of disability of sudden onset in paraplegia. *Paraplegia*, **10**, 94–102.

Kielhofner, G. (1993) Functional assessment: toward a dialectical view of person–environment relations. *American Journal of Occupational Therapy*, **47**(3), 248–51.

Krause, J.S. (1992) Employment after spinal cord injury. *Archives of Physical Medicine and Rehabilitation*, **73**, 163–9.

Krause, J. and Crewe, N. (1987) Prediction of long term survival among persons with spinal cord injury: an 11 year prospective study. *Rehabilitation Psychology*, **32**, 205–13.

Law, M. (1991) The environment: a focus for occupational therapy. *Canadian Journal of Occupational Therapy*, **58**(4), 171–9.

Law, M., Baptiste, S., Carswell-Opzoomer, A. *et al.* (1991) *Canadian Occupational Performance Measure*, Canadian Association of Occupational Therapists, Toronto, Ont.

Lundqvist, C., Siösteen, A., Blomstrand, C. *et al.* (1991) Spinal cord injuries: clinical, functional and emotional status. *Spine*, **16**, 78–83.

MacKenzie, E.J., Shapiro, S., Smith, R.T. *et al.* (1987) Factors influencing return to work following hospitalisation for traumatic injury. *American Journal of Public Health*, **77**, 329–34.

Maddox, S. (1987). *Spinal Network*, Spinal Network, Boulder, CO, pp. 114–74.

Madorsky, J.G.B. and Curtis, K.A. (1984) Wheelchair sports medicine. *American Journal of Sports Medicine*, **12**(2), 128–32.

Madorsky, J.G., Madorsky, A.G. and Ericksson, P. (1992) Sports for health, recreation and competition, in *Management of Spinal Cord Injury*, 2nd edn, (ed. C.P. Zejdlik), Jones and Bartlett, Boston, MA, pp. 523–45.

McKinnon, A.L. (1992) Time use for self care, productivity and leisure among elderly Canadians. *Canadian Journal of Occupational Therapy*, **59**(2), 102–10.

Morgan, D. and Jongbloed, L. (1990) Factors influencing leisure activities following a stroke: an exploratory study. *Canadian Journal of Occupational Therapy*, **57**(4), 223–9.

Morris, J. (1989) *Able Lives*, Spinal Injuries Association and Women's Press, London.

Mulcahey, M.J. (1992) Returning to school after a spinal cord injury: perspectives from four adolescents. *American Journal of Occupational Therapy*, **46**(4), 305–12.

NIDRR (1992) National Institute on Disability and Rehabilitation Research. Consensus statement. The prevention and management of urinary tract infections among people with spinal cord injuries, *Journal of the American Paraplegia Society*, **15**(3,), 194–204.

New Mobility (1992) News. Fall, p. 18.

Nilsen, R., Nygard, P. and Bjørholt, P.G. (1985) Complications that may occur in those with spinal cord injuries who participate in sports. *Paraplegia*, **23**, 152–8.

Oxelgren C., Harker, J., Hammell, I. and Boyes, B. (1992) *A New Beginning. Attendant Services Through Individualised Funding*, South Saskatchewan Independent Living Centre, Regina, Sas., pp. 2–3.

Pinkerton, A.C. and Griffin, M.L. (1983) Rehabilitation outcomes in females with spinal cord injury: a follow up study. *Paraplegia*, **21**, 166–75.

Rasmussen, L., Tate, D., Casoglos, T. *et al.* (1989) *Hospital to Community: a Collaborative Program for Independent Living and Medical Rehabilitation*, University of Michigan Medical Centre, Ann Arbor, MI.

Reed, K.L. and Sanderson, S.N. (1992) *Concepts of Occupational Therapy*, 3rd edn, Williams and Wilkins, Baltimore, MD, p. 64.

Rintala, D.H. and Willems, E.P. (1987) Behavioral and demographic predictors of post discharge outcomes in spinal cord injury. *Archives of Physical Medicine and Rehabilitation*, **68**, 357–62.

Rintala, D.H., Young, M.E., Hart, K.A. *et al.* (1992) Social support and the well being of persons with spinal cord injury living in the community. *Rehabilitation Psychology*, **37**(3), 155–63.

Rogers, J. and Figone, J. (1978) The avocational pursuits of rehabilitants with traumatic quadriplegia. *American Journal of Occupational Therapy*, **32**(9), 571–6.

Rohe, D. and Athelstan, G.T. (1982) Vocational interests of persons with spinal cord injury. *Journal of Counseling Psychology*, **29**, 283–91.

Rohe D.E. and Athelstan, G.T. (1985) Change in vocational interests after spinal cord injury. *Rehabilitation Psychology*, **30**(3), 131–43.

Schulz, R. and Decker, S. (1985) Long term adjustment to physical disability – the role of social support, perceived control and self blame. *Journal of Personality and Social Psychology*, **48**(5), 1162–72.

Siösteen, A., Lundqvist, C., Blomstrand, C. *et al.* (1990) The quality of life of three functional spinal cord injury subgroups in a Swedish community. *Paraplegia*, **28**, 476–88.

Staas, W.E., Formal, C.S., Gershkoff, A.M. *et al.* (1988) Rehabilitation of the spinal cord injured patient, in *Rehabilitation Medicine: Principles and Practice*, (ed. J.A. DeLisa), J.B.Lippincott, Philadelphia, PA, p. 653.

Stotts, K.M. (1986) Health maintenance: paraplegic athletes and non athletes. *Archives of Physical Medicine and Rehabilitation*, **67**(2), 109–14.

Stover, S.L. and Fine, P.R. (1986) *Spinal Cord Injury: the Facts and Figures*, University of Alabama, Birmingham, AL, p. 33.

Trieschmann, R.B. (1988) *Spinal Cord Injuries. Psychological, Social and Vocational Rehabilitation*, Demos, New York, NY, pp. 24, 252, 257–8.

Yerxa, E.J. and Locker, S.B. (1990) Quality of time use by adults with spinal cord injuries. *American Journal of Occupational Therapy*, **44**(4), 318–26.

Young, H. and Cocks, N. (1991) The ventilator-dependent spinal cord injured child: a new challenge for occupational therapists. *Australian Occupational Therapy Journal*, **38**(2), 101–3.

Zejdlik, C.P. (1992) Spinal cord injury in children, in *Management of Spinal Cord Injury*, 2nd edn, (ed. C.P. Zejdlik), Jones and Bartlett, Boston, MA, p. 553.

9

Long-term issues and ageing

> It is not by muscle, speed or physical dexterity that
> great things are achieved, but by reflection, force of
> character and judgement; in these qualities old age is
> usually not only not poorer, but is even richer.
>
> (*Cicero, 106–43 BC*)

INTRODUCTION

Previous chapters have examined concepts related to acute care, rehabilitation philosophies and re-engagement in productive, leisure and social occupations and activities. This chapter examines some of the issues that are important, not only in the early years following injury but also over the course of a lengthy lifetime of living with spinal cord injury.

SEXUALITY, SEXUAL FUNCTION AND FERTILITY

Although sufficient quantities of information exist to warrant a volume dedicated entirely to this important aspect of human behaviour and expression, it is important to outline highlights of such information here, to encourage rehabilitation professionals to provide accurate information to their spinal cord injured clients.

'Sexuality' refers to who we are and constitutes a separate issue from sexual function and fertility. Sexuality is connected with sexual identity – the sense of self as a man or woman and is contextual to the individual, based upon cultural influences, self-image and the attitudes of others. Spinal cord injury does not necessarily lead to changes in perceptions of sexuality and sexual identity. However, if those who surround the client (especially influential people such as healthcare workers and members of the rehabilitation team) convey the message that the individual is devalued and no longer a sexual being, these influences may be hard to resist. Cultural stereotypes of men as strong, independent and aggressive may lead some men with spinal cord injuries to review their sexual identity and definition of masculinity. A rehabilitation programme that encourages independent thought, competence and decision making, while discouraging passivity and compliance, will assist both men and women in asserting their sexuality and in viewing themselves as sexual beings.

It is unfortunate that spinal cord injury literature has focused predominantly upon performance dysfunctions rather than examining more fully the opportunities that exist for a wide range of sexual expression, sexual intimacy and sexual satisfaction.

Sexual function and fertility have been the subjects of numerous research studies. Considerable advances have been made in the understanding of sexual dysfunction following spinal cord injury and also how such problems may be overcome. It is strongly recommended that people who have sustained spinal cord injuries and their partners are given the opportunity to discuss their options with a knowledgeable sexual health practitioner. Many spinal cord injury clinicians have developed considerable expertise and sensitivity in this area and can provide appropriate and current information, advice and counselling. There can be few areas where it is more important for rehabilitation workers to acknowledge the limitations of their own knowledge and to refer the client to someone who can provide accurate information rather than risk provision of misleading or inappropriate information.

Rabin (1980) provided an excellent guide to sexual adjustment for people with spinal cord injuries. He outlines some sexual facts concerning spinal cord injury, which are adapted below. It is important that all personnel who are involved in the acute care, rehabilitation and continuing care of people with spinal cord injuries are aware of at least this basic information. Although serious counselling concerning sexual concerns is best handled by someone who has considerable knowledge to contribute to the discussion, any member of the care team may be approached for information by the spinal cord injured person or his or her partner. Avoidance of the subject, provision of misinformation or projection of one's own morals or religious ideas onto the patient will be extremely damaging and may have severe implications for the sexual relationship.

1. Interest in sexual activity is generally maintained following injury, for both men and women.
2. It is possible to experience orgasms after spinal cord injury.
3. Most spinal cord injured men can achieve erections, even when the spinal cord is completely severed. Erectile dysfunction has been treated using various methods, recently including intracavernous injections of vasoactive drugs.
4. The lower the spinal cord lesion, the less likely are erections and the more likely are (unassisted) ejaculations.
5. The higher the spinal cord lesion, the more likely erections become and the less likely are (spontaneous) ejaculations.
6. Sexual functioning (as any physical functioning) of any individual cannot be predicted accurately by level of lesion.
7. Erections may occur without awareness and may be due to touch or movement.
8. Many men with spinal cord injuries are able to father children and the outlook for having a child following spinal cord injury continues to improve with advancements in assisted technologies, particularly vibratory stimulation and electroejaculation (Stein, 1992).
9. Females with spinal cord injuries usually have no impairment in their ability to conceive and undergo pregnancy. Most are able to have vaginal deliveries.

A sexual counselling programme has been described as a 'mandatory part' of any rehabilitation programme following spinal cord injury. Therapists who advocate holistic treatment to assist the client in achieving a high level of functioning must therefore consider the interdependence of the client's sexuality. Contrary to Brown's premise (1992) that people with spinal cord injuries are unattractive prospects for potential partners, Stien (1992) advocates for clients to be helped to reject the idea that they are not sexual persons or unattractive. Open discussion should be initiated early, directed by someone who has 'a relaxed relationship to his/her own sexual life . . . embarrassed and red faced therapists should be replaced immediately' (Stien, 1992)!

A comprehensive rehabilitation programme which seeks to address the needs of clients and the multiplicity of sequelae and impairments following spinal cord injury will, by definition, include counselling regarding sexuality and sexual functioning. The goals of these services will include the dispelling of myths, increasing the client's freedom of choice and supporting the client's right to expression of feelings (Szasz, 1992). A positive relationship has been reported between the provision of helpful information given by healthcare professionals and reports of increased physical sexual activity (White *et al.*, 1992). However, although physical disability does not decrease sexuality and libidinous drive, rehabilitation programmes have an unauspicious record in responding to this fact with information or helpful assistance. In addition to counselling, services should also be provided to use techniques to overcome erectile dysfunction and enhance fertility.

Evidence suggests that rehabilitation counsellors have focused predominantly on the concerns of men with spinal cord injuries, believing that women have few or no concerns, because of continued fertility and a perception of passivity in sexual relations. A review of the literature concerning women with spinal cord injuries could lead to the erroneous conclusion that women's sexuality is defined solely by the ability to conceive and deliver babies. Charlifue and colleagues (1992) report that female sexuality has been equated with childbearing, with scientific interest being focused upon pregnancy and its complications. They propose further research into the specific needs and concerns of women with spinal cord injuries. It is also recommended that spinal cord injury unit staff are involved in postpartum care of women who have spinal cord lesions and that the spinal injury specialist is involved throughout pregnancy and delivery to ensure correct management of aspects such as skin care, autonomic hyperreflexia and urinary tract management (Verduyn, 1986).

There has been little or no help or information available for those individuals who are homosexual, yet the prevalence is presumably as high among the spinal cord injured population as among the general population from which they are drawn. Hence perceptions of alienation, isolation and stigmatization may be increased by the double discrimination of disability and homosexuality and by projection of the rehabilitation professionals' personal prejudices.

Although sexual dysfunction, altered abilities for sexual

expression and performance may create initial difficulties following spinal cord injury, it should be emphasized that, although many people achieve considerable satisfaction with their sex lives, a satisfying and fulfilling relationship is not based solely upon sexual performance. Sex acts comprise elements of emotional closeness and physical pleasure and are more complex than the motor and genital emphasis commonly revealed in the literature. Trieschmann (1988) suggests that a study of sexual function among people with spinal cord injuries must be broadened to include the multitude of sexual expression and acts which form a pattern of communication between two caring people. She further proposes that, following spinal cord injury, men have the opportunity to relax and really pay attention to the nuances of sexual activity that were not as important to them before. Grundy and Swain (1993) enunciate what others have noted, that: 'Some couples find that the extra time and effort required for sexual expression after one of them has suffered a spinal cord injury enriches their lives and results in a more understanding and caring relationship'.

More complete and thorough information is available in many sources, notably, Rabin (1980), Szasz (1987) and Stien (1992). Rehabilitation professionals are responsible for their own continuing education in this area of human performance and function.

MARRIAGE AND THE FAMILY

The onset of severe disability can have profound effects, not necessarily damaging, on existing personal relationships and on the formation of new relationships. . . . For many couples an active and satisfying sexual relationship will be possible, but it will be different. These changes, in addition to the feelings engendered by loss of function and its actual cause, are likely to have major repercussions.

(Grundy and Swain, 1993)

Someone who has sustained a spinal cord injury may suffer serious concerns about the impact of such a disability upon an existing personal relationship or upon the likelihood of forming close relationships in the future.

It is pertinent to study the relevant literature to research the impact which spinal cord injury has been found to have upon close relationships. This is especially important for rehabilitation personnel, who have not only held the belief that marriages are doomed to failure following spinal cord injury, but worse, have communicated that message to their clients. As the predictions of influential persons may easily become self-fulfilling prophecies, it is important to examine the findings of those who have researched this issue.

Abrams (1981) reviewed three decades of literature concerning marital adjustment and spinal cord injury, finding no significant impact on marital functioning to have been established. However, she indicates that, although divorce or separation may be reliable indicators of marital discord, non-termination is not a reliable measure of marital satisfaction. Troubled marriages may be maintained for several reasons, including children, finances, social and cultural pressures and lack of viable alternatives – just as they may for people who do not have a spinal cord injury. Abrams reports that studies of marital satisfaction suggest that companionship suffers when couples no longer share activities which are performed away from home.

Urey *et al.* (1987) examined predictors of marital adjustment among people with spinal cord injuries. Results indicated that, for both husbands and wives, the number of recreational and social activities engaged in with others was the strongest predictor of positive marital adjustment. Husbands and wives in distressed marriages engaged in significantly fewer leisure and social activities, both alone and as a couple. This provides a challenging mandate for the rehabilitation team. 'It seems possible that encouraging mutually enjoyable activities would enhance the marital relationship and thus have a favourable impact on long term outcome' (Urey and Henggeler, 1987).

In a further study, women were asked if anything positive had resulted from their experiences related to their partner's spinal cord injury – 92% said 'yes'. The majority of responses were related to changes in relationships with their partners and families, especially in regard to feeling closer to their partners, to having more communication and being grateful for the opportunity to spend more time together. Many women reported experiencing changes in values (Kester *et al.*, 1988).

Glass (1993) reports on a study of people with high spinal cord injuries and ventilator dependency who lived at home with their families. His findings present an optimistic perspective on the situation of this group of people following severe traumatic injury. The spinal cord injured subjects perceived their families as having high levels of interaction, clarity of communication, expressiveness and high levels of organization. Levels of conflict were reported at significantly lower levels than average. Similarly, the families perceived high levels of cohesion, and significantly higher than average scores for independent attributes, achievement orientation and moral/religious philosophies. Although this study examined a range of family relationships, the results are encouraging, most particularly in the light of the extreme severity of disability of the spinal cord injured subjects.

Brown (1992) speculates that an able-bodied person would not generally be expected to be attracted to someone who has a spinal cord injury. Fortunately, although this view is expressed by a spinal cord injury rehabilitation professional, such stigmatizing and discriminatory views are not universal – either in the rehabilitation professions or among the general public. A high proportion of people who sustain spinal cord injuries proceed to form short- and long-term relationships following injury, and to marry. Indeed, psychologists' assessment of marriages, based on interviews with spinal cord injured subjects and their spouses, revealed that post-injury marriages were happier than pre-injury marriages (Crewe *et al.*, 1979). Further, persons married after injury were found to be more often sexually active, more independent and more likely to be employed than couples who were married before injury. Divorce rates suggest that, although pre-injury marriages may be comparable to other marriages, post-injury marriages may be superior to others (Crewe *et al.*, 1979).

Further study by Crewe and Krause (1988) confirmed earlier findings. People married after injury reported greater satisfaction with their sex lives, living arrangements, social lives, health, emotional adjustment and with their control over their lives. Loneliness was reported as being less of a problem, and they were more likely to be employed and socially active outside their homes.

It is encouraging to note that, although some rehabilitation professionals are clearly unable to look beyond traditional stereotypes and the stigmatization of disability, other people not only do, but they also pursue intimate relationships with people who have spinal cord injuries, achieving significant fulfilment and satisfaction in their marriages.

Although several studies have investigated marital adjustment following spinal cord injury, few have examined parenthood. This has allowed the speculation to flourish that normal child development and adjustment will be compromised by the presence of a parent who has a disability. Buck and Hohmann (1981) provide the first major attempt to investigate empirically the relationship between spinal cord injury in fathers and the subsequent adjustment patterns of their children. They found that these children were well-adjusted, emotionally stable people, who had attained normal sex role identities. Health patterns, body image, recreational interests, interpersonal relationships and family relationships were not found to be adversely affected by their fathers' disabilities. The researchers indicate that rehabilitation professionals can offer the person with a spinal cord injury reassurance that parenthood can be undertaken successfully. They further encourage rehabilitation professionals to avoid allowing theoretical assumptions, generalizations and personal biases to dictate beliefs about psychosocial aspects of disability.

It is encouraging to note from these studies that, although spinal cord injury may cause significant stress and upheaval in the short term, there is no reason to assume that important role functions such as being a marital partner or a parent need be precluded because of a spinal cord injury.

INDEPENDENT LIVING OPTIONS

Most people with spinal cord injuries return to their own homes or to their families following discharge from the rehabilitation programme.

There remains a percentage of people, however, who may have high cord lesions, concomitant injuries or who have lost functional ability (and carers) due to ageing, for whom other independent living options must be examined.

Few people would choose nursing home or other institutional care as a realistic living option. Yet, even in the 1990s, people with spinal cord injuries in some countries are placed in predominantly geriatric facilities, where staff have little or no training in spinal cord injury management and where the individuals with cord injuries have little in common with their ageing companions. Weingarden and Graham (1992) clearly illustrate the inadequacies inherent in nursing home placement for young people with spinal cord injuries (i.e. under the age of 50). Nine of the 12 subjects under study were re-admitted to hospital a total of 21 times during their first year in nursing homes, mainly because of urinary tract infections and pressure sores. Four of these nine died before the end of the first year. The high mortality rate was not correlated with severity of injury. The researchers describe these subjects as a minimally visible population that lacks advocacy for change.

Spinal cord injuries affect predominantly young, predominantly male people. Nursing home populations are primarily female, and are the most cognitively impaired, frail and chronically ill of their age group. Hence, although physical needs may be similar, psychosocial needs are at great variance. Opportunities for engagement in productive activities, meaningful occupations, leisure activities, and for age-appropriate socialization are severely limited.

In the absence of advocacy by professionals, the Independent Living Movement has been at the forefront of development of alternatives for independent living options. Many individuals with high cord lesions, and those who are ageing with spinal cord injuries, express a strong desire to remain in their own homes, living independent and personally fulfilling lives, maintaining autonomy and directing their own attendant services. Many models of attendant care and living options exist, and Independent Living Resource Centres should be able to provide information regarding local solutions. No one arrangement will suit the need of every individual and much depends upon funding provisions. Nevertheless, numbers of people with spinal cord injuries are able to achieve independent living using informal carers and care attendants to provide assistance with daily living requirements.

INFORMAL CARERS AND PERSONAL CARE ATTENDANTS

Politicians, healthcare planners, social services staff and rehabilitation professionals all view community care as an attractive proposition. Institutional care is expensive, is rejected by the majority of people who have spinal cord injuries and is viewed negatively, as a means of segregating society.

However, community care services, despite the rhetoric, rarely intend to provide support to the level that is required by someone who has a high spinal cord injury and care is usually expected to be provided by a relative – usually the closest female relative. In the UK, at any given time, there are more women caring for elderly and disabled dependents than for 'normal' children (Briggs, 1981). Indeed, it is the availability of female relatives that often determines the location of care for someone who has a disability. It is further suggested that 'community care' policies represent a euphemism for under-resourced systems that place heavy burdens on individual members of the community, most of them women (Goodman, 1986).

The rehabilitation professions have often contributed to this problem. Discharge planning has frequently included the assumption that close family members will assume a caring role. Professionals assume that care will be provided and frequently, the very people to whom the caring burden will fall are excluded from the decision-making process involving discharge to the community of the individual who has sustained a spinal cord injury.

Discharge planning must make full consideration not only of the needs of the spinal cord injured client but also of the dynamics of his family relationships. The majority of people with spinal cord injuries below C6 can, and may wish to, live independently. For those people who will require personal assistance, the availability of relatives should not be an automatic predictor of discharge location. The spinal cord injured client may not have been living at his parental home before injury, for example, and may not wish to return there following discharge. Ageing parents may be unable to provide care. They may additionally have other plans for their own futures. Marriages are not all happy and fulfilling, hence spouses may not wish (or be able) to provide for all care requirements.

The rehabilitation team may have little concept of what demands are placed upon family members who provide care for 24 hours a day. 'Just as a day in a wheelchair is a salutary experience for an able bodied person, so a day as a carer would be a learning experience for those who have not been in this position' (Briggs and Oliver, 1985). Delargy *et al.* (1988) assessed the situation of family members who provided care for people with high-lesion quadriplegia. A total of 75% of their respondents indicated a significant level of psychological distress. Gardner *et al.* (1985) suggest that those professionals who make the decision to prolong life should also be prepared to ensure that support to the family is established and maintained following discharge.

To enable people with spinal cord injuries to choose how and with whom they will live, and who will provide care services, health professionals should advocate and lobby with their clients for adequate income levels to enable client-directed care support, provision of acceptable respite services, emergency support and the provision of the same services to married people as to single (Whalley Hammell, 1992).

Personal assistance services have been defined as essential components of Human Rights, by enabling people with disabilities to achieve quality living and full societal integration. The 'Strasbourg Resolution', (developed by disabled people from the Netherlands, United Kingdom, Denmark, Italy, Switzerland, Sweden, France, Austria, Finland, Belgium, USA, Hungary, Germany and Norway) states that no individual shall be placed in an institutionalized setting because of lack of resources or sub standard services. Rather, personal assistance services should be available for up to 24 hours a day to include assistance with each and every daily activity, determined by the client.

Personal assistance/attendant care services are those tasks performed by an attendant to assist someone with a disability in performing personal care activities such as bathing, grooming, dressing and toilet care. Additional help may be provided in activities such as food shopping, meal preparation, household chores, in enabling the disabled person to participate in productive occupations, social integration and leisure activities. The provision of care is directed by the consumer, who has the responsibility of recruiting, hiring, training and supervising the attendants. Attendant care has assumed premier significance among independent living advocates. The attendant care model incorporates the values and assumptions of civil rights, consumerism, self-help, de-medicalization and de-institutionalization movements. Attendant care allows relatively low-skilled individuals to provide personal care services in a community setting. The alternative is frequently institutionalization (DeJong and Wenker, 1979). Personal care attendants have been identified as the single most important factor in helping physically disabled people achieve independence and be in control of their own lives.

> Evidence is beginning to mount that medical rehabilitation may be futile if persons with severe disabilities do not have adequate personal assistance . . . to continue performing activities of daily living and maintaining health effectively after discharge. (Nosek, 1993)

Nosek indicates that personal assistance services are most often rendered informally by family members. However, reliance on family members alone was considered inadequate because of 'burn out', fatigue, exhaustion, emotional drain, guilt, role changes and economic strain. Nosek found a positive relationship between the adequacy of personal assistance and the ability of people with disabilities (including spinal cord injury) to maintain good physical and mental health. Persons with the best health combined assistance by relatives and unrelated persons. Nosek proposes that investments in improving the adequacy of personal assistance services for people with severe disabilities could yield healthcare savings in the billions. Prevention of medical complications, avoidance of institutional care, enhancement of work opportunities and engagement in productive occupations would have significant societal benefits in addition to enhancing quality of life and personal autonomy for the individual.

ATTENDANT MANAGEMENT

Personal assistance services may be provided by live-in, full-time, part-time or back-up attendants, in conjunction with, or as an alternative to, assistance from family members and friends. As personal assistance services are a function of independent living, a medical model of service provision is wholly inappropriate. Rather, consumers assume responsibility for managing and directing their own care attendant services. However, one of the most frequently cited problems in consumer-directed attendant services is the lack of effective management skills.

During the rehabilitation process, both before and following discharge, those individuals who have severe impairments and who require assistance with some aspects of daily living should be offered help in enhancing their attendant management skills. Many people will not require help, being already familiar with job description design, locating labour, interviewing, supervision and communication skills. For other individuals, it may be valuable to have the opportunity to develop a comprehensive needs inventory (personal care, transportation, household management, community management, work, education or social needs) and a lifestyle assessment (dietary preferences, personal habits and preferences) (Rasmussen, 1989). Other skills which may be required include determining a care proposal and accessing adequate funding, advertising, designing job descriptions and contracts, performing interviews, providing insurance, payment and providing appropriate and effective performance feedback. Independent Living Centres (see Chapter 8) may be able to provide assistance and information for someone who wishes to establish a care attendant scheme.

Throughout the period of hospitalization and rehabilitation, the person with a spinal cord injury should have been encouraged to express realistic and appropriate requests for help, to be a self-advocate and to be assertive in having needs met effectively. Individuals are ill-prepared for attendant management in the community if they have learned to be passive recipients of care in the institution. Trial periods at home will have enabled insight into the differences between 24-hour nursing care support and what can reasonably be expected of family members who also have other obligations to fulfil. Follow-up assessments should include consideration of the individual's support services.

Personal care attendants enable people with severe physical disabilities to lead independent and individual lifestyles in the community. It is suggested that effective attendant management skills can significantly contribute to the success of such a scheme, thereby enhancing autonomy, personal choice and quality of life.

DIET AND NUTRITION

Nutrition has been described as one of the most important aspects of care at the onset of spinal cord injury as well as throughout the life of the individual. Nutrition is a significant factor in maintaining ideal bodyweight, maintaining skin integrity, preventing urinary tract infections, promoting gastrointestinal function and preventing other secondary medical complications (Houda, 1993). Maintenance of optimal nutrition will enhance acute care and rehabilitation outcomes and will provide long-term resistance to infection and disease (Zejdlik, 1992).

Obesity is a significant contributor to the exacerbation of disability and the creation of handicap. Excess weight negatively correlates with engagement in productive, leisure and social activities. Ability to perform personal care tasks such as dressing is diminished, and functional mobility skills such as transfers, weight shifts and wheelchair propulsion are substantially reduced. The propensity to skin breakdown increases and pain may become disabling because of overstressed upper extremity joints and soft tissues. Obesity contributes to a negative body image, decreased self-esteem and to a reduction in the ability of attendants to provide care.

The rehabilitation process and continuing care services should emphasize that eating is not one of the only pleasures remaining in life (as some people with spinal cord injuries and their carers might believe) and should focus upon identifying pleasurable and meaningful activities that will not contribute to increased dependence, morbidity and mortality.

Although there appear to be no published weight standards for people with spinal cord injuries, Houda (1993) reports that people with paraplegia are recommended to achieve an ideal bodyweight of 4.5–6.8 kg below the guidelines for their height and frame size. For people with quadriplegia, the recommendation is for 6.8–9 kg below the guidelines for height and frame sizes.

Research indicates that people with spinal cord injuries consume energy at different rates to able-bodied people, therefore requiring a different (lower) calorie intake. It appears that people with spinal cord injuries have a reduction in their energy needs proportional to the amount of muscle that has been denervated. People with high-lesion quadriplegia have greatly reduced energy expenditure, reflecting their profound levels of motor loss and inactivity. People with low-lesion quadriplegia and with paraplegia will vary widely in their energy expenditure, dependent upon activity levels, physical abilities and interests.

Malnutrition is also common among people with spinal cord injuries, even during acute treatment. Zejdlik (1992) outlines some of the factors that may contribute to malnutrition among people with spinal cord injuries, including:

- chronic, inadequate nutritional intake
- chewing or swallowing difficulties
- depression
- difficulty (or embarrassment) with self-feeding
- assistance that is not relaxed or is antagonistic
- side effects from medications.

Malnutrition constitutes a significant problem to someone with a spinal cord injury, with the potential of impaired pulmonary function, reduced resistance to infection, increased risk of skin breakdown (especially over bony prominences), diminished wound healing and prolonged hospitalizations. (Prolonged hospitalization may itself be a significant contributor to malnutrition through inadequate nutritional support). Close collaboration between the client and team nutritionist will enable dietary recommendations to be generated which are appropriate to the cultural and religious practices of the individual, his family status and role, education, financial resources and dietary habits, both at home and away from home (Houda, 1993). The nutritionist should have particular knowledge regarding spinal cord injury and its management, the requirements for a high-fibre, high-fluid diet and the preventable medical complications for which excellent nutrition can play a significant prophylactic role.

PAIN

Although acute pain is experienced by everyone who sustains a spinal cord injury due to the mechanical or medical problem, chronic pain syndromes may create substantial disability and severely limit the level of activity of the individual. Chronic pain produces psychological and social handicaps and is negatively correlated with life satisfaction and quality of life.

However, it is also clear that the degree of incapacity produced by pain varies greatly between individuals so that some people are totally disabled by minor discomfort, although others will endure considerable pain to achieve their goals.

Fairholm (1992) outlines three groups of factors that may influence the degree of perceived pain and the individual's response to that pain.

- **Organic factors** include physiological contributors – mechanical, visceral, root and deafferentation factors.
- **Psychological factors** include anxiety, depression, dependency needs and stress.
- **Social factors** include relationships, social support, goals and occupations, and factors such as secondary gain, compensation and litigation.

Chronic pain may lead to depression, chemical dependency and suicide. It is thus important that chronic pain is neither ignored nor disbelieved.

A multifaceted, interdisciplinary approach to treatment of pain will consider the multifactorial nature of the problem and the factors that contribute to both the pain and the response to that pain. Importantly, management will be addressed within the context of a participatory planning process in which the client regains control and independence by setting goals, planning strategies to attain those goals and monitoring progress (Fairholm, 1992).

Two decades ago, Burke (1973) observed that the subject of pain following spinal cord injury had not attracted much attention in the professional literature. To date, this continues to be a largely neglected area of published research, indicating perhaps, the low level of importance of this issue in the minds of clinicians and researchers. Trieschmann (1988) indicates that a lack of understanding of pain among people with spinal cord injuries (particularly pain below the level of lesion) has been an excuse for not trying a variety of approaches to management. She suggests that, although we lack both good data on the incidence of pain among people with long-term spinal cord injuries and knowledge of the degree to which function is reduced, an integrated approach to management is still possible. In those instances where medical interventions are unable to eliminate the nociception and pain, individuals may learn to control the amount that they suffer.

Trieschmann's suggestions for a pain rehabilitation programme are closely correlated with the factors that contribute to effective rehabilitation for all people with spinal cord injuries, i.e. attention to increasing activity, to including and enhancing social supports, attending to depression and to re-introducing rewarding experiences into life. Further approaches to pain management in spinal cord injury are outlined by Ozer (1988), Segatore (1992) and Fairholm (1992) who also describes various types and features of pain that may follow spinal cord injury.

AGEING WITH A SPINAL CORD INJURY

Analysis of the medical and rehabilitation literature before 1990 could lead one to suppose that the person who has sustained a spinal cord injury requires excellent emergency and acute care, comprehensive in-patient rehabilitation and few further needs following discharge. Further, there is evidence to suggest that this has been the belief held by healthcare planners and professionals. However, it is proposed that the shifting demographics of the spinal cord injured population should be of considerable concern to healthcare planners.

In 1985, Eisenberg and Tierney observed that the majority of spinal cord injury treatment resources were expended to address problems during acute and early care following injury with major spinal cord injury research following this pattern. Until recently, spinal cord injury had been viewed as a static disability. Knowledge concerning spinal cord injury focused primarily upon acute and early care management and resided with specialists in neurosurgery, orthopaedics, urology and rehabilitation.

However, as one writer observed: 'The acute care period, albeit critical, represents only about 0.1 percent of the injured individual's remaining life span. After a relatively short period in a hospital, the injured individual must return to his old stomping grounds with some of his stomping equipment out of kilter' (Young, 1980).

Little is known about the quality of life that is experienced by people following spinal cord injury. Less is known about the long-term effects of the injury and the issues that arise for those who are ageing with spinal cord injuries.

Few primary care physicians are knowledgeable about the problems that may occur in those with this disability, or even about the unique sequelae and idiosyncracies of spinal cord injury and its impact upon multiple body systems. It is only comparatively recently that numbers of polio survivors have achieved an age at which symptoms of premature ageing ('post-polio syndrome') have been recognized. Similarly, people with spinal cord injuries of 30, 40 or 50 years' duration are only now coming to the attention of healthcare professionals in sufficient numbers for those professionals to recognize and identify trends and potential problems. Thus, the issue of ageing with a disability is a new problem for Western societies, 'one that has caught our healthcare system by surprise' (Trieschmann, 1987).

The medical and healthcare community has not been in the lead in the analysis of the needs of people who have spinal cord injuries and who are experiencing additional disabilities related to the ageing process. Rather, recent studies of the experience of ageing among people with spinal cord injuries have been spawned by the efforts of these individuals themselves. The British Spinal Injury Association, for example, became aware of some of the problems of ageing with a spinal cord injury through reports from their members. These reports indicated that problems experienced with ageing represented a potential threat to previously established ways of life. Zarb *et al.* (1990) note, however, that consultants in the spinal injury units were also finding that more and more of their former patients were returning to the spinal units to seek assistance with problems related to the ageing process. They further note that these specialized spinal units are set up to deal primarily with the treatment of acute admissions and the rehabilitation of newly injured people. They are less well equipped to deal with the long-term care needs of their clientele.

Despite this lack of planning, it is evident that the potential problems of ageing with a spinal cord injury are not in the future but are already present. In the USA, in 1988, it was estimated that 40% of people with spinal cord injuries were over the age of 45 (Berkowitz *et al.*, 1992). The majority of these people are likely to have already lived for close to a quarter century with their acquired impairments.

Evidence from Trieschmann (1987), Zarb *et al.* (1990) and, most recently from Whiteneck *et al.* (1993), indicates that the long-term consequences of living with a spinal cord injury may include an acceleration of the ageing process, decline in function and increased physical dependence upon others. It is also clear that professionals involved in spinal cord injury management have neither planned nor lobbied for the extensive additional services that this ageing population will require.

Those people who are experiencing problems related to ageing may have to demand the services they wish to see in place, such as follow-up at specialized clinics where doctors can gain enough experience to provide adequate care. There is a good research base to back up these demands, pointing to the superiority of specialist care for specialized conditions. When it was realised that polio survivors had not been prepared for additional disabilities associated with ageing, many survivors expressed bitterness that their original treating physicians and therapists had not prepared them for these changes. In view of their experience, 'it has become clear that spinal cord injury centres, treating teams, and individuals with spinal cord injury have a responsibility to evaluate aging and how it might affect spinal cord injury survivors' (Whiteneck *et al.*, 1993).

Much can be learned from the experience of polio survivors, and it is to be hoped that comprehensive services will quickly be established and expanded to meet the special needs of those who have survived spinal cord injury and are now ageing with the subsequent disability.

Changes associated with ageing

In the USA it is calculated that one in four spinal cord injured survivors is already over 20 years after injury. As 20 years after injury appears to be a point at which some of the problems of ageing become evident, a significant proportion of people with spinal cord injuries are likely to be experiencing additional impairment and disability (Menter, 1993a). Ageing may thus be related to the duration of disability rather than to chronological age.

Causes of morbidity and mortality more closely approximate those of the general population as years since injury increase. However, the illnesses and deaths among the survivors of spinal cord injury are occurring at younger ages than would be expected among the non-disabled population.

In the UK, recent estimates place between 15 500 and 20 500 people with spinal cord injuries of over 20 years' duration. Of these, between 6600 and 8900 are already over 60 years of age with a further 7000–9000 people reaching this age within the next 10 years (Zarb, 1993).

Healthcare professionals have accumulated little knowledge of the situation of people with spinal cord injuries living in the community or of the impact upon individuals of the accelerated ageing process. Follow-up services by spinal injury units in the UK are reportedly provided to only 30–75% of their original patients (Zarb, 1993). As approximately half those people who sustain spinal cord injuries are denied access to a specialized spinal injury unit in the UK, it can be assumed that the present knowledge base in the UK among healthcare personnel concerning the impact of ageing upon a person who has a spinal cord injury is based upon contact with only 15–37.5% of the total cord-injured population. With the low level of knowledge among healthcare personnel of the idiosyncracies of spinal cord injuries in general and the impact of ageing in particular, the majority of people with spinal cord injuries in the UK face a major void in terms of service provision related to their specific needs.

Someone who has lived for several decades with a spinal cord injury has already learned techniques of preventative medicine, self-diagnosis for common complaints and has experience of the relative effects of medications. Survival with a spinal cord injury requires acceptance of responsibility for health maintenance, hence the individual who has a long-term spinal cord injury is an expert in his own care and management, as is his spouse or partner. Trieschmann (1987) suggests that such individuals accept responsibility, make their own decisions and will not comply with healthcare decisions with which they disagree. Indeed, these characteristics have ensured survival. Healthcare providers cannot therefore, use a superior, domineering approach. Despite having achieved a certain degree of expertise within a given discipline, the professional does not have the level of individual expertise which has been achieved by the client. The client has long since achieved autonomy and healthcare personnel must become resources for the individual – partners in making decisions and care. This is a difficult concept for specialists in acute care medicine who are accustomed to making decisions on behalf of their clients in a paternalistic model of care (Menter, 1993b).

Menter (1993a) suggests that ageing involves at least three major, lifelong developmental processes which are distinct, yet overlap.

- **Physiologic changes** are the most evident and most commonly discussed elements of ageing. Loss of muscle mass results in decreased strength; osteoarthritis produces decreased range of motion, pain and reduced function. Skin may become more susceptible to pressure sores. There may be deterioration of genitourinary system function, decreased gastrointestinal function, deterioration of respiratory function, decreased cardiovascular capacity, endocrine changes, decreased resistance to infection and increased problems associated with the immune system.
- **Changing social roles** may result from growing older, to altered roles in family and community and to deaths of parents or the spouse.
- **Self-realization** includes those factors such as developing values, ethics and meaning in life which may serve to reduce the negative impact of physiological and sociological changes. Contrary to what might be expected, life satisfaction has been found to increase with advancing age and duration of spinal cord injury.

Menter proposes that, although a group of people of similar age and level of acute injury will present with similar, predictable levels of function and degrees of health impairments, there will be a tremendous variation between members of this group after many years. Individual patterns of ageing will occur in response to genetic variables, localized trauma, lifestyle factors, response to stress, relationships and interpersonal support. Hence, the impact of ageing with a spinal cord injury is complex and extremely variable from individual to individual.

The issues related to ageing with a spinal cord injury present a multiplicity of unanswered questions. However, the increased life expectancy and prevalence of people with spinal cord injuries of 20 or more years' duration cannot allow this state of ignorance to continue. Rather, there is an immediate need for full investigation and understanding of the needs of these people so that these needs can efficiently and competently be met.

Implications of ageing for rehabilitation professionals

Rehabilitation cannot be viewed as the time-limited period between acute care and hospital discharge. Long viewed as the process of maximizing function and increasing independence, rehabilitation programmes which seek to provide comprehensive services for people with spinal cord injuries must also teach people to adapt to deteriorating physical skills, reduced functional abilities and decreasing physical independence.

It is difficult for many individuals who have fought hard to achieve high levels of independence, mobility in a manual wheelchair and participation in competitive sports, employment and recreation to acknowledge that more equipment or help is required. Therapists will need to be sensitive, for example, to those for whom a powered wheelchair seems like an admission of defeat or failure after decades of physically demanding but independent self-propulsion. Ultimately, both care providers and survivors of spinal cord injury must recognize that changes in the musculoskeletal system with advancing age will produce changes in functional status.

> While it may seem desirable to a newly injured person to push to attain maximum levels of function and independence, survivors must be educated that high levels of function may not be maintained indefinitely.   (Waters *et al.*, 1993)

Menter *et al.* (1991) propose that healthcare providers need to be aware of the changing physical, psychosocial and socio-economic needs of people who are ageing with spinal cord injuries. Follow-up services should be directed towards early intervention rather than crisis management. There must be an awareness of the changing needs for equipment, support and attendant care services.

> Clinicians need to be aware of the potential declines their clients may experience and must be well versed in developing and offering compensating resources and lifestyle strategies that will allow individuals to maintain the quality of life they enjoyed in the early years after their injuries.
> (Menter *et al.*, 1991)

Corbet (1993) proposes that rehabilitation has an opportunity (one could add, a responsibility and a mandate) to reaffirm its original philosophy and then to expand it. An interdisciplinary approach to prevention, assessment and re-evaluation should be extended to people ageing with spinal cord injuries, not solely those with recent injuries.

Rehabilitation professionals will also need to recognize that they have more than one client. The needs for support and right to quality of life of the individual with a spinal cord injury cannot be championed at the expense of his spouse or informal care provider. The rehabilitation team have a shameful record of formulating care plans based upon the automatic assumption that the non-disabled partner will assume the caring role. As the disabled person becomes less able to achieve self-care tasks, the spouse, who is also ageing, is often expected to shoulder more and more of the care needs. There is a universal expectation, not least from the husband himself, that the wife will take on everything that is necessary. 'No consideration is usually given as to her own state of health, the other calls on her time and energies, or indeed, the state of her marriage' (Oliver, 1983).

It is further suggested that the support systems frequently relied upon by people with spinal cord injuries (spouses, parents, other family members) may become tenuous, as these people are also ageing and becoming increasingly less able to provide the level of care previously provided. Additionally, the level of assistance which is required may increase with advancing age.

Consideration of the needs of the population of people who are ageing with a spinal cord injury will involve again the concept of environmental interaction. The factors that contribute to 'handicap' following decades of living with a disability are not solely personal but will include variables related to the physical, social, economic and political environment. The person who ages with a supportive environment will be likely to experience less handicap and a higher quality of life than one who does not. Recent study has found that successful ageing and life satisfaction are not related to level or completeness of lesion; but rather to financial resources, physical health and emotional support (McColl *et al.*, 1993).

Individuals may experience difficulties in maintaining productive activities, employment and engagement in leisure pursuits because of increased fatigue and declining function. Zarb *et al.* (1990) propose that the outcome of the interaction of ageing and spinal cord injury will be an equation of personal resources, support services, finance, housing, employment, family situation and mobility. Hence, although medical problems will most appropriately be addressed in specialized centres where healthcare personnel have appropriate knowledge and expertise, other support services will most appropriately come from community services, social workers and therapists.

SELF-NEGLECT AND SUICIDE

Assessment of numbers of people with spinal cord injuries who had been discharged from hospital prompted Richards (1986) to comment: 'In an age when technologic advances in medicine are ensuring survival of persons who will be severely impaired for life, it is comforting to know that such persons as a group are able to adjust to their limitations in a way suggesting that quality of life is, in fact, possible'.

However, data from mortality and follow-up studies suggest that not everyone finds sufficient rewards in life after sustaining a spinal cord injury. Suicide rates following spinal cord injury appear to be significantly higher than among the general population.

Suicide has been reported to account for between 4% and 21% of all deaths among people with spinal cord injuries and has been shown to be one of the leading causes of death among people with traumatic paraplegia. Research showed that suicide was the leading cause of death for people with complete paraplegia and the second leading cause of death for those with incomplete paraplegia although the same trend has not been found among people with quadriplegias (DeVivo *et al.*, 1991).

> The psychosocial literature has consistently demonstrated this counter-intuitive lack of correlation between level of neurological loss and psychosocial adjustment. . . . It has been speculated that because less physical (and therefore social) support is provided to persons with paraplegia than those with quadriplegia, the burden of coping is greater.
>
> (DeVivo *et al.*, 1991)

Suicide is further reported to be one of the leading causes of death among younger people with spinal cord injuries, and is most common within five years of injury.

Suicide may be achieved by a deliberate, single act, or by a passive course of self-neglect, of evading responsibility and allowing medical problems to occur, to multiply and to deteriorate so that death occurs from seemingly 'legitimate' medical conditions (Trieschmann, 1987). Example may be found in the instance of pressure sores, which still account for numbers of deaths despite being wholly preventable and being overcome by conservative management if detected in the earliest stages. Recurrent and potentially avoidable hospitalizations, inattention to skin care, mismanagement of urinary tract care and substance abuse (including of medications) should alert healthcare personnel to the presence of self-neglectful behaviour which requires investigation and intervention (Macleod, 1988).

Suicide is considered to be under-reported, with deaths listed as being due to accidents or misadventure and to the effects of self-neglect, such as medical complications, alcohol and drug abuse. These latter forms of 'passive suicide' are frequently omitted from suicide statistics.

There may be instances in which it could be argued that a spinal cord injury was sustained in an attempt at suicide and hence that the subsequent risk of suicide will, by default, be higher than among the general population. However, it is tempting to attribute the high rates of substance abuse and suicide following traumatic spinal cord injury to defects and problems within the individual rather than examining the other variables that might be contributing factors.

> Despite our good intentions, it would appear that we are not successful at teaching people to live with their disabilities in their own environments in such a way that they can have the opportunity to find rewards and satisfactions in their lives. Our task must be not only to teach ADL [activities of daily living] and mobility techniques, but to teach a person to find a reason for getting out of bed in the morning. While we cannot give a person a reason to continue to live, perhaps we can teach him how to go about finding one for himself. (Trieschmann, 1988)

There is a considerable challenge for all members of the rehabilitation team and for community-based workers, to broaden the scope of intervention to incorporate those activities that have meaning for the individual. Clearly, quality of life issues fit more squarely into a model of practice that incorporates all aspects of adult occupations; productivity, leisure, socialization, within a psychosocial context, rather than into a physical/functional model. DeVivo *et al.* (1991) propose that the greatest results may be achieved by directing efforts towards mobilizing social support, improving coping skill and encouraging as rapid involvement in meaningful activities as possible.

Further, intervention must be directed not only towards an individual but also towards his environment and all its components. If the opportunity to participate in meaningful activities is prohibited by physical barriers, social stigmatization, poverty, discrimination and isolation, the skills learned during rehabilitation will appear worthless and substance abuse, passive or active suicide may become enticing forms of escape.

Is it possible that high rates of suicide among young people with recent spinal cord injuries reveal less about the individuals with those injuries than about the relevance of their rehabilitation programmes?

CONTINUING CARE SERVICES

'A spinal unit should ultimately be judged by the standard of its follow up system' (Bingley, 1990). People with spinal cord injuries may expect to have a near-normal lifespan and hence to encounter problems related to their acquired disability which could not have been anticipated during in-patient treatment. It is not sufficient to focus solely upon services required to save a life and to restoration of functional capacity. Rather there must be a commitment to long-term support services which can address issues as they arise, for example, for healthcare needs, vocational counselling, sexual counselling, or problems related to the premature ageing process.

Follow-up services have been described as an integral component of rehabilitation yet Zarb (1993) indicates that the spinal injury units in the UK provide an extremely variable level and quality of long-term support to an estimated 75–30% of former patients.

Brown *et al.* (1987) indicate, however, that the functions of a comprehensive spinal unit do not cease with the discharge of the patient from in-patient treatment after rehabilitation. The mandate of the specialized unit extends to aftercare in providing support, education, prevention and management of medical complications. They state that, although good continuing care services are demanding in terms of time, resources and money, they are cost effective in preventing repeat hospitalizations.

People with spinal cord injuries have a narrow margin of health and consume a disproportionately large share of health-care resources (DeJong and Batavia, 1991). DeJong and Batavia identify three health service issues that predominate among the spinal cord injured population following discharge:

- the very high rate of unscheduled rehospitalizations (see Chapter 5);
- the lack of access to primary care (see Chapter 5);
- the development of new problems associated with the ageing process.

They indicate that these problems require consideration of models of delivery of service which are targeted more carefully towards the needs of people with spinal cord injuries. Oliver *et al.* (1988) suggest that, although spinal cord injuries may present considerable problems of medical management, most of these can be overcome by skilled intervention and long-term monitoring from a specialized spinal unit. They advocate for spinal units to provide an 'accident to the grave' service, to keep medical problems to an absolute minimum and hence to reduce intrusion of complications into the life of the individual. However, it is evident that continuing care services are required which can address more than purely medical and healthcare needs. Services must be community centred, co-ordinated and allow equal access to all clients rather than using the medical model under which the physician is the 'gatekeeper' to every service, both medical and non-medical (Menter, 1993b).

The entire professional team must be available to provide numerous supportive services throughout the individual's life. Follow-up services should interact with community services and be based upon the needs of the disabled people it serves, the qualities and the resources of the facility and the qualities and resources of community services. Zejdlik (1992) indicates that the essential principles of specialized follow-up services include the provision of a wide range of services to address concerns which may include health issues, housing, attendant care, financial concerns, psychosocial issues, equipment, home modifications and drug and alcohol treatment.

Additionally, vocational issues may be addressed appropriately when the client is living in the community and has had time to assess his opportunities, goals and interests. Those essential activities of life that relate to productivity, leisure and social integration, sexual relationships and family relationships may all be addressed by appropriate continuing care services. Case management should facilitate co-ordination of services and ensure appropriate continuity of care by planning and arranging service delivery. The case manager who is able to perform this function and to interact and collaborate with the family is more appropriately a social worker, community nurse or occupational therapist than a physician. The aim is to eliminate fragmentation of care, enhance access and provide continuity and comprehensive service delivery.

Different centres follow various models of continuing care service delivery. Clearly, an annual review in the sterile environment of a special unit or hospital will be inadequate for all but a medical review. An understanding of the impact of the disability and its inherent problems will be gained in the community and the client's own environment, not in the confines of an in-patient facility (Bingley, 1990). Brown *et al.* (1987) propose that an effective aftercare service will link reviews to the home, community facilities and workplace by different members of the team. This enables an understanding by the team of the individual's unique situation and provides for more relevant problem solving and intervention. The visits will commonly involve the social worker, sexual counsellor, community nurse or occupational therapist, as appropriate. 'Such visits emphasize the problems related to the disability and the handicaps imposed by the outside environment, and not to illness; they are therefore best dealt with in the environment in which they occur' (Brown *et al.*, 1987).

Bingley (1990) reports that the Southport Spinal Injuries Unit in England has established a system of community-based surveillance located in the homes of the individuals with spinal cord injuries. The consultant physician, nurse in charge of co-ordination of care, clinical psychologist, local physicians and community nurses meet with the client, spouse and other carers. It is estimated that at least 20% of re-admissions have been avoided through the provision of this community-based service.

The function of continuing care services is not just to enable service provision appropriate and relevant to the needs of the individual. It is also an invaluable opportunity for all disciplines involved in the rehabilitation of people with spinal cord injuries to learn from their clients what it means to live with a disability in the context of their own environments. It is difficult for rehabilitation programmes to be made relevant to post-discharge needs if the staff are ignorant of the realities of life with a spinal cord injury in the community. An in-patient facility is not an optimal environment for learning about the community. 'Hospitals have been inward looking far too long. It is time we realized there is a very real world outside spinal injury centres' (Bingley, 1990).

People with spinal cord injuries who have returned to live in the community have commented that the therapists at the spinal unit knew nothing about what it means to live with a disability in the community (Hammell, 1991). Unit staff may be deluding themselves if they think they can learn about life with a spinal injury from the confines of an out-patient clinic. It is difficult to conceive how rehabilitation programmes can effectively be evaluated and modified when little meaningful contact exists between the rehabilitation centre staff and their former clients in the community. An athletic trainer, for example, would be viewed with great suspicion and scepticism if he developed intensive training programmes for his athletes and then failed to attend the meets to see those athletes perform and hence evaluate whether his training methods are suitable to competition conditions. Yet, rehabilitation outcomes have frequently been evaluated at discharge rather than by observing their effectiveness and appropriateness for people in their roles of worker, parent, partner, athlete, in an environmental context.

It may further be postulated that those personnel who see former clients in an out-patient clinic will be unlikely to see those individuals who have achieved high levels of productivity and societal re-integration, as these people will be the least able to adhere to clinic appointments (which are established to suit the desired work routines of the professionals, not their clients). This may contribute to the negative perception that some rehabilitation workers have of outcomes: of unemployment, of social isolation and lack of interests. A cycle is established by which therapists encourage future patients to establish low goals and expectations. Further, therapists may avoid discussion of future engagement in productive activities and occupations if they are unaccustomed to seeing people with spinal cord injuries who have jobs.

> Further research is needed which would focus on the disabled individual's experiences after discharge, not only to determine how rehabilitation programs might be made more effective, but to assess the limits of such programs and to aid the development of community programs which would ease the individual's return to the community.　　(Dew *et al.*, 1983)

QUALITY OF LIFE

Rehabilitation professionals frequently state that their primary goal is to improve their client's quality of life. Unfortunately, quality of life is difficult to define and conceptualize, and is infrequently studied.

If 'quality of life' is our primary goal, what do we know about what constitutes a life of quality and satisfaction following spinal cord injury – one that makes survival worthwhile? What do our former patients feel about what contributes to a life of quality? How do they perceive their own quality of life? If rehabilitation professionals wish to contribute to the enhancement of quality of life, they will surely need a clear understanding of what 'quality of life' means to people with spinal cord injuries.

Analysis of the literature would seem to suggest that medical and rehabilitation attention is not actually as preoccupied with quality of life following spinal cord injury as their rhetoric suggests. A cursory examination of the articles in the 1992 edition of *Paraplegia* – the prestigious, international journal of the spinal cord, for example, reveals four articles pertaining to quality of life following spinal cord injury, approximately 30 concerning rehabilitation (predominantly bioengineering and FES) and approaching 100 related to medical matters.

Despite the rhetoric among rehabilitation professionals which professes a primary focus upon goals and issues concerning quality of life, even the rehabilitation literature is not replete with such assessments. Most commonly, outcome measures that seek to judge rehabilitation interventions are expressed in terms of functional achievements; as if the ability to dress, transfer or increase one's range of motion constitute some form of enhanced quality of life. Eisenberg and Saltz (1991) indicate that, although such specific functional outcomes are important to measure and may indeed justify and validate a specific rehabilitation practice and intervention (which may provide the real motivation behind their measurement), it must be considered whether such an evaluation can be considered either complete or definitive.

Measures of quality of life lack a standardized conceptual definition of how such global assessments should be measured. However, the inherent difficulties in achieving a consensus on definition have not prevented researchers in other disciplines from assessing quality of life issues. Within the fields of medicine and surgery, researchers are using quality of life instruments to assess the effects of their interventions and the impact on quality of life of diseases such as diabetes, end-stage renal failure, hearing impairment, HIV and AIDS. Studies have sought assessments of quality of life to justify and validate such interventions as bone marrow or kidney transplantation, dialysis and amputation.

If the interventions of the rehabilitation team do indeed aim to enhance the quality of life of people who have been injured, it should surely be a priority among rehabilitation professionals to use assessments of quality of life both in research and clinical practice.

Rehabilitation following spinal cord injury is financially expensive and frequently lengthy. Any analysis of outcome to assess the benefits of treatment and rehabilitation which fails to include 'quality of life' provides information that is incomplete and misleading (Niemi *et al.*, 1988).

Although quality of life must be defined by the subjective experience and report of the individual, there is general consensus that the components which contribute to perceived quality of life are:

- standard of living/financial security/material wellbeing;
- productivity/job/work/occupation/personal development and fulfilment/engagement in interesting, worthwhile, rewarding, productive activity;

- physical wellbeing/satisfaction with health/safety;
- level of activity/use of spare time/active leisure pursuits, sports, social and recreational activities;
- learning/education/personal development;
- family life/marriage/friends/social support/interpersonal relationships/close relationship with partner;
- degree and quality of social and community interaction;
- psychological wellbeing and sense of self-worth;
- sexual satisfaction;
- housing/physical environment;
- creative expression;
- satisfaction with role functioning. ('Life satisfaction' encompasses many of these concepts.) (Flanagan, 1982; Bowling, 1991; Wood-Dauphinee and Küchler, 1992).

Although measurement of quality of life may have appeared too complex for rehabilitation researchers, it is clear that few research attempts have been made to investigate even components of quality of life, or life satisfaction.

If rehabilitation workers and researchers accept the premise that the above factors do indeed comprise a large part of perceived quality of life, close scrutiny must again be focused upon the inconsistencies in this belief – and the content of traditional rehabilitation programmes. Although perception of quality of life is clearly personal and subjective, if it consists of even half the above components, it is evident that a physical/functional approach to rehabilitation must be seen as being inconsistent with its stated goals.

It could further be proposed that once the elements of 'quality of life' are identified, rehabilitation programmes should be directed towards enhancement of these elements. Close collaboration with the client will enable the therapist to identify what 'quality of life' means to each individual. This will require an understanding of the individual's beliefs and values, economic and cultural background, his social environment and his life stage. Analysis of the possible components of quality of life outlined above will suggest that they are all potentially amenable to intervention during the rehabilitation process and through community-based services. Appropriate referrals to occupational therapists, social workers, psychologists, community workers and Independent Living Centres should enable the rehabilitation team to provide relevant assistance to the individual in addressing his priorities and concerns.

Rehabilitation workers should also be aware of what has been discovered, to date, about the perceptions of the quality of a life with a spinal cord injury.

Review of studies on quality of life following spinal cord injury

Fuhrer *et al.* (1992) assessed the relationship between life satisfaction and impairment, disability and handicap among persons with spinal cord injury living in the community. In common with other researchers, perceived quality of life was not found to be predicted by impairment – that is, the level of injury (assessed by the ASIA total motor score). Further, no significant association was established between life satisfaction and a measure of disability (the self-report version of the functional independence measure, FIM).

> The question then becomes: if life satisfaction is not correlated with extent of disability, what factors explain it? And, if predictors of life satisfaction can be found, can points of intervention also be identified? (DeVivo and Richards, 1992)

Fuhrer did observe relationships between life satisfaction and each of three dimensions of handicap – social integration, occupation and mobility. In all three instances, greater life satisfaction was associated with lesser handicap.

Several studies in the USA have indicated that people with spinal cord injuries who are living in the community generally report a lower level of life satisfaction than do people in the general population. However, the impact of a disabling environment again requires careful scrutiny. Several studies in Sweden have found that perception of quality of life among people with spinal cord injuries (and other severe mobility impairments) did not differ from control population samples (e.g. Siösteen *et al.*, 1990).

Hence, it seems evident that it is not the innate qualities of the individual's disability which serves to limit life opportunities but the failure of social policies to meet the needs of those citizens who have mobility impairments. 'Quality of life is a product of the interaction of personal attributes and resources with environmental resources' (DeVivo and Richards, 1992).

Life satisfaction among people with spinal cord injuries has been found to be significantly related to social integration, mobility, occupation, social support, perceived control and self-assessed health status (Fuhrer *et al.*, 1992).

It is striking that most studies concerning quality of life have been published during the 1990s. Decades from the 1940s onwards have been preoccupied with increasing survival rates for people with increasingly higher levels of injury. It is hoped that these studies on quality of life are a prelude to a more complete understanding of the quality of the lives that have been saved and the perceptions of life satisfaction among those who have survived traumatic spinal cord injuries.

Although rehabilitation programmes have primarily focused upon prevention of impairments and upon reduction of disability, it is becoming clear from studies of life satisfaction that perceptions of quality of life are most strongly associated with reduction of handicap.

There is an intriguing implication in these findings for all who are involved in the rehabilitation of people with spinal cord injuries. For over 50 years, rehabilitation professionals have sought to teach each individual client physical and functional skills following a spinal cord injury, with the commendable aims of increasing independence and reducing the effects of disability.

However, if it is indeed true that it is the impact of a disabling physical, social, cultural, economic, legal and political environment which limits mobility, social integration, economic self-sufficiency and productivity (thus increasing handicap and reducing quality of life), a single question remains. Has the rehabilitation industry played an effective role in intervening to improve quality of life through reduction of handicap, by forcing changes in legal, political and social policies?

As DeVivo and Richards (1992) query: 'If predictors of life satisfaction can be found, can points of intervention be identified?' If predictors of life satisfaction are indeed found among dimensions of handicap such as social integration, productivity/occupation and mobility, as recent studies suggest (Siösteen *et al.*, 1990; Fuhrer *et al.*, 1992; Kinney and Coyle, 1992) does the rehabilitation industry as a whole; and do rehabilitation professionals as individuals, have the courage to intervene in arenas which do not have an individualistic focus?

Is 'quality of life' truly our ultimate goal in the rehabilitation of people with spinal cord injuries? If it is, then our assessments, our interventions and our outcome measures should surely be re-aligned to correlate more positively with our stated goals.

REFERENCES

Abrams, K.S. (1981) Impact on marriages of adult onset paraplegia. *Paraplegia*, **19**, 253–9.

Berkowitz, M., Harvey, C., Greene, C.G. and Wilson, S.E. (1992) *The Economic Consequences of Traumatic Spinal Cord Injury*, Demos, New York, NY, p. 54.

Bingley, J.D. (1990) Rehabilitation after spinal cord injury: the Southport experience. *Nursing Standard*, **4**(38), 27–30.

Bowling, A. (1991) *Measuring Health: a Review of Quality of Life Rating Scales*, Open University, Milton Keynes, pp. 1–11.

Briggs, A. (1981) *Equal Opportunities Commission Report*, EOC, Manchester.

Briggs, A. and Oliver, J. (1985) *Caring: Experiences of Looking After Disabled Relatives*, Routledge and Kegan Paul, London, p. x.

Brown, J.F. (1992) Another ethical issue without a resolution. . .to some. *SCI Psychosocial Process*, **5**(2), 42–3.

Brown, D.J., Judd, F.K. and Ungar, G.H. (1987) Continuing care of the spinal cord injured. *Paraplegia*, **25**, 296–300.

Buck, F.M. and Hohmann, G.W. (1981) Personality, behavior, values and family relations of children of fathers with spinal cord injury. *Archives of Physical Medicine and Rehabilitation*, **62**, 432–8.

Burke, D. (1973) Pain in paraplegia. *International Journal of Paraplegia*, **10**, 297–313.

Charlifue, S.W., Gerhart, K.A., Menter, R.R. *et al.* (1992) Sexual issues of women with spinal cord injuries. *Paraplegia*, **30**(3), 192–9.

Cicero, (106–43 BC) On old age VI, in *Medical Quotations*, (eds J. Daintith and A. Isaacs), (1989), Collins, London, p. 152.

Corbet, B. (1993) What price independence?, in *Aging with Spinal Cord Injury*, (eds G.G. Whiteneck, Charlifue, S.W., Gerhart, K.A. *et al.*), Demos, New York, NY, p. 227.

Crewe, N.M., Athelstan, G.T. and Krumberger, J. (1979) Spinal cord injury: a comparison of pre injury and post injury marriage. *Archives of Physical Medicine and Rehabilitation*, vol. 60, pp. 252–6.

Crewe, N.M. and Krause, J.S. (1988) Marital relationships and spinal cord injury. *Archives of Physical Medicine and Rehabilitation*, **69**, 435–8.

DeJong, G. and Batavia, A.I. (1991) Toward a health services research capacity in spinal cord injury. *Paraplegia*, **29**, 373–89.

DeJong, G. and Wenker, T. (1979) Attendant care as a prototype independent living service. *Archives of Physical Medicine and Rehabilitation*, **60**, 477–82.

Delargy, M., Parry, H. and Burt, A. (1988) Quadriplegic care: an assessment of the impact on the carer. *International Disability Studies*, **10**(4), 145–7.

DeVivo, M.J., Black, K.J., Richards, J.S. and Stover, S.L. (1991) Suicide following spinal cord injury. *Paraplegia*, **29**(9), 620–7.

DeVivo, M.J. and Richards, J.S. (1992) Community reintegration and quality of life following spinal cord injury. *Paraplegia*, **30**(2), 108–12.

Dew, M.A., Lynch, K., Ernst, J. and Rosenthal, R. (1983) Reaction and adjustment to spinal cord injury: a descriptive study. *Journal of Applied Rehabilitation Counseling*, **14**, 32–9.

Eisenberg, M.G. and Saltz, C.C. (1991) Quality of life among aging spinal cord injured persons: long term rehabilitation outcomes. *Paraplegia*, **29**(8), 514–20.

Eisenberg, M.G. and Tierney, D.O. (1985) Changing demographic profile of the spinal cord injury population: implications for health care support systems. *Paraplegia*, **23**, 335–43.

Fairholm, D. (1992) Managing pain, in *Management of Spinal Cord Injury*, 2nd edn, (ed. C.P. Zejdlik), Jones and Bartlett, Boston, MA, pp. 594–601.

Flanagan, J.C. (1982) Measurement of quality of life: current state of the art. *Archives of Physical Medicine and Rehabilitation*, **63**, 56–9.

Fuhrer, M.J., Rintala, D.H., Hart, K.A. *et al.* (1992) Relationship of life satisfaction to impairment, disability and handicap among persons with spinal cord injury living in the community. *Archives of Physical Medicine and Rehabilitation*, **73**, 552–7.

Gardner, B.P., Theocleous, F., Watt, J.W.H. and Krishnan, K.R. (1985) Ventilation or dignified death for patients with high tetraplegia. *British Medical Journal*, **291**, 1620–2.

Glass, C.A. (1993) The impact of home based ventilator dependence on family life. *Paraplegia*, **31**(2), 93–101.

Goodman, C. (1986) Research on the informal carer: a selected literature review. *Journal of Advanced Nursing*, **11**, 705–12.

Grundy, D. and Swain, A. (1993) *ABC of Spinal Cord Injury*, 2nd edn, British Medical Journal, London, pp. 43, 53.

Hammell, K.R.W. (1991) *An Investigation into the Availability and Adequacy of Social Relationships Following Head Injury and Spinal Cord Injury: a Study of Injured Men and their Partners*, MSc thesis, (Rehabilitation Studies), University of Southampton, Southampton.

Houda, B. (1993) Evaluation of nutritional status in persons with SCI: a prerequisite for successful rehabilitation. *SCI Nursing*, **10**(1), 4–7.

Kester, B.L., Rothblum, E.D., Lobato, D. and Milhous, R.L. (1988) Spouse adjustment to spinal cord injury: long term medical and psychosocial factors. *Rehabilitation Counseling Bulletin*, **32**, 4–21.

Kinney, W.B. and Coyle, C.P. (1992) Predicting life satisfaction among adults with physical disabilities. *Archives of Physical Medicine and Rehabilitation*, **73**, 863–9.

Macleod, A.D. (1988) Self neglect of spinal injured patients. *Paraplegia*, **26**, 340–9.

McColl, M.A., Rosenthal, C., Tonak, M. (1993) Resource needs for aging with a spinal cord injury. *Journal of the American Paraplegia Society*, (abstract), **16**(2), 93.

Menter, R.R. (1993a) Issues of aging with spinal cord injury, in *Aging with Spinal Cord Injury*, (eds G.G. Whiteneck, Charlifue, S.W., Gerhart, K.A. *et al.*), Demos, New York, NY, pp. 1, 4–5.

Menter, R.R. (1993b) Changing rehabilitation philosophy for aging, in *Aging with Spinal Cord Injury*, (eds G.G. Whiteneck, Charlifue, S.W., Gerhart, K.A. *et al.*), Demos, New York, NY, pp. 327–32.

Menter, R.R., Whiteneck, G.G., Charlifue, S.W. *et al.* (1991) Impairment, disability, handicap and medical expenses of persons aging with spinal cord injury. *Paraplegia*, **29**(9), 620–7.

Niemi, M.L., Laaksonen, R., Kotila, M. and Waltimo, O. (1988) Quality of life 4 years after stroke. *Stroke*, **19**, 1101–7.

Nosek, M.A. (1993) Personal assistance: its effects on the long term health of a rehabilitation hospital population *Archives of Physical Medicine and Rehabilitation*, **74**, 127–32.

Oliver, J. (1983) The caring wife, in *A Labour of Love: Women, Work and Caring*, (eds J. Finch and D. Groves), Routledge and Kegan Paul, London, p. 73.

Oliver, M., Zarb, G., Silver, J. *et al.* (1988) *Walking into Darkness: the Experience of Spinal Cord Injury*, Macmillan, Basingstoke, p. 33.

Ozer, M.N. (1988) *The Management of Persons with Spinal Cord Injury*, Demos, New York, NY, pp. 97–104.

Rabin, B.J. (1980) *The Sensuous Wheeler*, Rabin, Long Beach, CA.

Rasmussen, L., Tate, D., Casoglos, T. *et al.* (1989) *Hospital to Community: a Collaborative Program for Independent Living and Medical Rehabilitation*, University of Michigan, Ann Arbor, MI, pp. 104–7.

Richards, J.S. (1986) Psychologic adjustment to spinal cord injury during first post discharge year. *Archives of Physical Medicine and Rehabilitation*, **67**, 362–5.

Segatore, M. (1992) Deafferentation pain after spinal cord injury, Part II. Management. *SCI Nursing*, **9**(3), 72–8.

Siösteen,A., Lundqvist, C., Blomstrand, C. *et al.* (1990) The quality of life of three functional spinal cord injury subgroups in a Swedish community. *Paraplegia*, **28**, 476–88.

Stien, R. (1992) Sexual dysfunction in the spinal cord injured. *Paraplegia*, **30**(1), 54–7.

Szasz, G. (1987) Sexual management, in *Physical Management for the Quadriplegic Patient*, 2nd edn, (eds J.R. Ford and B. Duckworth), F.A. Davis, Philadelphia, PA, pp. 377–96.

Szasz, G. (1992) Sexual health care, in *Management of Spinal Cord Injury*, 2nd edn, (ed. C.P. Zejdlik), Jones and Bartlett, Boston, MA, p. 187.

Trieschmann, R.B. (1987) *Aging with a Disability*, Demos, New York, NY, pp. 1, 4, 107–11.

Trieschmann, R.B. (1988) *Spinal Cord Injuries. Psychological, Social and Vocational Rehabilitation*, 2nd edn, Demos, New York, NY, pp. 168, 174, 273–9, 285.

Urey, J.R. and Henggeler, S.W. (1987) Marital adjustment following spinal cord injury *Archives of Physical Medicine and Rehabilitation*, **68**, 69–74.

Urey, J.R., Viar, V. and Henggeler, S.W. (1987) Prediction of marital adjustment among spinal cord injured persons. *Rehabilitation Nursing*, **12**(1), 26–7, 30.

Verduyn, W.H. (1986) Spinal cord injured women, pregnancy and delivery. *Paraplegia*, **24**, 231–40.

Waters, R.L., Sie, I.H. and Adkins, R.H. (1993) The musculo-skeletal system, in *Aging with Spinal Cord Injury*, (eds G.G. Whiteneck, Charlifue, S.W., Gerhart, K.A. *et al.*), Demos, New York, NY, p. 70.

Weingarden, S.I. and Graham, P. (1992) Young spinal cord injured patients in nursing homes: rehospitalisation issues and outcomes. *Paraplegia*, **30**(12), 828–33.

Whalley Hammell K.R. (1992) The caring wife: the experience of caring for a severely disabled husband in the community. *Disability, Handicap and Society*, **7**(4), 349–62.

White, M.J., Rintala, D.H., Hart, K.A. *et al.* (1992) Sexual activities, concerns and interests of men with spinal cord injury. *Archives of Physical Medicine and Rehabilitation*, **71**, 225–31.

Whiteneck, G.G., Charlifue, S.W., Gerhart, K.A. *et al.* (eds). (1993) *Aging with Spinal Cord Injury*, Demos, New York, NY.

Wood-Dauphinee, S. and Küchler, T. (1992) Quality of life as a rehabilitation outcome: are we missing the boat? *Canadian Journal of Rehabilitation*, **6**(1), 3–12.

Young, J.S. (1980) Follow up care. *SCI Digest*, **1**(4), 2.

Zarb, G. (1993) Changes in health care: a British perspective, in *Aging with Spinal Cord Injury*, (eds G.G. Whiteneck, Charlifue, S.W., Gerhart, K.A. *et al.*), Demos, New York, NY, pp. 313, 320.

Zarb, G.J., Oliver, M.J. and Silver, J.R. (1990) *Ageing with Spinal Cord Injury: the Right to a Supportive Environment?*, Thames Polytechnic and the Spinal Injuries Association, London, pp. 2–4, 34.

Zejdlik, C.P. (1992) *Management of Spinal Cord Injury*, 2nd edn, Jones and Bartlett, Boston, MA, pp. 332, 346, 674–89.

10

The way forward

The reasonable man adapts himself to the world; the
unreasonable one persists in trying to adapt the
world to himself. Therefore, all progress depends on
the unreasonable man.

(G.B. Shaw, 1903)

After 50 years of formal rehabilitation services for people with
spinal cord injuries it is time to re-evaluate what is being
attempted, what is being achieved and what should be the way
forward.

PREVENTION

Prevention of spinal cord injury must remain the top priority.
Education and legislation may help to reduce the numbers of
preventable injuries, such as many sporting injuries and some
motor vehicle accident injuries.

There is a major, worldwide cause of spinal cord injuries that
is clearly preventable – but unlikely to be prevented: war.
Recognition of this fact has led disabled peoples' groups in
countries such as Lebanon and South Africa to become politi-
cally active in the movement to prevent war and violence, which
conspire to create tens of thousands of disabilities.

However, the spinal cord is vulnerable to injury from many
unpreventable causes, such as earthquakes and falls. Treatment
and rehabilitation for people with spinal cord injuries must still
remain a worldwide concern.

REHABILITATION RESEARCH

Research in rehabilitation is a comparatively recent phenomenon and remains a largely underdeveloped area of professional
practice.

Spinal cord injury research has focused upon seeking a cure for spinal cord damage and, although this remains outside the skills of therapists, it is clearly the most important issue for people with spinal cord injuries.

However, although some progress has been made, a cure, if ever found, is likely to be decades away and, at best, is unlikely to provide a solution for every form of damage to the spinal cord (Bedbrook, 1992). Rehabilitation following traumatic (and non-traumatic) spinal cord injury is therefore to be considered a future reality.

It is important to identify what issues concerning rehabilitation are of prime concern to people with spinal cord injuries – in both the acute stage, formal rehabilitation and in community living. Research must be appropriate to the skills and education of the researcher and the goals of the spinal cord injured community. In the future it has been suggested that people with disabilities will no longer co-operate with research studies which do not address their needs, concerns and priorities.

Functional electrical stimulation (FES, see Chapter 5) for example, has been a high priority for researchers for over 20 years yet it remains a low priority for the majority of people with spinal cord injuries. The latter view this intervention as impractical, inaccessible for most people with spinal cord injuries and above all, not 'functional'.

It is proposed that, if improvement in quality of life is an important goal of rehabilitation, it should be included as an outcome in rehabilitation research – a rare phenomenon to date. Future research must also consider the impact of a disabling environment upon the opportunity for social interaction and for engagement in meaningful occupations for people with spinal cord injuries (Jongbloed and Crichton, 1990). Future development of alternative models of service delivery will include examination of how the client's role demands and unique environment can be incorporated into the rehabilitation equation.

Outcome measurement requires an effective measure of handicap. Assessment commonly focuses upon impairment and disabilities, documenting limitations in physical, cognitive and psychosocial functions rather than examining handicap – the individual's interactions with environmental and social barriers (Batavia, 1992). The long-term goals of rehabilitation, however, must be the reduction of handicap. 'Handicap' is the disadvantage that limits fulfilment of roles such as occupation, social integration, family and community involvement. Many rehabilitation outcome measures have superficially used 'return to work' as an assessment of outcome, yet use of a sensitive measure of handicap will allow assessment of the real impact of the rehabilitation programme upon an individual's ability to achieve full re-integration to the community. Clearly an effective measure of handicap is only measurable after discharge, as it is not applicable to the environment of the rehabilitation facility.

Rehabilitation professionals have directed considerable attention to measuring impairments and disabilities, reflecting the prevailing medical model of care, rather than that espoused by rehabilitation practitioners. To map the effects of the rehabilitation programme in terms of the individual's full integration into society, productivity and enlargement of opportunities, sensitive measurements of handicap must be developed (Whiteneck, 1987).

COMMUNITY-BASED SERVICES

Institutions have been the traditional location of care for people with spinal cord injuries. This is totally appropriate for emergency and acute care needs and early therapy services. A spinal cord injury centre is an ideal place to build up muscle strength, learn techniques such as transfers, early wheelchair mobility and self-care skills such as catheterizations and dressing. Indeed, research studies have indicated that people who receive their care in a specialized spinal unit suffer less complications and have more successful outcomes from their rehabilitation process than those who are treated at general hospitals or rehabilitation units. Patients cared for in district general hospitals have reported inadequate care from unknowledgeable and poorly trained staff.

Healthcare professionals have also tended to have an affection for employment in institutions. There is professional support, comradeship, a sense of shared, rather than personal responsibility, team work and often a sense of control, if not power.

The hospital environment, however, has tended to isolate both healthcare professionals and their clients from an intimate knowledge of the environment to which the newly disabled person will return. People with spinal cord injuries have commented that they felt their real rehabilitation occurred only after they left the rehabilitation facility and re-entered their own sociocultural and physical environments. They also thought that their therapists and other healthcare workers did not have sufficient insight into the barriers to full community participation to be able to assist the disabled person to adapt and learn appropriate skills. People with spinal cord injuries have expressed frustration at the predominant interest in physical and functional aspects of the injury and neglect of psychosocial aspects of adult functioning. Many units do not address fully the exploration of opportunities and options for leisure activities and for meaningful occupation, whether in paid employment, or in other occupations which provide satisfaction and fulfilment. The message is therefore transmitted: 'You will do nothing more fulfilling or useful in your life than wash, dress and perform range-of-motion exercises'!

It is clear that each person with an acute spinal cord injury should have access to excellent and knowledgeable care, that this has proved more satisfactory in specialized units (Carvell and Grundy, 1989) and that quality care will be needed throughout life. What is equally clear is that many people will not be allowed access to such specialized units, because of the lack of beds, the geographical location and the selection criteria maintained by many special units.

There is a need for an expanded focus upon community-based services, not just follow-up at a distant clinic or rehabilitation centre. Research studies have suggested that there is a need for continuing support services for both the person with the spinal cord injury and his partner following discharge to the community. This would allow resolution of problems as they were identified. These might be in the area of social skills, in resolving environmental barriers, in psychological counselling, in identifying meaningful occupations in the context of the local environment or in solving physical/functional difficulties related to a particular activity or location.

Follow-up services related to cardiopulmonary status, urodynamics, pressure clinics, assessment of mobility and strength, vocational aptitude or sexual concerns may all be appropriately addressed in the rehabilitation facility. This is the location of choice when specialized equipment and facilities and a multi-disciplinary team are indicated.

For the individual concerns that arise after discharge to the community, solutions such as a telephone 'hot line' to a nurse specialist, or an invitation to return to a specialized unit – perhaps hundreds of miles away, are simply not adequate to the task. Specialized knowledge concerning spinal cord injury is crucial to excellence in management, prevention of unnecessary complications and in facilitating the adaptation to the injury in all arenas of life – physical, social, emotional and cultural. However, when faced with the problems of living with a disability in one's own environment, people with spinal cord injuries have commented that it is the domiciliary (community) occupational therapist who knows more, not about spinal cord injury, but about what it means to be disabled in the community and hence how to address the difficulties encountered (Hammell, 1991).

If more contact was facilitated between rehabilitation centre therapists and people with spinal cord injuries who are living in the community, more insight could be gleaned into how to adjust the overall rehabilitation programme to suit the needs of the clients. 'A spinal unit should ultimately be judged by the standard of its follow up system. Casual 'review' in the sterile environment of a hospital contributes little to the serious study of long-term implications of spinal cord injury' (Bingley, 1990).

Out-patient services may be appropriate in some instances for people who live close to a rehabilitation facility, thereby enabling the client to seek help with problems from knowledgeable professionals. This may also be viewed as a transition period from full institutional care to full community living. However, frequent out-patient services will not be appropriate for people who live long distances from the facility or who have transportation difficulties. Moreover, if they have employment or educational commitments, these may prevent participation in out-patient programmes which have been designed to suit the desires of professionals for Monday to Friday, nine-to-five type work schedules, rather than the need for flexible services to meet their client's own agendas.

More effort must be directed towards establishing new models of service delivery, to enable responsive professional support in the community. These should be appropriate to the

sociocultural and physical environment of each disabled client
and conversant with the unique problems and idiosyncracies
associated with spinal cord injury.

The needs for these services are expanding because of the
incidence and prevalence of spinal cord injury. It is estimated
that only about half the people with new spinal cord injuries
in the UK will receive treatment at a specialized spinal unit;
the remainder attend a general hospital. In the USA, 50–70%
of people with traumatic spinal cord injuries are treated in
community facilities, not in the Department of Veterans'
Affairs Spinal Cord Injury Centres, or the Model Spinal Cord
Injury System (Zejdlik, 1992). As the population of people
with spinal cord injury ages, demands will be placed upon
the specialized units which cannot be met even for their former patients. The community is the location for living with a
spinal cord injury and it is likely to become increasingly the
location for caring for problems related to physical disability
and the ageing process.

> No compassionate society should be content providing just
> hospital care without continuing responsibility for the safety
> and full restoration of quality of life for a group of disabled
> people. Hospitals have been inward looking for too long. It is
> time we realized there is a very real world outside spinal
> injury centres.
>
> (Bingley, 1990)

It is time to ensure that community-based services are in
place, that they are responsive to the needs of people with
spinal cord injuries and that they are available in the
environments in which the people with spinal cord injuries
are living, working and engaging in leisure and social
activities.

If rehabilitation is indeed the process of learning to live with a
disability in the context of one's own environment, then it may
be postulated that true adaptation to the disability is not complete at discharge but rather, this is when the real learning
process begins. Professional rehabilitation services must identify ways in which they can be responsive to, and facilitate this
process, working with the client and his family in their own
environment to achieve again a life that has meaning, quality
and purpose.

ADVOCACY AND SOCIAL CHANGE

For over 50 years, rehabilitation professionals have sought to teach each individual client to adjust to an inaccessible environment following a spinal cord injury. Finally, we are coming to realize what these individuals have long recognized – that the problems which may be associated with disability are not solely the results of any personal, physical limitation but are the consequences of a disabling environment (Jongbloed and Crichton, 1990).

It is time for rehabilitation professionals to leave the security of the rehabilitation facility and to work alongside their clients to achieve an environment that is accessible to all the members of that community. It is especially time for us to advocate on behalf of clients whose ability to do so may be compromised.

Therapists continue to try to adjust each client to an inaccessible environment and have failed in the attempt to re-integrate many of them. We aim to place 'empowerment', 'quality of life', and 'meaningful occupation' firmly on the rehabilitation agenda yet have failed to address directly the societal barriers which may prevent attainment of those very goals.

Rehabilitation professionals who have focused on the medical aspects of disability, on function and self-care activities have paid less attention – if any – to the more personally meaningful activities of socialization, productivity and leisure. This approach ignores both the impact that spinal cord injury has on many complex areas of living and also the satisfaction of full participation in society, as an adult. Further, this approach fails to accord with the priorities of our clients, the consumers, who demand full participation in society, increased community-based supports and express the need to engage in more meaningful roles and activities (Pentland *et al.*, 1992).

Law (1991) has proposed that 'health is determined by an individual's purposeful engagement in occupation and by a balance of self-care, productivity and leisure'. Pentland's group propose that people with physical disabilities who live in the community will face considerable barriers to achieving such a balance. Rehabilitation staff are employed to assist the transition from acute care dependency to full community living. We fail in our responsibilities on two counts: if we focus upon only one component in the equation – self-care activities, and if we fail to address the community barriers that mitigate against a balanced equation.

In reality, the inaccessible society to which we return our clients has not been a burning issue among rehabilitation professionals. Jongbloed and Crichton (1990) argue convincingly for rehabilitation professionals to move beyond an individual focus on disability to improving the circumstances of all people with disabilities through changes in law or social policies. This requires involvement in economic, social and political issues that currently prevent full societal participation by our clients. Such strategies are now being advocated by some organizations of healthcare professionals. The Canadian Association of Occupational Therapists, for example, advocates a greater emphasis on changing environments such as workplace conditions, public policies, attitudinal barriers, community resources, social supports and socioeconomic conditions. This widens the focus of environmental intervention, from a specific, physical environmental adaptation, such as installing a ramp, to effecting change in the broader environment to enhance occupational performance for the client population as a collective group (CAOT, 1991).

Jongbloed and Crichton (1990) suggest that rehabilitation professionals have an unauspicious record in the struggle for removal of architectural barriers and in civil rights for people with disabilities. In many instances, we have also exported our professional alienation from such issues to developing countries, further reinforcing the powerlessness of people with disabilities throughout the world.

Law (1991) affirms that, if we recognize that environments have the potential to foster dependency and increase the problems associated with disability, solutions must focus predominantly upon modification of those environments. She proposes that either locally, for an individual client, or more globally, for all people with disabilities, we must help to shape social policy and community planning to ensure that public transportation and buildings are accessible. She foresees a future in which occupational therapists work together with their clients and others to resolve environmental problems.

In countries that do not provide that most basic of human rights for its citizens – healthcare – it is incumbent upon the healthcare professionals to advocate on behalf of their clients. In

Chapter 6 it was suggested that saving a life but denying the equipment necessary to sustain quality of that life is an exercise in technology and not of humanity. Garber *et al.* (1988) indicate that, in the USA, 25–50% of people with high-lesion quadriplegias are unable to obtain powered wheelchairs, because of funding restrictions. It could be suggested that this is enabled by the silent collusion of professional organizations with insurance companies and governments. Hence, once these people's lives have been dramatically saved, up to half are denied any opportunity of independent mobility but are condemned to sit in one spot until moved. This can hardly constitute quality of life or even humane treatment. The sensory deprivation, lack of choice and control could rather be regarded as 'cruel and unusual punishment'. It follows from this policy that access to the community, to an environmental control system or to a computer will be severely compromised. These issues too must be addressed in the future. It is not appropriate for healthcare professionals to acquiesce to such scenarios as acceptable social norms.

This is a challenge for professionals who have been content with a non-confrontational existence, with regular working hours, in a familiar institutional environment. Advocacy and political involvement will not permit an individualistic focus which ignores the reality of the societies to which our clients return.

In the presence of a supportive environment and positive social provisions, a study in Sweden found no difference in perceived quality of life between groups of people who had complete C6 quadriplegias, complete paraplegias, incomplete (ambulant) paraplegias or who were in the control population (Siösteen *et al.*, 1990). This positive outcome following spinal cord injury and its resultant impairments must be examined in the context of a society which has been committed to offering people with disabilities equal opportunities and the same living standards as able-bodied people. This national standard of equality and the recognition of individual rights is proof of what may be accomplished, in the presence of political will and social commitment. The member countries of the United Nations have stated that these rights exist, yet the vast majority have failed to translate their rhetoric into reality.

Perhaps in the future we will see therapists employed not

solely to provide individual client intervention but also to act for disabled people as a group in areas of community access, employment rights and economic marginalization.

Politicians and social leaders should hear from rehabilitation professionals not solely when we perceive our professions as being under threat but when the lives of our clients are compromised. Jongbloed and Crichton (1990) point out that, although the 1980s witnessed an increased involvement in political activity by healthcare professionals, this was primarily focused upon increasing their own power, rather than advocating for and with their clients. This approach will do little to enhance the credibility of our professions with our consumers – people with disabilities.

Rehabilitation can no longer be viewed as a comfortable 8-hour job but as a commitment to improving quality of life and assisting disabled people in removing the environmental barriers that prevent attainment of their goals. It is time for all rehabilitation professionals to broaden their horizons and accept more wholeheartedly their mandate to facilitate full community re-integration for their clients. This cannot be fully achieved from within the walls of an institution and it will not be accomplished without considerable effort in the social, economic and political arenas of our communities.

People with disabilities in developed and developing countries are demanding full human rights – full participation in society, self-determination and the equalization of opportunities. They view the barriers to the attainment of those rights as being erected by cultures, societies, economies and physical environments. In this, 'the last civil rights movement' (Driedger, 1989), rehabilitation professionals will be judged by the stand they take on these issues. Those who are not actively addressing solutions are identified as being part of the problem.

> In an oppressive society, unless you are actively countering the oppression you are perpetuating it. There is no neutral ground. (Read (cited in French), 1992)

REFERENCES

Batavia, A.I. (1992) Assessing the function of functional assessment: a consumer perspective. *Disability and Rehabilitation*, **14**(3), 156–60.

Bedbrook, G. (1992) Fifty years on fundamentals in spinal cord injury care are still important. *Paraplegia*, **30**(1), 10–13.

Bingley, J. (1990) Rehabilitation after spinal cord injury. *Nursing Standard*, **4**(38), 27–30.

CAOT (1991) *Occupational Therapy Guidelines for Client Centred Practice*, Canadian Association of Occupational Therapists and the Health Services Directorate, Health Services and Promotion Branch, Health and Welfare Canada, Toronto, Ont., p. vii.

Carvell, J. and Grundy, D. (1989) Patients with spinal cord injuries. Early transfer to a specialist centre is vital *British Medical Journal*, **299**, 1353–4.

Driedger, D. (1989) *The Last Civil Rights Movement. Disabled Peoples' International*, C. Hurst, London.

French S. (1992) Health care in a multi ethnic society. *Physiotherapy*, **78**(3), 174–80.

Garber, S.L., Lathem, P. and Gregorio, T.L. (1988) *Specialized Occupational Therapy for Persons with High Level Quadriplegia*, Institute for Rehabilitation and Research, Houston, TX.

Hammell, K.R.W. (1991) *An Investigation into the Availability and Adequacy of Social Relationships Following Head Injury and Spinal Cord Injury: a Study of Injured Men and their Partners*, MSc thesis (Rehabilitation Studies), University of Southampton, Southampton.

Jongbloed, L. and Crichton, A. (1990) A new definition of disability: implications for rehabilitation practice and social policy. *Canadian Journal of Occupational Therapy*, **57**, 32–8.

Law, M. (1991) The environment: a focus for occupational therapy. *Canadian Journal of Occupational Therapy*, **58**(4), 171–9.

Pentland, W., Krupa, T., Lynch, S. and Clark, C. (1992) Community integration for persons with disabilities: working together to make it happen. *Canadian Journal of Occupational Therapy*, **59**(3), 127–30.

Shaw, G.B. (1903) Maxims for revolutionists. *Man and Superman*, III, Penguin, London.

Siösteen, A., Lundqvist, C., Blomstrand, C. *et al.* (1990) The quality of life of three functional spinal cord injury subgroups in a Swedish community. *Paraplegia*, **28**, 476–88.

Whiteneck, G.G. (1987) Outcome analysis in spinal cord injury rehabilitation, in *Rehabilitation Outcomes: Analysis and Measurement*, (ed. M.J. Fuhrer), Brookes, Baltimore, MD, pp. 221–31.

Zejdlik, C.P. (1992) *Management of Spinal Cord Injury*, 2nd edn, Jones and Bartlett, Boston, MA, p. 7.

Bibliography

Ford, J. and Duckworth, B. (1987) *Physical Management for the Quadriplegic Patient*, 2nd edn, F.A. Davis, Philadelphia, PA.

Ozer, M.N. (1988) *The Management of Persons with Spinal Cord Injury*, Demos, New York, NY.

Somers, M.F. (1992) *Spinal Cord Injury Functional Rehabilitation*, Appleton and Lange, East Norwalk, CT.

Trieschmann, R.B. (1987) *Aging with a Disability*, Demos, New York, NY.

Trieschmann, R.B. (1988) *Spinal Cord Injuries. Psychological, Social and Vocational Management*, 2nd edn, Demos, New York, NY.

Whiteneck, G.G., Adler, C., Carter, R.E. *et al.* (eds) (1989) *The Management of High Quadriplegia*, Demos, New York, NY.

Whiteneck, G.G., Charlifue, S.W., Gerhart, K.A. *et al.* (eds) (1993) *Aging with Spinal Cord Injury*, Demos, New York, NY.

Zejdlik, C.P. (1992) *Management of Spinal Cord Injury*, 2nd edn, Jones and Bartlett, Boston, MA.

Grundy, D. and Swain, A. (1993) *ABC of Spinal Cord Injury*, 2nd edn, British Medical Journal, London. (Of limited value for rehabilitation topics but clear information on medical management and acute care.)

Books related to disability, rather than just spinal cord injury

Coleridge, P. (1993) *Disability, Liberation and Development*, Oxfam, Oxford.

Swain, J., Finkelstein, V., French, S. and Oliver, M. (1993) *Disabling Barriers – Enabling Environments*, Open University and Sage, London.

Appendix A: Resource list

UNITED KINGDOM

Spinal Injuries Association, Newpoint House, 76 St James's Lane, London N10 3DF

International Spinal Research Trust, Nicholas House, River Front, Enfield, Middx EN1 3TR

CANADA

Canadian Paraplegic Association, 1500 Don Mills Road, Suite 201, Don Mills, Ont. M3B 3K4

Disabled Peoples' International (Headquarters), 101, 7 Evergreen Place, Winnipeg, Man. R3L 2T3

Canadian Association of Occupational Therapists, 110 Eglinton Avenue West, 3rd Floor, Toronto, Ont. M4R 1A3

(Publishers of: *Occupational Therapy Guidelines for Client-centred Practice (1991)* and *Canadian Occupational Performance Measure (1991)*)

AUSTRALIA

Australian Quadriplegic Association, 1 Jennifer Street, Little Bay, NSW, 2036.

USA

International Ventilator Users Network, Gazette International Networking Institute, 5100 Oakland Avenue, No. 206, St Louis, MO 63110–1406.

National Spinal Cord Injury Association, 600 West Cummings Park, Suite 2000, Woburn, MA 01801.

Paralyzed Veterans of America, 801 18th Street NW, Washington DC 20006

Appendix B: Suppliers

Obus, vacuum wand, birdbeak, card holder, bookstands, keyguards, mobile arm supports, scoop dish, plate guards, swivel cutlery
Fred Sammons Inc., 1224 Dundas Street E, Unit 5, Mississauga, Ont. L4Y 4A2, Canada

Sumed bath cushion
Sumed International Ltd, 11 Beaumont Business Centre, Beaumont Close, Banbury, Oxon OX16 7TN, UK

ROHO
ROHO Raymar, PO Box 16, Henley on Thames, Oxon RG9 1LL, UK
ROHO Inc., PO Box 658, Belleville, IL 62222, USA
Sunrise Medical, 265 Hood Road, Unit 3, Markham, Ont. L3R 4N3, Canada.

Jay, Quickie
Gerald Simmons, 9 March Place, Gatehouse Way, Aylesbury, Bucks, HP19 3UG, UK

Newspaper stand
Nottingham Rehabilitation, Ludlow Hill Road, West Bridgford, Nottingham NG2 6HD, UK
Physio ERP, 1170 Burnhamthorpe Road W, No. 32, Mississauga, Ont. L5C 4E6, Canada

Posturite book ledger
Posturite (UK) Ltd, PO Box 468, Hailsham, East Sussex BN27 4LX, UK

Vaperm system
Slumberland Medicare Ltd, Bee Mill, Shaw Road, Royton, Oldham, Lancs OL2 6EH, UK

Ulti-mate
Special Health Systems Ltd, 225 Industrial Parkway South, Aurora, Ont. L4G 3V5, Canada

Index

Page numbers appearing in **bold** refer to figures.

Abdominal binders 96, 101–2
Accessing community resources
    161–2
Accountability 18–19
Activated patients 20–2, 238–9
Activity, in-patient 266
Acute care 75–93
    family involvement 78–80
    neuropsychological deficits
        43–4
    sensory deprivation 77–8
Adjustment, *see* Psychological
    adaptation
ADL (Activities of Daily Living)
    assessment scales 11
Adolescents and spinal cord injury
    276–7
Advocacy 148, 282–3, 296, 298,
    333–6
Aetiology
    children 274–5
    elderly 277
    non-traumatic lesions 66–7
    traumatic injuries 54–6
Ageing with a spinal cord injury
    304–11
    changes 306–8
    implications for rehabilitation
        309–11
Air travel 160–1
Ambulation 149–56
    FES (Functional electrical
        stimulation) 153–6
    see also Gait training
Americans With Disabilities Act
    (1990) 161
Anterior cord syndrome 60–1

Assessment
    ADL scales 11
    client centres 10–12
    COPM 12
    impairments 5–10, 61–2
    motivation 25–6
    motor 62–3
    problem oriented 11–12
    process 12
    sensory 63–4
Assisted cough 102
Attendant care 299–300
    see also Personal Care Attendants
Autonomic dysreflexia, *see*
    Autonomic hyperreflexia
Autonomic hyperreflexia 96–9, 106
Autonomic nervous system 68–9

Ball bearing feeders, *see* Mobile arm
    supports
Body temperature regulation 99–100
Body weight 301
Bowel management 106–7
Breathing exercises 102–3
Brown–Séquard syndrome 60

Canadian Model of Occupational
    Performance 2–3
    assessment process 10–12
    performance components 3, 10
Canadian Occupational
    Performance Measure (COPM)
    12, 185
Cardiovascular disease 263
Caregiver/spouse 268, 269, 310
Carers
    informal 296–9

Carpal tunnel syndrome 156–7
Case management 315
Catheter
  indwelling 105
  intermittent 104–5
  self-intermittent 104–5
Cauda equina lesions 61
Central cord syndrome 60, 124–5
Centres for Integrated Living, *see*
  Independent Living Centres
Children and spinal cord injury
  274–6
Chronic overuse syndromes 156–7
Client centred assessment 248
Client centred practice 1, 270–1, 279
  assessment 10–12
  education 36
Client centred research 328
Communication 158
Community
  activity levels 265–6
  based services 329–32
  care 297
  health nurses 166, 315
  management 157–65
  support services 218, 311
  visits 158–9
Compliance 19–20
  education 38–9
  outcomes 251
  psychological adaptation 237–8
Computers 213–15
Concomitant head injury 43–4, 80–1
Continuing care services, *see* Follow
  up services
Contractures 85–6, 92–3
Conus medullaris syndrome 61
COPM, *see* Canadian Occupational
  Performance Measure
Crisis 225–6
Cultural environment 270–1
Cure 328
Cushions, *see* Wheelchair cushions

Deep vein thrombosis, prevention
  94–5
Denial 225–6, 229
Dependent oedema management
  93–4
Depression 228–33
  assessment 230
  leisure 259
  social support 236
Depressive illness 230
Dermatome 63–4

Developing countries 56, 147–8,
  334, 336
Diet 300–2
Disability
  definition 2
    see also ICIDH
  life satisfaction 320
  quality of life 321
  reduction 93–113
Disability rights 252
Disability rights movement 154
Disabled Peoples' International 162
  definition of handicap 2
Disabling Professions
  the medical model 9
Discharge planning 165–7, 297
Diving as a cause of SCI 58
Driving 159–60

Education
  adult 36
  employment 253–4
  problem solving 40–2
  rehabilitation team 33–4
  see also Learning
Elderly and spinal cord injury 277–9
Emergency management 69–71
Employment 247, 253–7
  high lesion quadriplegia 219–20
Empowerment 20–2, 333
  learning 39–40
  motivation 24, 25
  see also Rehabilitation,
    empowerment
Energy expenditure 301–2
Enhancer cushion 133
Environment 2
  accessibility 158–9
  adaptation 235–6
  ageing 310
  assessment 10
  barriers 158–9, 162–5, 166, 252–3,
    330
  empowerment 21
  change 282
  children 275
  cultural 270–1
  disabling 6, 266, 320, 321, 328,
    333
    employment 255
    and quality of life 321
    suicide 313
  employment 257
  follow up services 315
  handicap 26, 282–3, 321

Environment *contd*
  IL philosophy 281
  impact on health 169
  influence 6
    see also Environment, disabling
  in-patient 266, 329–30
  intervention 144, 259–60, 265, 334
    productivity 255
  person match 267–8
  occupational performance 3, 10,
    265
  psychological reaction 78
  rehabilitation 241
  self care 119, 137
  self care outcome 140
  service delivery 331–2
  social 235–6
  socialization 265
  supportive 219–20, 241, 253, 270,
    335
  treatment 217
  women 272
Environmental control
  acute care 82
  high lesion quadriplegia 180–1
Environmental control systems
  209–13
Experiential learning 282
  see also Learning

Families 237, 269, 292–5, 297–8
  adaptation 235–6
  attendant care 299
  involvement in acute care 78–80
  involvement in learning 48–9
  psychological adaptation 228
Fertility 289, 290
Flexor hinge splints 129–30
Follow up services 250, 309, 313–17,
    330–2
  see also Community based
    services
Functional assessment 138–9,
    175
Functional Electrical Stimulation
    (FES) 153–6, 251, 328
  incomplete lesions 153
Functional expectations 65
Functional levels 119–24
Functional mobility 141–56
  community barriers 251–3
  the elderly 278
Functional Neuromuscular
  Stimulation, *see* Functional
  Electrical Stimulation (FES)

Gait
  expectations 151–2
  training 149–56
Goals
  adolescents 276
  behaviour 237
  choices 238
  client centred 249
  collaborative planning 14–15
  definition 15
  education 38, 47–8
  motivation 25
  pain management 303
  personal care 139
  physical 251
  setting 13–15
  staff expectations 250–1
  women with SCI 274

Handicap 328–9
  ageing 310
  definition 2
    see also ICIDH; Disabled
      Peoples' International
  environmental barriers 252–3
  outcome measurement 328–9
  quality of life 320, 321
Health care needs 168
Head injury, *see* Concomitant head
    injury
Helplessness
  employment 254
    see also Learned helplessness
Heterotopic ossification 88–90
High cervical lesions, *see* High
    lesion quadriplegia
High lesion quadriplegia 6, 174–220,
    293–4
  ADL scores 11
  blowdarts 197–8
  bookstands 196
  cassette tape books 196
  children 276
  community care 297
  community management 216–19
  computers 213–15
  definition 178
  disabling society 335
  drinking 198–200
  early intervention 178–85
  employment 219–20
  equipment and training 186–98
  functional activities 186–7
  functions 121
  hunting, shooting and fishing 197

hypothesis of reduced emotions 233
incidence 177
independence 125–6
learning 45
leisure activities 194–8
living options 296
mobility 181–2
music 197
occupational performance 185
orthotics 178–9, **180**
personal care 125–6
photography 196
physical independence 6
postural hypotension 182
productivity 190–4
reading 194–6
rehabilitation 177–8
remote control vehicles 197
respiratory care 103, 183–4
self care 198–202
self feeding 200–2
sensory and motor stimulation 184–5
spotting scope 196–7
staff attitudes 176
teaching 48
telephones 213
wheelchairs, manual 203–5
wheelchairs, powered 205–9
wheelchair trays 203
word processing 193–4
work stations 215–16
Hip guidance orthosis (HGO) 152
Historical perspective 52–3
Homosexuality 291
Household management 247, 248

ICIDH
and Model of Occupational Performance 2, 3
Impairments 60–9
assessment 61–2
definition 2
see also ICIDH
incidence 53–4
quality of life 320, 321
Incidence and prevalence 53–4
Independence
definition 3–4
education 34
physical 6
physical skills 6
Independent living
therapy practice 282–3

Independent Living (IL) Centres 280–2, 300
Independent Living (IL) Movement 168, 279–83, 296
Independent living options 295–6
Interdependence 6, 228
Intermittent catheterisation 104–5
International Classification of Impairments, Disabilities and Handicaps, *see* ICIDH
Institutionalization 280
Institutional living 217, 295–6, 297, 298

Jay cushion 134–5

Learned helplessness 22
elderly patients 278
locus of control 23
motivation 24
Learning
barriers to 43–5
empowerment 39–40
experiential 36–7
family involvement 48–9
how do we 36–7
Maslow's hierarchy 45–7
neuropsychological deficits 43–4
reflection 36
role of peers 42–3
problem based 35–6
process 34
theories 35–6
see also Education
Learning theory in rehabilitation 37–8
Leisure 3, 247, 258–64
the elderly 279
high lesion quadriplegia 186
outcome measurement 266–7
see also Model of Occupational Performance; Recreation; Socialization
Level of injury
depression 230
employment 253
implications 121–4
incidence 65–6
productivity 251
quality of life 246, 320
Life satisfaction 240, 246, 281, 320, 321
ageing 308, 310
mortality 112–13
pressure sores 110

Life satisfaction *contd*
  social support 268
  see also Quality of life
Living options 295–6
Locus of control
  adaptation 234
  employment 254
  learning 37
  motivation 24–5
  theory 22–3
Lower motor neurone lesions 61

Malnutrition 302
Marriage 292–5
Maslow's hierarchy 13
  learning 45–7
Mattresses 136–7
Medical model of rehabilitation 7–9,
  270–1, 299, 329
  assessment of performance
    components 10
  follow-up services 314
  motivational theory 24
Mobile arm supports 200–2
Model of Occupational
  Performance, *see* Canadian
  Model of Occupational
  Performance
Morbidity 306
Mortality 111–13
  elderly 278
Motivation 24–6
Motor examination (ASIA) 62–3
Motor vehicle accidents
  as cause of SCI 57–8
Mouthstick activities 190–3
Mouthstick design 187–90
Myotome 62

Neurogenic bladder 103–4
Neurological classification of injury
  65
Nursing homes 278–9, 295–6
  see also Institutionalization;
    Institutional living
Nutrition 300–2

Obesity 301
Objectives
  accountability 18–19
  definition 15
  establishing 15–17
  identifying attainment 17–18
Occupational Performance 3, 249
  assessment 12

high lesion quadriplegia 185–6
  see also Canadian Model of
    Occupational Performance
Occupational therapist 315
  community 166, 331
Occupational therapy
  IL paradigm 282
  Canadian Model of Occupational
    Performance 10
  goals 13–14
  high lesion quadriplegia 179, 181,
    185–98
  upper limb reconstruction 131
Occupations, *see* Leisure;
    Productivity; Self care
Oedema, *see* Dependent oedema
    management
Opponens splint
  long 179, **180**
  short 83, **84**
Orthoses
  gait 152–6
Orthostatic hypotension 95–6
  see also Postural Hypotension
Orthotics, *see* Splinting the hand
Outcome 247–8
  adjustment 235–6
  learning process 49
Outcome measurement 247–8,
    317–19, 328–9
  accountability 18–19
  achievement of objectives 17–18
  assessment of physical skills 7
  cultural context 271
  education 33
  environment 258
  leisure 266–7
  performance components 19
  personal care 138–9
  productivity 258
  quality of life 18
  rehabilitation 138–9
  self care 140–1
Out patient services 239, 331
Oxbow transfer board 142–3

Page turners 195–6
Pain, chronic 302–4
Paraplegia
  functions 123–4
  high lesion, functions 123
Parenthood 295
Peer counselling 274, 280
Peer learning
  high lesion quadriplegia 217

Peers
    adolescent 276
    education 42–3
Personal care 125–9
    assistance 140
    C5 126–7
    C6 127–8
    C7 128
    long term engagement 137–40
Personal Care Attendants 119, 166,
    218–19, 296–9
Personality
    adaptation 234
Philosophy
    Independent Living (IL) 279,
    281
    rehabilitation 5–9, 281
Physiotherapist 183
Physiotherapy 100
    high lesion quadriplegia 184–5
Play 275
Poikilothermia 68, 99
Positioning 101–2
    bed 93
Post polio syndrome 305, 306
Postural hypotension 182
    see also Orthostatic hypotension
Powerlessness, *see* Learned
    helplessness
Powered wheelchairs, *see*
    Wheelchairs
Pressure sores
    athletes 264
    prevention 107–11
Prevalence 53–4
Prevention of spinal cord injury
    56–9, 327
Primary care, *see* Health care needs
Problem solving
    education 40–2
Productivity 3, 247–58
    high lesion quadriplegia 185–6
    outcome measurement 258
    transportation 251–2
    see also Employment; Household
    management; Model of
    Occupational Performance,
    Play; School
Psychological adaptation 224–41
    challenge to stages 228
    sociological theories 235–6
    stage theories 226–8
Psychological care, acute 77
Psychological distress
    staff perceptions 227, 228–33

Psychological theories of adaptation
    224–33, 239–40
Public transport 161
Pulmonary embolism, prevention
    94–5
Pushing mitts 148–9

Quadriplegia
    acute shoulder pain 86–9
    arm positioning 88, **89**
    functions 122–3
    high lesions, *see* High lesion
    quadriplegia
Quality of life 3, 240, 246, 269,
    312–13, 317–22, 328, 333, 336
    attendant care 299
    high lesion quadriplegia 175,
    176
    measurement 317–19
    outcome measurement 18
    pain 302
    pressure sores 110
    studies 320–2
    survival 112–13

Range of motion
    acute care 85–6
    acute shoulder pain 87–8
    contractures 92
    deep vein thrombosis 95
    heterotopic ossification 90
    high lesion quadriplegia 183
    spasticity 91–2
Readmission to hospital 167–9
Reciprocating Gait Orthoses (RGO)
    152
Recreation
    active 260–3
    quiet 260
Reduction of disability 74–5
Rehabilitation
    children 275
    definition 7
    educational approach 9
    empowerment 20–2
    implications of ageing 309–11
    mandate 333–6
    medical model 7–9
    productivity 250
    women 272–3
Rehabilitation outcomes 5, 177–8,
    316, 329
    staff attitudes 233
    high lesion quadriplegia 175
Rehabilitation philosophies 5–9

Rehabilitation programmes 241
    leisure 259
    quality of life 319–20
    psychological adaptation 238–41
    social support 268–9
Rehabilitation research 327–9
Rehospitalization 34
    see also Readmission to hospital
Research 327–8
    women 272
Respiratory care
    acute 100–3
    high lesion quadriplegia 183–4
Respiratory therapist 183
Respiratory therapy 100
Respite care 218, 276
Resting splint 179, **181**
Robotics 216
ROHO cushion 132–4
Role demands 328
Roles
    assessment process 11
    COPM 12

School 275
Self care 3, 247
    activities 119
    elderly 278
    handicap 11
    high lesion quadriplegia 185
    skills 125–9
    time spent 6
    see also Community management;
        Functional mobility; Model of
        Occupational Performance;
        Personal care
Self neglect 311–13
Sensation seeking traits 227
Sensory deprivation 77–8, 225–6
    overcoming 179
Sensory examination (ASIA) 63–4
Sexual function 288–92
Sexual issues 288–92
Sexuality 288–9
Shoulder pain
    acute quadriplegia 86–9
    chronic 156–7
Smoking
    deep vein thrombosis 95
    lung function 103
    pressure sores 110
Social adjustment 235–6
Social change 333–6
Social environment 163
Socialization 264–5

Social policy 251–2, 255, 257, 282–3,
    320, 321, 334
Social skills 162–5
Social support 236, 267–9
Social workers 218, 311, 315
Society
    inaccessible 334
Sociological theory of adaptation
    235–6
Spasticity management 90–2
Specialized spinal injury unit 71,
    305, 313–14, 329, 330, 332
    high lesion quadriplegia 175–6
Spinal cord injury
    complete 60
    incomplete 60
    neurological levels 62
    skeletal levels 62
Spinal shock 75–6
Spinal Units, see Specialized spinal
    injury unit
Splinting the hand 82–5
    dynamic 129–30
Sport
    activities 261–2
    injuries 264
    recreation, as cause of SCI
        58–9
Spouse/carer 268, 269, 310
Staff
    attitudes 288–9
    perceptions of psychological
        adaptation 239, 240
    role in psychological adaptation
        236–7
    women with SCI 272–3, 274
Standing 151
Strasbourg Resolution 298
Stryker frame 76, 179
Suicide 111, 303, 311–13
    women 273
Sumed bath cushion 136
Survival 111–13

Tenodesis 83–4
Tetraplegia, see Quadriplegia
Therapist/client relationship 26–9
    non dependent 21
Therapy practice and IL paradigm
    282–3
Time use 247, 248, 258
    elderly people 279
    personal care 138
Transfer boards 142–4
Transfers 142–4

Transportation 159–61, 266
    productivity 251–2

Ultimate cushion 135–6
Upper limb reconstruction 130–1
Upper motor neurone lesions 61
Urinary tract infections 106, 247
Urinary tract management 103–6
    complications 106
    external collection systems 105–6

Ventilators
    and communication 184
    see also High lesion quadriplegia
Vocational interests 255–6
Vocational rehabilitation 254–5,
    256–7

Walking programmes 149–56,
    251
Wheelchairs
    choice 145–8
    control options 207–9
    cushions 131–6, 205
    developing countries 147–8
    high lesion quadriplegia 203–5
    powered 205–9
    shoulder pain 156–7
    skills 144–5
Women and spinal cord injury
    271–4
    sex 291
    vocational interests 255–6
Workplace spinal cord injuries
    59